AACN Certification and Core Review for High Acuity and Critical Care

6th Edition

Edited by

JoAnn Grif Alspach, RN, MSN, EdD, FAAN

Consultant, Nursing Staff Development, Preceptor Development and
Competency-Based Perfomance Appraisal Systems

Editor, *Critical Care Nurse*
Annapolis, Maryland

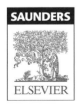

SAUNDERS

ELSEVIER

AMERICAN
ASSOCIATION
of CRITICAL-CARE
NURSES

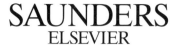

SAUNDERS
ELSEVIER

11830 Westline Industrial Drive
St. Louis, Missouri 63146

AACN Certification and Core Review for High Acuity
and Critical Care, Sixth Edition

ISBN-13: 978-1-4160-3592-3
ISBN-10: 1-4160-3592-3

Notice

Knowledge and best practice in this field are constantly changing. As new research
and experience broaden our knowledge, changes in practice, treatment and drug
therapy may become necessary or appropriate. Readers are advised to check the most
current information provided (i) on procedures featured or (ii) by the manufacturer
of each product to be administered, to verify the recommended dose or formula, the
method and duration of administration, and contraindications. It is the responsibility
of the practitioner, relying on their own experience and knowledge of the patient,
to make diagnoses, to determine dosages and the best treatment for each individual
patient, and to take all appropriate safety precautions. To the fullest extent of the
law, neither the Publisher nor the Authors assumes any liability for any injury and/
or damage to persons or property arising out or related to any use of the material
contained in this book.

The Publisher

Previous editions copyrighted   1998, 1991, 1985

ISBN-13: 978-1-4160-3592-3
ISBN-10: 1-4160-3592-3

Executive Publisher: Barbara Nelson Cullen
Senior Developmental Editor: Jennifer Ehlers
Publishing Services Manager: John Rogers
Designer: Margaret Reid

Printed in the United States of America

Last digit is the print number: 9 8 7 6 5 4 3 2 1

Contributors

CARING AND ETHICAL PRACTICE

Sonya R. Hardin, RN, PhD, CCRN
Associate Professor, School of Nursing
University of North Carolina
Charlotte, North Carolina

Roberta Kaplow, RN, PhD, AOCNS, CCNS, CCRN
Clinical Nurse Specialist
DeKalb Medical Center
Decatur, Georgia

CARDIOVASCULAR

Karen L. Cooper, RN, MSN, CCRN, CNS, WOCN
Clinical Nurse Specialist, ICU, Telemetry, Medical-Surgical
Kaiser Permanente
Sacramento, California

PULMONARY

Karen L. Cooper, RN, MSN, CCRN, CNS, WOCN
Clinical Nurse Specialist, ICU, Telemetry, Medical-Surgical
Kaiser Permanente
Sacramento, California

Christine A. Cottingham, RN, MS, CCRN
Clinical Nurse Specialist, Critical Care and
Trauma, Harborview Medical Center
Clinical Faculty, University of Washington School
of Nursing
Seattle, Washington

Patricia A. Radovich, RN, MSN, CNS, FCCM
Clinical Nurse Specialist, Hepatology, Liver
Transplant
Loma Linda University Medical Center
Loma Linda, California

Kyla F. Snyder, RN, MN, CCRN
Staff Nurse, Trauma Intensive Care Unit
Harborview Medical Center
Adjunct Faculty, Seattle Pacific University
Clinical Faculty, University of Washington School
of Nursing
Seattle, Washington

NEUROLOGIC

Lori K. Madden, MS, RN, ACNP, CCRN, CNRN
Nurse Practitioner III, Department of Neurological
Surgery, University of California–Davis
Sacramento, California
Assistant Clinical Professor, Department of
Physiological Nursing
University of California
San Francisco, California

RENAL

Ann E. Keane, RN, MSN, MA, CCRN
Director of Nursing, Acute Care
Sound Shore Medical Center
New Rochelle, New York

ENDOCRINE

Shelba D. Durston, RN, MSN, CCRN
Staff Nurse, Intensive Care Unit, San Joaquin
General Hospital
French Camp, California
Nursing Instructor, San Joaquin Delta College
Stockton, California

HEMATOLOGY/IMMUNOLOGY

Shelba D. Durston, RN, MSN, CCRN
Staff Nurse, Intensive Care Unit, San Joaquin
General Hospital
French Camp, California
Nursing Instructor, San Joaquin Delta College
Stockton, California

GASTROINTESTINAL

Patricia A. Radovich, RN, MSN, CNS, FCCM
Clinical Nurse Specialist, Hepatology, Liver
Transplant
Loma Linda University Medical Center
Loma Linda, California

MULTISYSTEM

Leslie A. Collins, RN, APN-CNS, CCRN-CSC, CCNS
Clinical Nurse Specialist, Cardiothoracic Surgery
Northwest Community Hospital
Arlington Heights, Illinois

Preface

As a dynamic specialty nursing organization, the American Association of Critical-Care Nurses (AACN) continually evolves to better meet the needs of its members and the patients they serve. As the healthcare industry, healthcare services, and the traditional boundaries of healthcare institutions have been altered so rapidly and pervasively over recent years, AACN has continued its vital growth and development in order to remain at the forefront of these changes.

Quality care of the critically ill patient requires that the nurse be competent in critical care nursing practice. AACN denotes competency in critical care nursing by means of its CCRN certification program. Certification in critical care nursing demands both a clinical practice requirement as well as the successful completion of the CCRN examination, a written test on the cognitive elements that underlie critical care nursing practice. AACN's *Core Curriculum for Critical Care Nursing* defines the knowledge base for critical care nursing, and *AACN Certification and Core Review for High Acuity and Critical Care* provides a means to verify acquisition of that knowledge base.

In addition to its usefulness as a study guide for critical care nursing practice, the *Core Review* is also designed to assist nurses who are preparing to take the Adult CCRN certification examination administered by the AACN Certification Corporation. Each CCRN certification examination is based on a job analysis study that defines the dimensions of acute and critical care nursing practice. Using the AACN Synergy Model for Patient Care as an organizing framework, those dimensions of care are then reviewed in order to define the knowledge, skills, and abilities required for critical care nursing practice. CCRN certification examinations are based on these skills and abilities and the knowledge necessary to perform them. The *Core Review* provides three complete practice CCRN examinations based on the latest edition of the *AACN Core Curriculum*. The test items in this book evaluate the knowledge, skills, and abilities identified as crucial for nursing care of patients with acute and life-threatening health problems. Achievement of

these dual purposes necessitates retention of many aspects of the prior edition of this work as well as inauguration of some new features.

Similarities with the fifth edition include comprehensive coverage of topics contained in the most recent version of the *Core Curriculum*. This edition of the *Core Review* is based on the sixth edition of the *Core Curriculum*. As with prior versions of the *Core Review*, test items cover revised, continued, expanded, additional, and updated content from the most recent *Core Curriculum* and integrate psychosocial aspects of care. The test items still consist of four-option multiple-choice questions with explanations for both correct and incorrect answers, and the test items are again segregated into three separate practice CCRN examinations. Content areas and their distributions precisely match those detailed in the adult version of the CCRN examination blueprint–adult version (available at www. aacn.org/certcorp/). Feedback on answers is again located at the end of each examination so that test completion and timing are not disrupted and item responses may more closely resemble completion of the actual CCRN examination. References for each correct answer and annotated bibliographies are again provided to assist readers in identifying relevant references for each content area in the CCRN examination blueprint.

Most of the new features of this edition of the *Core Review* were introduced to ensure that each practice examination matches the content areas, content distribution, item numbers, cognitive levels, and format used in the actual CCRN examination. Content new to this edition includes areas embraced within the *Core Curriculum*'s new chapter on Professional Caring and Ethical Practice as well as its new chapter on special populations such as bariatric, geriatric, sedated, and high-risk obstetric patients. Content distributions precisely match those designated in the latest blueprint for the adult CCRN examination, including 80% of items pertaining to the nurse competency of Clinical Judgment and 20% of items now related to the other seven nurse competencies (Advocacy–Moral Agency, Caring Practices, Collaboration, Systems Thinking,

Response to Diversity, Clinical Inquiry, and Facilitation of Learning) grouped under the umbrella of Professional Caring and Ethical Practice. Because the CCRN examination now tests critical thinking using higher cognitive levels, the majority of items contained in the *Core Review* now test at the application or analysis cognitive level. Consistency with the actual CCRN examination is also the rationale for including 150 rather than 200 items per test and for no longer incorporating use of clinical scenarios that apply to more than one test item. The accompanying CD-ROM includes 50 extra examination questions and provides the ability to review body systems and to take the examinations electronically.

Although these review tests are intended to simulate the CCRN examination, none of the test questions were or will be actual CCRN examination items. Because changes in the CCRN examination occur from time to time, candidates preparing for this examination are strongly encouraged to contact the AACN Certification Corporation and check its website (www.certcorp.org) to obtain the current CCRN certification examination handbook and blueprint that will be in effect for the date on which they plan to take the examination.

The contributors to this book have made every attempt to provide a study guide that is helpful in validating a nurse's ability to apply the content of the *Core Curriculum* to critical care nursing practice and in assisting nurses to prepare for the CCRN certification examination. We welcome your comments regarding how well we have achieved these objectives.

Grif Alspach, RN, MSN, EdD, FAAN
Editor-in-Chief, *Core Curriculum* Series
Annapolis, Maryland

Instructions

Each of the three tests in this book consists of 150 four-option multiple choice questions. To simulate taking a CCRN examination, mark your answer to each question on the reproducible answer sheet and allow a maximum of 3 hours to complete each test. After you have completed each test, compare your answers to those that appear in the answer key that follows that test.

ADDITIONAL STUDY REFERENCES

A list of additional study references is provided for you in the annotated bibliographies for each content area of the CCRN certification examination. These bibliographies are located after the last of the three tests and are subdivided by topic area.

Core Review Test
Answer Sheet

1. ❑ A ❑ B ❑ C ❑ D   26. ❑ A ❑ B ❑ C ❑ D   51. ❑ A ❑ B ❑ C ❑ D

2. ❑ A ❑ B ❑ C ❑ D   27. ❑ A ❑ B ❑ C ❑ D   52. ❑ A ❑ B ❑ C ❑ D

3. ❑ A ❑ B ❑ C ❑ D   28. ❑ A ❑ B ❑ C ❑ D   53. ❑ A ❑ B ❑ C ❑ D

4. ❑ A ❑ B ❑ C ❑ D   29. ❑ A ❑ B ❑ C ❑ D   54. ❑ A ❑ B ❑ C ❑ D

5. ❑ A ❑ B ❑ C ❑ D   30. ❑ A ❑ B ❑ C ❑ D   55. ❑ A ❑ B ❑ C ❑ D

6. ❑ A ❑ B ❑ C ❑ D   31. ❑ A ❑ B ❑ C ❑ D   56. ❑ A ❑ B ❑ C ❑ D

7. ❑ A ❑ B ❑ C ❑ D   32. ❑ A ❑ B ❑ C ❑ D   57. ❑ A ❑ B ❑ C ❑ D

8. ❑ A ❑ B ❑ C ❑ D   33. ❑ A ❑ B ❑ C ❑ D   58. ❑ A ❑ B ❑ C ❑ D

9. ❑ A ❑ B ❑ C ❑ D   34. ❑ A ❑ B ❑ C ❑ D   59. ❑ A ❑ B ❑ C ❑ D

10. ❑ A ❑ B ❑ C ❑ D   35. ❑ A ❑ B ❑ C ❑ D   60. ❑ A ❑ B ❑ C ❑ D

11. ❑ A ❑ B ❑ C ❑ D   36. ❑ A ❑ B ❑ C ❑ D   61. ❑ A ❑ B ❑ C ❑ D

12. ❑ A ❑ B ❑ C ❑ D   37. ❑ A ❑ B ❑ C ❑ D   62. ❑ A ❑ B ❑ C ❑ D

13. ❑ A ❑ B ❑ C ❑ D   38. ❑ A ❑ B ❑ C ❑ D   63. ❑ A ❑ B ❑ C ❑ D

14. ❑ A ❑ B ❑ C ❑ D   39. ❑ A ❑ B ❑ C ❑ D   64. ❑ A ❑ B ❑ C ❑ D

15. ❑ A ❑ B ❑ C ❑ D   40. ❑ A ❑ B ❑ C ❑ D   65. ❑ A ❑ B ❑ C ❑ D

16. ❑ A ❑ B ❑ C ❑ D   41. ❑ A ❑ B ❑ C ❑ D   66. ❑ A ❑ B ❑ C ❑ D

17. ❑ A ❑ B ❑ C ❑ D   42. ❑ A ❑ B ❑ C ❑ D   67. ❑ A ❑ B ❑ C ❑ D

18. ❑ A ❑ B ❑ C ❑ D   43. ❑ A ❑ B ❑ C ❑ D   68. ❑ A ❑ B ❑ C ❑ D

19. ❑ A ❑ B ❑ C ❑ D   44. ❑ A ❑ B ❑ C ❑ D   69. ❑ A ❑ B ❑ C ❑ D

20. ❑ A ❑ B ❑ C ❑ D   45. ❑ A ❑ B ❑ C ❑ D   70. ❑ A ❑ B ❑ C ❑ D

21. ❑ A ❑ B ❑ C ❑ D   46. ❑ A ❑ B ❑ C ❑ D   71. ❑ A ❑ B ❑ C ❑ D

22. ❑ A ❑ B ❑ C ❑ D   47. ❑ A ❑ B ❑ C ❑ D   72. ❑ A ❑ B ❑ C ❑ D

23. ❑ A ❑ B ❑ C ❑ D   48. ❑ A ❑ B ❑ C ❑ D   73. ❑ A ❑ B ❑ C ❑ D

24. ❑ A ❑ B ❑ C ❑ D   49. ❑ A ❑ B ❑ C ❑ D   74. ❑ A ❑ B ❑ C ❑ D

25. ❑ A ❑ B ❑ C ❑ D   50. ❑ A ❑ B ❑ C ❑ D   75. ❑ A ❑ B ❑ C ❑ D

Core Review Test
Answer Sheet *(Continued)*

76.	❑ A	❑ B	❑ C	❑ D	101.	❑ A	❑ B	❑ C	❑ D	126.	❑ A	❑ B	❑ C ❑ D
77.	❑ A	❑ B	❑ C	❑ D	102.	❑ A	❑ B	❑ C	❑ D	127.	❑ A	❑ B	❑ C ❑ D
78.	❑ A	❑ B	❑ C	❑ D	103.	❑ A	❑ B	❑ C	❑ D	128.	❑ A	❑ B	❑ C ❑ D
79.	❑ A	❑ B	❑ C	❑ D	104.	❑ A	❑ B	❑ C	❑ D	129.	❑ A	❑ B	❑ C ❑ D
80.	❑ A	❑ B	❑ C	❑ D	105.	❑ A	❑ B	❑ C	❑ D	130.	❑ A	❑ B	❑ C ❑ D
81.	❑ A	❑ B	❑ C	❑ D	106.	❑ A	❑ B	❑ C	❑ D	131.	❑ A	❑ B	❑ C ❑ D
82.	❑ A	❑ B	❑ C	❑ D	107.	❑ A	❑ B	❑ C	❑ D	132.	❑ A	❑ B	❑ C ❑ D
83.	❑ A	❑ B	❑ C	❑ D	108.	❑ A	❑ B	❑ C	❑ D	133.	❑ A	❑ B	❑ C ❑ D
84.	❑ A	❑ B	❑ C	❑ D	109.	❑ A	❑ B	❑ C	❑ D	134.	❑ A	❑ B	❑ C ❑ D
85.	❑ A	❑ B	❑ C	❑ D	110.	❑ A	❑ B	❑ C	❑ D	135.	❑ A	❑ B	❑ C ❑ D
86.	❑ A	❑ B	❑ C	❑ D	111.	❑ A	❑ B	❑ C	❑ D	136.	❑ A	❑ B	❑ C ❑ D
87.	❑ A	❑ B	❑ C	❑ D	112.	❑ A	❑ B	❑ C	❑ D	137.	❑ A	❑ B	❑ C ❑ D
88.	❑ A	❑ B	❑ C	❑ D	113.	❑ A	❑ B	❑ C	❑ D	138.	❑ A	❑ B	❑ C ❑ D
89.	❑ A	❑ B	❑ C	❑ D	114.	❑ A	❑ B	❑ C	❑ D	139.	❑ A	❑ B	❑ C ❑ D
90.	❑ A	❑ B	❑ C	❑ D	115.	❑ A	❑ B	❑ C	❑ D	140.	❑ A	❑ B	❑ C ❑ D
91.	❑ A	❑ B	❑ C	❑ D	116.	❑ A	❑ B	❑ C	❑ D	141.	❑ A	❑ B	❑ C ❑ D
92.	❑ A	❑ B	❑ C	❑ D	117.	❑ A	❑ B	❑ C	❑ D	142.	❑ A	❑ B	❑ C ❑ D
93.	❑ A	❑ B	❑ C	❑ D	118.	❑ A	❑ B	❑ C	❑ D	143.	❑ A	❑ B	❑ C ❑ D
94.	❑ A	❑ B	❑ C	❑ D	119.	❑ A	❑ B	❑ C	❑ D	144.	❑ A	❑ B	❑ C ❑ D
95.	❑ A	❑ B	❑ C	❑ D	120.	❑ A	❑ B	❑ C	❑ D	145.	❑ A	❑ B	❑ C ❑ D
96.	❑ A	❑ B	❑ C	❑ D	121.	❑ A	❑ B	❑ C	❑ D	146.	❑ A	❑ B	❑ C ❑ D
97.	❑ A	❑ B	❑ C	❑ D	122.	❑ A	❑ B	❑ C	❑ D	147.	❑ A	❑ B	❑ C ❑ D
98.	❑ A	❑ B	❑ C	❑ D	123.	❑ A	❑ B	❑ C	❑ D	148.	❑ A	❑ B	❑ C ❑ D
99.	❑ A	❑ B	❑ C	❑ D	124.	❑ A	❑ B	❑ C	❑ D	149.	❑ A	❑ B	❑ C ❑ D
100.	❑ A	❑ B	❑ C	❑ D	125.	❑ A	❑ B	❑ C	❑ D	150.	❑ A	❑ B	❑ C ❑ D

Contents

Core Review Test 1

1-1. A patient admitted with shortness of breath demonstrates the following findings: temperature 36.8° C, HR 120/min sinus tachycardia, BP 130/76 mm Hg, RR 36/min with SpO_2 91%. Breath sounds reveal inspiratory crackles and rhonchi in all lung fields. The chest x-ray report states that there are Kerley B lines, enlargement of the peribronchial hilar spaces, and enlarged cardiac silhouette. These findings are consistent with which of the following?

A. Pericardial tamponade
B. Pulmonary edema
C. Pneumonia
D. Acute inferior wall MI with right ventricular failure

1-2. A research study is being conducted in the ICU and telemetry units to look at the effectiveness of steroid use prior to cardiac catheterization. A 56-year-old telemetry patient is approached by one of the research staff; the patient's nurse, outside the room, overhears their conversation. The staff member asks the subject if he would like to enroll in the study because it is a quick way to make $100. The patient asks whether any risk is involved, and the staff member says, "Not really. All you have to do is sign this form." How should the patient's nurse respond?

A. Report what was overheard to the ethics committee

B. Contact the primary investigator on the study
C. Enter the room and review the protocol with the patient
D. Recognize that the staff member is a volunteer interested in gathering data for this important study

1-3. A patient is hospitalized for severe fractures of the pelvis and left femur. Two hours after the initial patient assessment, the nurse notes the following findings: increased anxiety and confusion, BP unchanged at 148/84 mm Hg, HR increased from 120 to 146/min, respiratory rate increased from 18 to 44/min. Pulmonary artery pressures are 55/28 mm Hg, and cardiac output is decreased from 4 to 2.3 L/min. The nurse's intervention at this point should be to

A. Reassess all parameters in 1 hour
B. Initiate sequential compression device
C. Administer oxygen and prepare for intubation
D. Administer thrombolytic medication

1-4. A patient undergoes emergency CABG surgery after failed thrombolysis and a percutanous coronary intervention in which coronary artery dissection occurred. Prior to surgery, the patient was alert and able to give verbal consent. Mediastinal and pleural chest tubes are present with moderate drainage. Moderate oozing is also present at the sternotomy and saphenous vein graft incisions and at the right groin sheath site. The patient has a PA catheter, an NG tube, and a urinary catheter in place. Frequent assessments by the nurse for this patient should include which of the following?

A. Hourly pupil checks to determine if intracranial bleeding has occurred
B. Inspecting the patient's back hourly for signs of retroperitoneal bleeding
C. Hourly groin palpation and neurovascular checks of the leg used for PCI
D. Hourly auscultation of bowel sounds to determine if gastric bleeding is present

1-5. For a patient admitted to the hospital after a motor vehicle crash, which of the following assessment components would the critical care nurse expect to perform at the bedside *immediately* upon arrival?

A. Breathing, circulation, and vital signs
B. Airway, breathing, and circulation
C. Disability, head-to-toe examination, and exposure
D. Vital signs, circulation, and inspection

1-6. A patient in the ICU was admitted for acute coronary artery syndrome. Which of the following leads is recommended for ST segment monitoring?

A. II
B. V_6
C. I
D. V_3

1-7. Which of the following vasopressors is indicated in low cardiac output syndrome when the desired effect is vasoconstriction without tachycardia?

A. Norepinephrine (Levophed)
B. Phenylephrine (Neosynephrine)
C. Dopamine
D. Epinephrine

1-8. A patient with urosepsis was admitted to the ICU 12 hours ago, has received 6 L of fluid thus far, and is receiving levophed to maintain her systolic BP >90 mm Hg. She is on assist-control ventilation with a rate of 12, tidal volumes of 8 mL/kg, PEEP of +5, and FiO_2 of .50. Over the past 2 hours, her oxygen saturation has been slowly decreasing from 99% to 90% despite increasing her

FiO_2 to .80. Her most recent ABG shows a pH of 7.30, $PaCO_2$ of 55 mm Hg, and PaO_2 of 60 mm Hg. Her pulmonary pressures are increasing, and her static pressure is now 40. What ventilator changes does the nurse anticipate?

A. Increase the PEEP to +10 and reevaluate O_2 saturation and ABG
B. Switch to a pressure support mode for greater patient comfort
C. Increase the set respiratory rate to normalize the pH
D. Decrease tidal volumes to 6 mL/kg and maintain minute ventilation.

1-9. A patient is admitted to the ICU after sustaining a concussion and blunt abdominal trauma to the right upper quadrant in a domestic dispute. The patient's vital signs are BP 145/86 mm Hg, pulse 86 beats/min, respiration 15 breaths/min, and temperature 98.8° F. The nurse is monitoring the patient's bowel sounds, abdominal tenderness, and abdominal girth frequently. Which of the following laboratory parameters is especially important for the nurse to closely monitor for bleeding in this patient?

A. Platelet count
B. Protime
C. Hematocrit
D. Mean corpuscular volume

1-10. A patient is admitted for elective craniotomy and clipping of a posterior communicating artery aneurysm. On the initial ICU assessment, the nurse notes that the patient's Glasgow Coma Scale (GCS) score is 15 with no focal weakness. The patient has a large, nonreactive pupil as well as ptosis in the left eye. The nurse's best course of action at this point would be to

A. Call the neurosurgeon immediately, as the aneurysm may have ruptured
B. Prepare the patient for an anticipated STAT head CT scan to evaluate for expansion of the aneurysm
C. Review the medical record to identify the patient's presenting symptoms and examination prior to admission
D. Call anesthesia STAT for emergent intubation in response to the altered level of consciousness

1-11. Approximately 3 minutes after the first CRRT treatment is begun, a patient complains of severe back pain and itching. The patient's vital signs are BP 84/50 mm Hg, HR 115 beats/min, RR 26/min. The nurse's initial intervention for this patient would be to

A. Administer 100 mL normal saline fluid bolus

B. Check for bleeding at the access site

C. Administer diphenhydramine (Benadryl) 12.5 mg IV

D. Disconnect the patient from the machine

1-12. The alarm on a patient's monitor sounds, and the nurse immediately responds to assess the patient. The patient denies chest pain but complains of palpitations. The nurse places oxygen on the patient and obtains the following vital signs: BP 120/70 mm Hg and respiratory rate 22/min. The nurse then obtains the 12-lead ECG below. The most appropriate immediate intervention for the nurse would be to

A. Have the patient perform a vagal maneuver

B. Administer adenosine 6 mg IV rapidly

C. Administer diltiazem 0.25 mg/kg IV over 2 minutes

D. Perform immediate synchronized cardioversion

1-13. Bedside transesophageal echocardiography reveals a dissecting aortic aneurysm with pericardial effusion in a patient with a blood pressure of 80/50 mm Hg. Prior to transferring the patient to the operating room, which of the following does the nurse need to prepare for?

A. Immediate pericardiocentesis to relieve tamponade

B. Administration of labetolol to decrease afterload and contractility

C. Administration of norepinephrine at 4 mcg/min to raise BP

D. Insertion of two large-bore IVs to obtain laboratory samples and administer fluids

1-14. After a patient has received an implantable cardioverter defibrillator (ICD), one of the most common psychological problems the patient may experience is

A. Fear of being shocked by the device

B. Anxiety over being awakened from sleep by the device

C. Worry that physical exertion will trigger the device

D. Depression over dependence on the device

1-15. A patient admitted for acute alcohol ingestion was intubated by paramedics at the scene because of a decreased level of con-

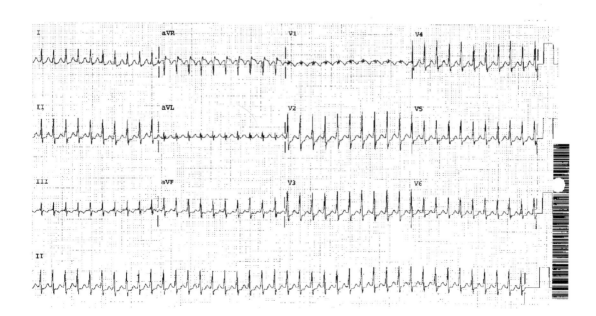

sciousness. The paramedics reported that the patient vomited a large amount of emesis during the intubation. On admission to the ICU, the patient's vital signs are as follows: temperature 38.5° C, HR 120/min, BP 90/60 mm Hg, RR 28/min, S_aO_2 94% on FiO_2 100%. A chest x-ray shows infiltrates in the patient's right lower lobe. Which of the following interventions should the critical care nurse anticipate?

A. Aggressive broad-spectrum antibiotics
B. Bronchoalveolar lavage to clear the distal airways
C. Steroid therapy to mitigate the inflammatory cascade
D. Aggressive pulmonary hygiene and culturing

1-16. Recent research has found that African Americans experiencing myocardial infarction are likely to delay treatment if they are single, widowed, or divorced, because they do not view their symptoms as life-threatening or serious. A nurse is now planning care for a 56-year-old African-American patient who delayed coming into a small community hospital for chest pain and experienced a myocardial infarction without the opportunity to receive thrombolytics. The nurse's plan of care for this patient should include

A. Teaching the patient about thrombolytic agents
B. Obtaining an emergency call device so help can be summoned immediately if chest pain recurs
C. Educating the patient and family regarding early interventions
D. Admonishing the patient for the delay in response so it does not happen again

1-17. A patient is admitted to the critical care unit from the general surgical floor after an episode of vomiting. The patient developed respiratory distress secondary to aspiration pneumonia and required intubation for refractory hypoxia and airway management. During the past week, the patient has remained hypoxic despite aggressive pulmonary support and has developed acute tubular necrosis and hepatic failure. To establish appropriate priorities of care for this patient, the nurse needs to plan care for a patient with which of the following conditions?

A. Systemic inflammatory response syndrome (SIRS)
B. Septic shock
C. Bacteremia
D. Multiple organ dysfunction syndrome (MODS)

1-18. A patient admitted 2 weeks ago for bilateral flail chest injuries associated with a motor vehicle collision had chest tubes inserted and has been intubated and mechanically ventilated throughout that period. His left chest tube demonstrates persistent bubbling during inspiration and expiration, although his breath sounds are clear bilaterally and the drainage system is working properly. Which of the following interventions should the critical care nurse consider next?

A. Monitor tidal volumes
B. Obtain a STAT chest x-ray
C. Assess the patient for tracheal deviation
D. Place the left chest tube to water seal

1-19. The critical care nurse is performing peritoneal dialysis on a patient with end-stage renal disease (ESRD). Following the inflow period, the patient complains of severe shoulder pain. The critical care nurse should immediately

A. Drain the effluent with the patient in the knee-chest position
B. Change the patient's position to right side-lying
C. Ensure that all future infusions are warmed to body temperature
D. Increase the dwell time

1-20. A patient is admitted following involvement in a multi-vehicle collision. The patient's urine output has increased from 125 mL to 1000 mL over the last 2 hours. Which of the following is the most important assessment the nurse should make at this time?

A. Abdominal girth measurement
B. Urine specific gravity
C. Capillary blood glucose level
D. Potassium level

1-21. A patient is intubated for acute respiratory failure. The patient has no history of cardiac disease, and there is no evidence of peripheral edema. Upon admission to the ICU, diagnostic testing reveals the following:

12-lead ECG demonstrating sinus tachycardia at 120 beats/min with atrial premature contractions and 1-mm ST segment depression in leads V_3, V_4, V_5, V_6

CPK-MB 5%

Troponin 0.3 ng/mL

BNP 598 pg/mL

These findings are most consistent with

A. Acute MI with cardiogenic shock
B. Pericarditis
C. Acute heart failure
D. Tricuspid valve insufficiency

1-22. A patient recently treated for deep vein thrombosis is now admitted to the ICU. The patient is pale and complains of dizziness, chest pain, and shortness of breath. During the review of medications, the nurse learns that the patient has been on heparin therapy. Which of the following laboratory tests would be most important for determining whether this patient is experiencing heparin-induced thrombocytopenia (HIT)?

A. Enzyme-linked immunosorbent assay and platelet count
B. International normalized ratio and prothrombin time
C. Complete blood count with manual differential
D. Arterial blood gas and mixed venous blood gas

1-23. A 42-year-old man is admitted to the ICU with severe abdominal pain, elevated lipase levels, and no prior history of alcoholism. A tentative diagnosis of pancreatitis has been made. The patient states that he never wants to suffer this way again. How can the nurse best assist this patient in better understanding his diagnosis to meet his goal?

A. Discuss the etiology of this disorder
B. Provide information on how to regain weight
C. Assess the patient's food preferences
D. Ask if a living will is on file

1-24. Pulmonary edema is most likely to develop when

A. Right atrial pressure exceeds 18 mm Hg
B. Cardiac output is 4 L/min or less
C. PCWP exceeds 20 mm Hg
D. Systemic blood pressure exceeds 180/110 mm Hg

1-25. A patient who has been hospitalized for several weeks with a severe pelvic fracture is readmitted to the ICU with hypotension, chest pain, and shortness of breath. His BP is now 88/54 mm Hg, down from 128/77 mm Hg in the emergency department; pulse is 74 beats/min, and respiratory rate is 28 breaths/min. The patient does not exhibit edema, pulses are 2+, and extremities are warm. The most likely cause of this patient's hypotension is

A. Increased afterload
B. Peripheral vasodilatation
C. Cardiomyopathy
D. Reduced preload

1-26. A patient admitted to the ICU after endovascular repair of an abdominal aortic aneurysm (AAA) has the following assessment findings: BP 120/74 mm Hg, HR 90/min, RR 20/min, temperature 36° C. Distal pulses are 2+, capillary refill is 2 seconds, and the groin site demonstrates no evidence of hematoma. Urine output is 20 mL/hr for 2 hours. The most likely cause of decreased urine output is

A. Renal toxic effects of contrast agents
B. Occlusion of the renal artery by the endograft
C. Hypovolemia due to operative blood loss
D. Hypovolemia due to retroperitoneal bleeding

1-27. A patient is in the ICU after undergoing a gastric resection for stomach cancer and has been started on a regular diet prior to transfer out of the unit. Within minutes of eating, the patient develops diaphoresis, weakness, cramping, and palpitations, BP is 102/70 mm Hg, pulse is 96 beats/min, and respirations are 22 breaths/min. Which of the following conditions best explains these clinical findings?

A. Myocardial infarction

    B.   Pulmonary embolism
    C.   Severe rebound hyperglycemia
    D.   Dumping syndrome

1-28. An 88-year-old woman is admitted to the ICU with electrolyte imbalance, malnutrition, and chest pain. Upon receiving the patient from the emergency department, the ICU nurse notices the residue from a tape mark across the patient's mouth, which was documented in the patient's ED assessment. After the two nurses discuss this finding, what should be considered as the next best course of action?

    A.   Make a report to adult protective services
    B.   Carefully document assessment and patient response to tape marks
    C.   Call the physician to report these findings
    D.   Discuss these findings with the family in order to gain more information

1-29. A patient who is 32 weeks' pregnant is admitted with pre-eclampsia and generalized edema. BP is 210/128 mm Hg, pulse is 120 beats/min, RR is 36/min. The chest x-ray shows evidence of pulmonary edema. Prior to transfer to the ICU, 40 mg of furosemide (Lasix) is administered to the patient. Which of the following medications would be used to reduce blood pressure and prevent potential harm to the fetus?

    A.   Sodium nitroprusside (Nipride) titrated to achieve a systolic BP of 150 mm Hg
    B.   Nitroglycerin titrated to achieve a systolic BP of 150 mm Hg
    C.   Captopril (Capoten) 100 mg PO
    D.   Phentolamine (Regitine) 5 mg IV

1-30. A patient in the ICU is intubated and mechanically ventilated on the following settings: tidal volume 600 mL, rate 12/min, FiO_2 70%, PEEP 15 cm H_2O. The peak inspiratory pressure is 50 cm H_2O, and the patient's respiratory rate is 12/min. Arterial blood gas values include pH 7.25, PaO_2 60 mm Hg, $PaCO_2$ 48 mm Hg. Which of the following findings would best indicate clinical improvement in this patient?

    A.   Peak inspiratory pressure 43 cm H_2O
    B. $PaCO_2$ 45 mm Hg

    C. PaO_2 62 mm Hg
    D.   Respiratory rate 14/min

1-31. In caring for a patient who is mechanically ventilated, the critical care nurse will best implement evidenced-based recommendations for the prevention of ventilator-associated pneumonia (VAP) and possible development of bacteremia and sepsis by

    A.   Elevating the HOB 30 to 45 degrees
    B.   Providing oral care every 4-6 hr
    C.   Changing ventilator circuit every 24 hr
    D.   Keeping oral mucosa dry

1-32. Upon arrival to the critical care unit after coronary artery bypass graft surgery, the patient has a BP of 180/110 mm Hg, a heart rate of 70 beats/min 100% paced, a RAP of 6 mm Hg, a PAD of 10 mm Hg, a temperature of 36° C, and cardiac output of 3.5 LPM. Urine output for the first hour is 60 mL. Which of the following interventions should the nurse perform first?

    A.   Bolus the patient with 250 mL to increase the RAP and PAD
    B.   Increase the nitroglycerin infusion by 6.6 mcg/min to decrease BP
    C.   Increase the pacing rate to 75 to improve cardiac output
    D.   Administer propranolol 1 mg IV to decrease blood pressure

1-33. A 30-year-old patient with longstanding asthma was admitted to the ICU with a severe asthma attack. Her work of breathing has been increasing, and her most recent ABG results on 40% facemask are pH 7.25, PCO_2 65 mm Hg, PO_2 60 mm Hg, and HCO_3 25 mEq/L. Based on these findings, which of the following interventions should the critical care nurse anticipate?

    A.   Addition of steroids to the bronchodilator regime
    B.   Changing from beta-agonists to leukotriene inhibitors
    C.   Initiation of inhaled nitric oxide
    D.   Immediate intubation

1-34. Ventilator-associated pneumonias (VAP) result in approximately 6 more days in the ICU, and $10,000 to $40,000 per episode in costs. Your facility has decided to focus on decreasing VAP. Which of the following interventions would provide the farthest-reaching impact on this health problem?

   A. Adherence to handwashing and sterile technique

   B. Prophylaxis antibiotics for ventilator patients

   C. Pneumococcal vaccines for patients older than 65 years

   D. DVT prophylaxis

1-35. The patient admitted with a presumptive diagnosis of acute myocardial infarction has an insulin drip infusing. Over the past 30 minutes, the patient has become agitated and irritable. Which of the following should the nurse do first?

   A. Assess breath sounds

   B. Administer an anxiolytic medication

   C. Measure capillary glucose

   D. Provide milk and crackers

1-36. A patient about to receive a bone marrow transplant is in strict isolation and expressing feelings of anxiety. Nursing measures appropriate to this situation include

   A. Playing music the patient enjoys and allowing photographs at the bedside

   B. Allowing the patient's cat to visit for a pet therapy session

   C. Encouraging the patient's school-aged grandchildren to visit

   D. Asking family members to bring in fresh produce as comfort food

1-37. The nurse should immediately perform which of the following interventions for a patient with chest pain, hypotension, and tachycardia at a rate of 180 beats/min?

   A. Administer amiodarone 150 mg IV over 10 minutes

   B. Administer adenosine 6 mg. rapid IV push

   C. Perform synchronized cardioversion

   D. Defibrillate with 300 joules

1-38. During a staff meeting, the unit-based performance improvement nurse provides data on stress-related mucosal disease (SRMD) in the ICU. Data for 3 months suggest that, on average, 20 of the monthly census of 100 patients are developing SRMD. The nurse asks her colleagues for suggestions to decrease the incidence of SRMD. One good suggestion would be to

   A. Develop a prevention protocol for high-risk patients in the ICU

   B. Add a proton pump inhibitor to the standing orders for all patients

   C. Deliver the data to physicians on the medical ICU committee for their consideration

   D. Continue data collection to ensure sufficient evidence exists before a response is made

1-39. After cardiac catheterization with percutaneous balloon angioplasty, a patient develops a paradoxical pulse. The most likely cause for this finding is

   A. Pericardial tamponade

   B. Coronary artery spasm

   C. Dysrhythmia

   D. Vasovagal reaction

1-40. A postoperative abdominal surgery patient weighing 700 lb (318 kg) develops acute onset of dyspnea and chest pain. Arterial blood gas values are pH 7.35, PaO_2 is 74 mm Hg, $PaCO_2$ is 30 mm Hg, and O_2 is saturation 90%. Chest x-ray demonstrates an enlarged cardiac silhouette, a prominent pulmonary artery, and mild right pleural effusion. The 12-lead ECG demonstrates T wave inversions in the anterior leads. These findings suggest that this patient has most likely developed which of the following?

   A. Aspiration pneumonia

   B. Pulmonary embolism

   C. Acute myocardial infarction

   D. Pneumothorax

1-41. A patient with chronic renal failure presents to the ED with severe itching, abdominal cramps, nausea, and diarrhea. The patient's serum calcium is 6.2 mg/dL. Which of the following needs to be administered for management of this patient?

   A. IV potassium supplement

   B. Oral phosphate supplement

   C. Oral aluminum hydroxide

   D. IV sodium bicarbonate

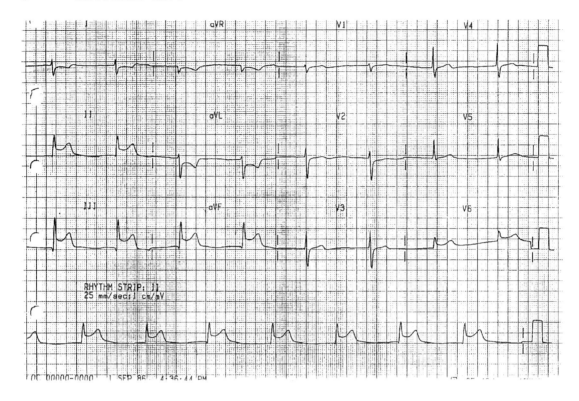

1-42. The 12-lead ECG above is obtained on a patient experiencing chest pain. The nurse administers 1/150 grains of sublingual nitroglycerin, and the patient's BP drops from 130/80 mm Hg to 80/50 mm Hg. The most likely cause of the decrease in blood pressure for this patient is

A. Hypersensitivity to nitroglycerin
B. Right ventricular MI
C. Papillary muscle rupture
D. Rupture of the ventricular free wall

1-43. A patient had an upper esophagogastroduodenoscopy (EGD) 30 minutes ago and is drowsy. As the patient is slowly waking up, he asks, "Can I have a drink of water?" The nurse's best response would be to say

A. If you can swallow, you can have something to drink.
B. You cannot have anything until your gag reflex returns.
C. Try to rest for now; you need to recover from the procedure.
D. Now that you're thirsty, we can order your lunch tray for delivery in 30 minutes.

1-44. A multiple trauma patient with a grade IV liver laceration is re-admitted to the ICU from the operating room after having the liver packs replaced for the third time. The patient has been on mechanical ventilation for 5 days and maintenance of the ventilator equipment is now being considered. Which of the following measures for prevention of ventilator-associated pneumonia is indicated at this time?

A. Replacing the humidifier
B. Changing all flexible ventilator tubing
C. Discarding condensate in ventilator tubing
D. Changing all ventilator circuit components

1-45. When a patient with an implanted cardioverter defibrillator develops rapid atrial fibrillation that results in inappropriate delivery of defibrillation shocks, the nurse's first intervention should be to

A. Perform overdrive pacing with a transcutaneous pacemaker
B. Place a pacemaker magnet over the pacemaker generator
C. Administer diltiazem 15 mg IV over 2 minutes

D. Administer amiodarone 150 mg IV over 10 minutes

1-46. A patient has been receiving intravenous steroids to treat an acute exacerbation of asthma. While previously alert and oriented, this morning the patient is obtunded, and morning labs reveal a serum glucose of 624 mg/dL with no other notable findings. In planning care for this patient, which of the following conditions should the nurse now anticipate needing to manage?

A. Diabetes insipidus
B. Type 1 diabetes mellitus
C. Hyperglycemic, hyperosmolar, nonketotic coma
D. Polycythemia vera

1-47. Classic echocardiographic features of diastolic dysfunction in patients diagnosed with heart failure would include which of the following?

A. Ejection fraction 55% and decreased early diastolic filling time
B. Ejection fraction 50% and increased late diastolic filling time
C. Ejection fraction 60% and prolonged left ventricular ejection time
D. Ejection fraction 35% and shortened left ventricular ejection time

1-48. A nurse in a 16-bed ICU that is managed with a shared governance model is currently the chair of a multidisciplinary committee that evaluates use of medical devices for attriutes such as unit costs, type, infection rate, and malfunction rate. The committee is notified that a new cardiologist coming in a few months will be implanting cardioverter-defibrillator devices, so the hospital would like the committee to develop a tool to be used to evaluate outcomes related to this device, similar to a registry (log of positive and negative outcomes). As the leader of this multidisciplinary group, how should the nurse proceed to investigate this device?

A. Contact the sales representative from a company selling ICDs
B. Research the current registries to identify variables measured
C. Modify the current evaluation tool for use with the ICD

D. Consider obtaining a consultant to help the committee with this task

1-49. An ICU nurse caring for a patient admitted with severe abdominal discomfort and fatigue notes that the patient tested positive for *Helicobacter pylori* and has a history of cigarette smoking. The patient develops nausea and abdominal tenderness. His vital signs are BP 123/80 mm Hg, pulse 89 beats/min, respirations 15 breaths/min. Within 15 minutes, the patient vomits, and his emesis contains coffee grounds. His vital signs are BP 100/68 mm Hg, pulse 120 beats/min, respirations 24 breaths/min. Which of the following medical orders for this patient merits the nurse's immediate attention?

A. Secure initial coagulation study findings and monitor each shift
B. Insert large-bore IV
C. Upright KUB
D. Monitor fluid balance closely

1-50. A patient with community-acquired pneumonia has an advanced directive stating no intubation. The patient's spouse, who is also the Durable Power of Attorney (DPA) for the patient, wishes to have the patient intubated. The patient is in obvious respiratory distress, on BiPAP, but he remains alert and oriented. The nurse caring for the patient should

A. Inform the spouse that the DPA is not in effect until the patient is no longer able to make decisions
B. Encourage the patient to consider intubation as his spouse desires
C. Inform the patient of the spouse's concerns and ask if the patient wishes to be intubated for a trial period
D. Encourage the patient to discuss intubation with his spouse

1-51. Coronary artery spasm after percutaneous coronary atherectomy is best prevented with administration of

A. Nitroglycerin
B. Calcium channel blockers
C. Heparin
D. Glycoprotein IIb/IIIa inhibitors

1-52. A patient with a ruptured cerebral aneurysm may develop hydrocephalus because

   A. Blood in the subarachnoid space blocks reabsorption of cerebrospinal fluid (CSF) in the arachnoid villi
   B. A thrombus may form and obstruct flow of CSF out of the ventricles
   C. Cerebral edema may lead to a mass effect that blocks CSF flow
   D. Vasospasm may limit the flow of CSF

1-53. Which of the following is the earliest clinical sign of impending hypovolemic shock?

   A. Systolic BP less than 90 mm Hg
   B. Capillary refill time greater than 4 seconds
   C. Decreased urine output
   D. Tachycardia greater than 120 beats/min

1-54. A 75-year-old patient presents to the ED following a head-on motor vehicle collision where he was a belted driver. He is alert and oriented with stable vital signs and complains of mild pain to his right chest. During his trauma workup, he suddenly develops shortness of breath, his oxygen saturation drops to 85%, and his heart rate and blood pressure elevate slightly from baseline. He has decreased breath sounds in his right lung fields, and his trachea is midline. What is the most appropriate nursing action at this time?

   A. Secure a chest tube insertion kit and notify the physician that the patient may have a pneumothorax
   B. Administer oxygen via a nasal cannula and notify the physician about these assessment findings
   C. Obtain an order for and administer STAT a narcotic analgesic
   D. Document the assessment findings and prepare the patient for prompt admission to ICU

1-55. A nurse would like to start drawing blood for aPTT samples from heparin wells to aid in decreasing patients' pain from frequent venipunctures. What should the nurse do next to implement this change?

   A. Identify key stakeholders in this proposed change of practice

   B. Specify the intended change in bedside practice
   C. Modify the nursing flowsheet to accommodate the change
   D. Evaluate the success of the change in procedure

1-56. Two hours after coronary artery bypass graft surgery, a patient has the following assessment findings:

   Heart rate 80/min, 100% paced

   BP 80/62 mm Hg, MAP 68 mm Hg

   RAP 15 mm Hg

   PAD 14 mm Hg

   CO 3.0 L/min

   Chest tube output has been 50 mL per hour for 2 hours. These findings are consistent with which of the following?

   A. Normal postoperative course after open heart surgery
   B. Myocardial stunning
   C. Cardiac tamponade
   D. Perioperative myocardial infarction

1-57. In caring for a patient admitted from the ER with a diagnosis of ingestion of N-methyl-D-aspartate (Ecstasy), the critical care nurse observes that the patient has cola-colored urine with a specific gravity of 1.028. These findings are consistent with the development of rhabdomyolysis. One of the most important interventions to prevent renal failure in patients with rhabdomyolysis includes

   A. Maintaining a urine pH <5.0
   B. Inserting an indwelling urinary catheter
   C. Maintaining urine output >150 mL/hr
   D. Monitoring hemodynamics closely

1-58. Which of the following testing methods is most helpful in diagnosing myocardial ischemia in a patient with left bundle branch block (LBBB) and peripheral vascular disease?

   A. Exercise treadmill stress test
   B. SPECT perfusion imaging with technetium-99m sestamibi
   C. Dipyridamole stress test
   D. Magnetic resonance imaging (MRI)

1-59. A 29-year-old man is admitted to the telemetry unit with a diagnosis of unstable angina. The patient has had numerous admissions over the past year with a history of cocaine abuse and demanding demeanor. As soon as he is admitted, he asks for pain medication and for lunch. He states that his pain is midsternal and that its level is 6 on a scale of 1 to 10. The patient has NTG SL and morphine 2 mg IV ordered for pain. The charge nurse tells the nurse assigned to this patient, "Just give him the morphine; you know that is what he wants." What should the staff nurse do?

A. Give the NTG SL X 3 before administering the morphine
B. Administer morphine 2 mg IV
C. Inform the patient that he will have to wait 30 minutes until morphine can be given
D. Discuss treatment options with the patient

1-60. A patient with a known history of asthma is admitted with status asthmaticus. When planning care for this patient, the critical care nurse must keep in mind that the goals of mechanical ventilation for this patient will include use of

A. Low tidal volumes and minimal PEEP
B. High tidal volumes and low PEEP
C. Low respiratory rate and high tidal volumes
D. High PEEP and low FiO_2.

1-61. After aortofemoral bypass surgery for acute arterial occlusion, the patient's CPK is elevated, and his serum potassium level is 5.9 mEq/L. Arterial blood gas values include PaO_2 90 mm Hg, p_aCO_2 24 mm Hg, and HCO_3 19 mm Hg. This patient is at risk for developing

A. Dysrhythmias
B. Graft occlusion
C. Pulmonary embolus
D. Heart failure

1-62. A patient has just been admitted to the ICU from the emergency room with a diagnosis of gastrointestional bleeding. She is alert and oriented, however very nauseated and adamant about needing to call her son. The nurse says that she will call the son to notify him of his mother's admission. During the admission history, the nurse would like to assess the patient's beliefs related to her admitting diagnosis. Which question will provide the nurse with information for understanding her patient's cultural beliefs related to her diagnosis?

A. When do you experience your first symptoms?
B. Does anyone else in your family have this bleeding problem?
C. Do you consume alcohol on a regular basis?
D. Why do you think you are sick?

1-63. A patient with long-standing history of COPD is admitted for worsening dyspnea and desaturation. She is on home oxygen therapy at 2 lpm. Her admission VS are temperature 38.2° C, HR 104/min, BP 130/60 mm Hg, RR 28/min, SaO_2 88%. For this patient, the nurse knows that increasing the FiO_2 should

A. Improve the patient's oxygenation
B. Only be done on the basis of ABG results
C. Be avoided because it may weaken the patient's respiratory drive
D. Only be used as a last resort because it may increase hypoxemic vasoconstriction

1-64. A patient with acute pancreatitis is admitted to the ICU following respiratory arrest. The critical care nurse observes twitching of the patient's upper lip, increased peak airway pressure, and wheezing on auscultation. Which initial drug therapy would the critical care nurse anticipate administering via IV?

A. Magnesium sulfate 25 mEq in 1000 mL D5W
B. Plicamycin 1050 mcg in 1000 mL NS
C. Vasopressin 100 units in 250 mL D5W
D. Calcium chloride 1000 mg in 1000 mL NS

1-65. A 33-year-old male is brought to the emergency department by a family member after vomiting blood at home. He had been drinking and his alcohol history includes a 6 pack of beer on weekends. He also has a history of chronic back pain. He is admitted to the

ICU with a diagnosis of upper gastrointestinal bleeding. His vital signs are BP 110/50 mm Hg; pulse 94 beats/min; respiratory rate 12 breaths/min. Initial results show a blood alcohol level of 0.10 mg/dL. After 30 minutes, the nurse notes that he is lethargic, pale, and diaphoretic; BP is now 94/60 mm Hg, heart rate 134 beats/min with thready pulses, respiratory rate 20 breaths/min, and urine output 25 cc/hr. His abdomen is tender to palpation in the left upper quadrant, and bowel sounds are hyperactive. Which of the following conditions is likely contributing to this patient's current findings?

A. Pulmonary embolism with hypoxemia
B. Erosive gastritis with 25% blood volume loss
C. Intracranial hypertension
D. Dehydration owing to alcohol abuse

1-66. A patient admitted with hypertensive crisis has been on an intravenous nitroprusside (Nipride) infusion for 3 days. Systolic BP has been maintained at less than 150 mm Hg. The patient is becoming increasingly confused and combative. Vital signs include heart rate of 110/min sinus tachycardia, respiratory rate of 22/min with an SpO$_2$ of 96% on 3 L oxygen by nasal cannula. The likely cause of the patient's symptoms is which of the following?

A. Stroke
B. Acute MI
C. Thiocyanate toxicity
D. Encephalopathy

1-67. The patient in septic shock may present with a variety of clinical manifestations that may change dramatically as the condition progresses. Which physiologic symptoms best describe the clinical manifestations associated with septic shock?

A. ↑ temperature and ↑ urine output
B. ↓ systemic vascular resistance (SVR) and ↓ cardiac output (CO)
C. ↑ mixed venous oxygen saturation (SVO$_2$) and ↑ heart rate (HR)
D. ↑ right atrial pressure (RAP) and ↑ respiratory rate (RR)

1-68. Recent research supports the provision of oral care to reduce hospital-associated pneumonia among ventilated patients. What would be the best approach for the nurse to use in implementing oral care on the unit?

A. Place oral care kits at the bedside of every ventilated patient
B. Establish a new multidisciplinary team for this purpose
C. Hold a staff meeting to elicit colleagues' views on this issue
D. Include "oral care every 2 hours" on the standing orders for ventilated patients

1-69. A patient with heart failure is receiving diuretics, beta blockers, and ACE inhibitors. The patient has a weight gain of 2 kg and severe shortness of breath. BP is 120/76 mm Hg, HR 70/min, RR 26/min. The nurse anticipates administering 40 mg IV furosemide (Lasix) and

A. Discontinuing beta blocking medications
B. Decreasing beta blocker dosage
C. Administering an additional dose of beta blocker
D. Administering an additional dose of ACE inhibitor

1-70. The physician orders a trial of noninvasive ventilation (NIV) for a COPD patient with worsening arterial blood gases. The nurse knows that for this COPD patient, NIV

A. Will require fairly heavy sedation to enable the patient to tolerate this therapy
B. May be helpful in reducing the need for endotracheal intubation
C. Needs to be used with caution because it increases work of breathing
D. Needs to be administered via nasal pillows rather than a full mask

1-71. The patient's wife asks how her husband could have developed diabetic ketoacidosis, since he has been so careful to manage his diabetes properly these past 10 years. Which of the following represents the best explanation the nurse could provide to this question?

A. "Your husband must have been cheating on his diet or skipping insulin doses."

B. "In times of stress, the body produces more cortisol than normal, and blood sugar increases."

C. "Diabetic ketoacidosis is the result of a genetic abnormality affecting every other generation."

D. "Your husband recently started a daily exercise routine without consulting his primary care provider."

1-72. During fluid resuscitation for hypovolemic shock, the following laboratory values are obtained:

pH 7.28

PaO_2 80 mm Hg

PCO_2 24 mm Hg

Hemoglobin 12.0 g

Hematocrit 30%

Nursing management of this patient needs to include

A. Administration of sodium bicarbonate

B. Administration of one unit of packed red blood cells

C. Administration of crystalloid 200 mL per hour

D. Endotracheal intubation

1-73. A patient is admitted to the ICU after falling from a roof and sustaining fractures of the first three ribs on the right side. The patient is dyspneic and complains of hoarseness, and subcutaneous emphysema can be palpated. The patient is placed on 50% FIO_2 by facemask, and his oxygen saturation is 80%. The only notable findings on chest x-ray are the rib fractures and the presence of mediastinal subcutaneous emphysema. Auscultation reveals equal breath sounds bilaterally and a crunching sound during systole. Within a few minutes, the patient develops increasing respiratory distress. The next intervention the nurse should anticipate is

A. Increasing the FIO_2 to 80%

B. Inserting a right chest tube

C. Intubating the trachea

D. Repeating the chest x-ray

1-74. The best way for nurses to facilitate provision of a "good death" for a patient whose life is ending would be through

A. Having the same nurse assigned to care for the patient

B. Allowing unrestricted visiting for the patient.

C. Encouraging hope in the face of futile care

D. Managing the patient's pain and discomfort

1-75. A patient is admitted with a diagnosis of pulmonary edema. The patient has a bounding carotid pulse, systolic ejection murmur, hypotension, and tachypnea. Chest x-ray shows cardiomegaly and interstitial pulmonary edema. ECG demonstrates bradycardia, left ventricular hypertrophy, and left bundle branch block. Which of the following is the most likely etiology of these findings?

A. Aortic regurgitation

B. Mitral valve stenosis

C. Tricuspid regurgitation

D. Pericardial effusion

1-76. A patient was admitted to ICU yesterday evening after being found on the pavement following an apparent assault. The patient has not yet been identified, and his medical history is unknown. He has been clinically stable and maintained on mechanical ventilation with satisfactory ABGs. During a mid-morning assessment, the nurse notes that the patient demonstrates a rhythmic movement of his extremities and begins clenching his jaw on the endotracheal tube. He has not demonstrated this type of activity since admission but was placed on prophylactic anticonvulsants after traumatic brain injury. The nurse hypothesizes that the patient is most likely experiencing

A. Hypoxia

B. Delirium tremens

C. Substance withdrawal

D. Post-traumatic seizures

1-77. When caring for a patient admitted to the ICU following ingestion of 50 tablets of acetaminophen, the critical care nurse recognizes that hepatic encephalopathy with progressive symptoms occurs approximately 48 to 96 hours after ingestion and can develop an appropriate plan of care to prioritize patient management. What physiologic process contributes to the patient's progressive response to the toxic ingestion of acetaminophen?

   A. Clearance
   B. Absorption
   C. Distribution
   D. Chelation

1-78. In a coronary care unit in which medications are not permitted to be left at the bedside and the crash cart with monitor/transcutaneous pacemaker/defibrillator is outside the central nurses' station, an intubated patient on mechanical ventilation develops third-degree AV block at a rate of 35 beats/min with signs of poor tissue perfusion. The most appropriate initial intervention for the nurse assigned to this patient would be to

   A. Initiate transcutaneous pacing
   B. Administer atropine 0.5 mg IV
   C. Initiate an infusion of epinephrine at 5 mcg/min
   D. Initiate an infusion of dopamine at 5 mcg/min

1-79. In which cultural group is the nuclear family the most common form of family organization?

   A. Asian
   B. Anglo-American
   C. African American
   D. Native American

1-80. A patient is admitted to the ICU after a motor vehicle crash in which the air bag was deployed. The initial assessment of the patient reveals the following findings: heart rate 120 beats/min, blood pressure 90/76 mm Hg, respiratory rate 28, SpO_2 94%. Breath sounds are equal bilaterally and shallow. The patient has bulging jugular veins, and heart tones are distant. Which of the following interventions is most appropriate to relieve the patient's condition?

   A. Prepare for chest tube insertion
   B. Prepare for endotracheal intubation
   C. Prepare for pericardiocentesis
   D. Prepare for needle thoracostomy

1-81. A patient is admitted to the ICU with thoracic and facial bruises and abrasions sustained earlier that day in a motor vehicle crash. The patient was unrestrained in the car and indicates that he hit the steering wheel at the time of the incident. He complains of chest pain and has a respiratory rate of 33 breaths/min. His arterial blood gases on room air are pH 7.44, $PaCO_2$ 32 mm Hg, PaO_2 53 mm Hg, HCO_3 24 mEq/L. Which of the following findings indicate a potentially life-threatening emergency for this patient?

   A. Decreased breath sounds in both lung bases
   B. Inspiratory wheezing that clears with coughing
   C. Decreased breath sounds over right lung fields
   D. Absent breath sounds over right lung fields

1-82. A patient is admitted to the medical ICU with decompensated cirrhosis. He is encephalopathic with splenomegaly, ascites, and portal hypertension on CT scan. Portal hypertension places this patient at risk for gastrointestinal bleeding owing to the

   A. Development of right sided heart failure
   B. Excessive circulating blood volume associated with cirrhosis
   C. Fibrotic nature of the hepatic tissue
   D. Elevated pressure in esophageal veins

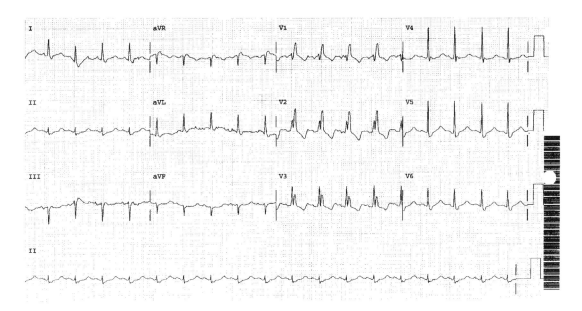

1-83. The 12-lead ECG above demonstrates which of the following?

    A. Right bundle branch block
    B. Left bundle branch block
    C. Sinus tachycardia
    D. Anterior wall myocardial infarction

1-84. When providing postoperative nursing care for a patient recovering from frontal craniotomy, optimal patient positioning will

    A. Maximize jugular venous outflow
    B. Decrease CPP
    C. Facilitate the flow of CSF
    D. Immobilize the surgical site

1-85. Which of the following findings indicates acute dissection of an aortic aneurysm?

    A. Difference in systolic BP between left and right arms exceeding 10 mm Hg and facial edema
    B. Visible pulsation in the abdomen and abdominal bruit
    C. Sudden onset of back pain and syncope
    D. Hypertension and renal insufficiency

1-86. When treating a patient with an acute COPD exacerbation, the critical care nurse can anticipate administering a variety of different pharmacologic agents, including

    A. Bronchodilators and antiviral agents
    B. Prostacycline and oxygen

    C. Mucolytic therapy and antibiotics
    D. Glucocorticoids and cholinergic agents

1-87. A patient's 12-lead ECG shows sinus bradycardia at 40 beats/min and ST segment elevation in leads II, III, and aVF. Which of the following should the nurse anticipate using as definitive treatment for bradycardia in this patient?

    A. Percutaneous coronary intervention
    B. Temporary transvenous pacing
    C. Transcutaneous pacing
    D. Administration of atropine

1-88. A 45-year-old patient with stage 3 heart failure, a 1-month history of frequent episodes of ventricular tachycardia, and an ejection fraction less than 35% is returned from the OR after implantation of an ICD (implantable cardioverter-defibrillator). The patient was unsure about getting the device and hesitantly signed the consent form. For 3 hours after admission to ICU, his vital signs are stable, and ECG monitoring shows normal sinus rhythm. The patient suddenly develops pulseless ventricular tachycardia, codes, and receives 45 minutes of resuscitation efforts with no improvement. Given that the ICD did not operate during a sustained period of ventricular tachycardia, what step(s) should the nurse caring for this patient take now?

A. Document the resuscitation effort in detail since litigation will likely occur
B. Provide emotional support to the family given the poor outcome
C. Complete an incident report and notify administration
D. Design an inservice on ICD malfunctions for the nursing staff.

1-89. A 60-year-old patient is admitted to the ICU with a 3-day history of nausea, vomiting, and persistent diarrhea. Past medical history is significant for coronary artery disease and hypertension. Admitting vital signs reveal the following: temperature: 102° F; HR: 110/min, sinus tachycardia; BP: 90/40 mm Hg; RR: 30/min. Laboratory values from ER are as follows: WBC: 20,000/mm³; hemoglobin: 10.0 g/dL; BUN: 80 mg/dL; creatinine: 2.5 mg/dL; serum lactate: 6 mmol/L. Cultures (blood, urine, sputum, and stool) have been sent, and antibiotic therapy has been initiated. The critical care nurse should expect the patient's immediate treatment to include the following:

A. Inotropic support
B. IV fluid bolus
C. Blood transfusion
D. β-blocker therapy

1-90. A patient in cardiogenic shock is in the ICU on vasopressor and intra-aortic balloon pump support. Which of the following assessment findings most reliably indicates that the current therapy is appropriate?

A. HR 100 BPM, MAP 66 mm Hg, SVR 1200 dynes/sec/cm⁻⁵
B. HR 117 BPM, MAP 53 mm Hg, SVR 1900 dynes/sec/cm⁻⁵
C. HR 110 BPM, MAP 70 mm Hg, SVR 2800 dynes/sec/cm⁻⁵
D. HR 117 BPM, MAP 53 mm Hg, SVR 2400 dynes/sec/cm⁻⁵

1-91. A 49-year-old man is admitted with exacerbation of COPD. The physician orders a genetic test for alpha-1 antitrypsin protein. The nurse knows that the result for this test was positive. The patient asks the nurse if his test results have returned. The nurse's best response would be to say

A. "Do you want to receive this information when you are alone or with your family?"
B. "The physician will need to provide you with those results."
C. "Would you like to have the chaplain present when you get the results?"
D. "Your family should be present when we discuss the results."

1-92. A patient has been admitted for an exacerbation of COPD. When taking this patient's history, which of the following should the critical care nurse focus on as the most likely cause of moderate to severe exacerbations of COPD?

A. Inspissated secretions
B. Infectious processes
C. Inflammatory processes
D. Excessive sputum production

1-93. A postoperative patient with a heart rate of 126 beats/min, blood pressure 80/68 mm Hg, and PCWP 5 mm Hg would benefit most from which of the following interventions?

A. Administration of a 250 mL bolus of normal saline
B. Administration of one unit of packed cells
C. Initiation of a dopamine infusion at 10 mcg/kg/min
D. Vasopressin 40 units IV push

1-94. On postoperative day 3 a patient (status: post roux-en-y gastric bypass) is admitted to the ICU with a diagnosis of sepsis secondary to gastric perforation. On postoperative day 5, the patient's weight increases by 10 kg, urine output is less than 325 mL/day for the last 3 days, and there are crackles bilaterally on lung auscultation. The patient's BP is 94/40 mm Hg, HR 140 bpm, RR 38/min, CVP 22 cm H_2O, PAOP 25 mm Hg. The patient's current laboratory values are Na 123 mEq/L, potassium 9.2 mEq/L, phosphorus 6.0 mg/dL, calcium 4.7 mg/dL, BUN 148 mg/dL, and creatinine 7.4 mg/dL. Based on these findings, nursing management of this patient will need to include

A. Continued administration of fluid boluses

B. Hemodialysis

C. Continuous renal replacement therapy

D. Peritoneal dialysis

1-95. A patient with heart failure is being transferred from the ICU to telemetry after an acute episode of pulmonary edema. The nurse is talking with him about signs and symptoms that should be reported to his health care provider once he is back home. What should the nurse say to the patient to avoid a readmission?

A. Report a weight gain of greater than 3 pounds over 3 days

B. Report fatigue and take an iron supplement to prevent anemia

C. Be compliant with all scheduled appointments.

D. Limit your fluid intake to prevent shortness of breath

1-96. A patient who has completed a course of chemotherapy for lung cancer is admitted to the ICU with a diagnosis of syncope. Physical examination reveals HR 134/min, BP 80/66 mm Hg, sinus tachycardia, RR 30 shallow BPM. Breath sounds are decreased on the side of previous thoracotomy but otherwise clear. A pericardial friction rub and JVD are present. An arterial line is inserted, and the waveform shows a decrease of 10 mm Hg with inspiration. Which of the following conditions has this patient most likely developed?

A. Hypovolemia

B. Pericardial tamponade

C. Tension pneumothorax

D. Superior vena cava syndrome

1-97. A 40-year-old patient who presents with nausea, vomiting, jaundice, and severe abdominal pain is diagnosed with acute pancreatitis. In this disorder, autodigestion of the pancreas causes release of cytokines and kinins, which alter capillary wall permeability and the vascular vasoactive properties. As the nurse anticipates potential complications that may result from these changes, which of the following interventions is most important to institute at this point?

A. Monitoring of QT intervals and seizure precautions

B. Monitoring for Cullen's sign and measuring abdominal girth

C. Fluid restriction and pain control

D. Auscultation of bowel sounds and peripheral pulses

1-98. A patient is admitted to the ICU following surgery to repair a tracheo-esophageal fistula. Her vitals are stable, and she is being mechanically ventilated via a low pressure cuff airway. She is receiving enteral feeds via a nasally inserted post-pyloric feeding tube. On postoperative day 2, the patient begins to cough up secretions resembling tube feeds. Which of the following is the highest priority nursing action?

A. Stop the tube feeding

B. Administer metoclopramide

C. Prepare the patient for bronchoscopy and/or endoscopy

D. Check placement of the feeding tube by auscultating an air bubble and aspirating residual

1-99. Which of the following nursing assessment findings would best indicate that therapy for acute pulmonary edema has been effective?

A. Respiratory rate on BiPAP is less than 30 breaths/min

B. The patient has diuresed 3000 mL

C. Heart rate is sinus rhythm at a rate less than 100 beats/min

D. Systolic blood pressure is less than 150 mm Hg

1-100. In SIRS/MODS, cytokines are responsible for the massive inflammatory response that can lead to multiple organ dysfunction. The critical care nurse recognizes the hemodynamic response to cytokine production as evidenced by

A. SVR: 1500 dynes/sec/cm^{-5}; CVP: 16 mm Hg; SVO$_2$: 50%

B. SVR: 400 dynes/sec/cm^{-5}; CVP: 12 mm Hg; SVO$_2$: 70%

C. SVR: 500 dynes/sec/cm^{-5}; CVP: 4 mm Hg; SVO$_2$: 80%

D. SVR: 1350 dynes/sec/cm^{-5}; CVP: 2 mm Hg; SVO$_2$: 55%

1-101. Which of the following findings best indicates that a postoperative coronary artery bypass patient requires return to the operating room?

    A. Chest tube output greater than 200 mL per hour for 2 consecutive hours

    B. MAP 50 mm Hg for 2 hours despite dopamine infusion at 10 mcg/kg/min

    C. Cardiac output 1.9 L/min

    D. PCWP 25 mm Hg

1-102. While orienting a new nurse to the ICU, the orientee's patient experiences cardiac arrest and requires resuscitation. The preceptor arrives and sees that the orientee has placed the patient in Trendelenburg position. Which of the following represents the best response the preceptor could make to afford instruction for this new nurse?

    A. Immediately begin chest compressions.

    B. Initiate the unit's code blue response.

    C. Reposition the patient supine

    D. Set up suction apparatus

1-103. Which of the following medications may worsen symptoms of heart failure associated with hypertrophic cardiomyopathy?

    A. Calcium channel blockers

    B. Beta blockers

    C. Nitroglycerin

    D. Amiodarone

1-104. For a patient with disseminated intravascular coagulopathy (DIC), the primary goal of medical treatment is to

    A. Accurately administer intravenous drip heparin to prevent "using up" clotting factors

    B. Administer subcutaneous fibrinolytics to dissolve clots formed in the microvasculature

    C. Identify and treat the underlying conditions that lead to the development of DIC

    D. Provide supportive care as needed until the DIC subsides

1-105. A critically ill patient is admitted to the ICU with a diagnosis of septic shock. After insertion of a pulmonary artery catheter, the initial set of hemodynamic measurements are as follows: PAP: 25/10 mm Hg; CVP: 8 mm Hg; PCWP: 12 mm Hg; CO: 8 L/min; CI: 3.0 L/min/cm²; SVR: 500 dynes/sec/cm⁻⁵; DO_2: 600 mL/min; VO_2: 100 mL/min. These findings indicate that the patient is demonstrating which of the following pathophysiological effects of septic shock on the cardiovascular system?

    A. Vasoconstriction

    B. Maldistribution of blood flow

    C. Myocardial excitability

    D. Hypervolemia

1-106. A young patient is admitted to the ICU after a motorcycle accident involving the center median of the freeway in which she sustained blunt head and chest trauma. Within minutes of arrival on the unit, the patient complains of dysphasia and is coughing. She develops upper airway obstruction unrelieved by oxygen, becomes cyanotic, and has palpable subcutaneous emphysema near the sternal notch. For which of the following interventions should the nurse prepare?

    A. Intubation and mechanical ventilation

    B. Fiberoptic bronchoscopy

    C. Emergent tracheostomy

    D. Initiation of cardiac compressions for CPR

1-107. A thin, elderly patient is admitted to the emergency department with sudden onset of a decrease in level of consciousness and left-sided paralysis. Head CT scan reveals a 2.5×2 cm deep, right hemispheric hemorrhage. The patient is on warfarin for atrial fibrillation with an INR of 6.7. Which of the following describes the most appropriate course of action for the nurse to anticipate with this patient?

    A. Urgent preparation for neurosurgery to evacuate the clot

    B. Aggressive correction of coagulopathy with vitamin K, fresh frozen plasma, and recombinant factor VIIa

    C. Urgent brain MRI to rule out other potential etiologies for these findings

    D. Immediate infusion of EACA to correct coagulopathy

1-108. An 85-year-old man who had a cerebrovascular accident 2 years ago is cared for at home by his wife owing to his limited functional ability. He is currently in the ICU on Bi-PAP for community-acquired pneumonia. His wife states that she is unsure if she can take him back home this time, as the workload of his care is increasingly draining her. She states that her preference would be to bring her husband home when he is better, but for now, feels she must place him in a nursing home. What would be the nurse's best response to the wife's comment?

A. "I will be glad to contact the ethics committee for you to help resolve this dilemma."
B. "There are some health care resources available to help you provide care in your home."
C. "You should feel hopeful because your husband is getting better."
D. "You sound as though the future is uncertain."

1-109. Which of the following laboratory results should the nurse report to the cardiologist for a patient with acute coronary syndrome who is scheduled to go for cardiac catheterization and possible PCI in 1 hour?

A. aPTT 65 sec
B. Troponin 0.2 ng/mL
C. Serum potassium 4.9 mEq/L
D. Serum creatinine 2.3 mg/dL

1-110. A patient with a 4-day history of "influenza" is admitted to the ICU with diabetic ketoacidosis. The patient stopped taking his routine dose of 45 units of Humulin 70/30 three days ago, stating he was "not able to eat because of nausea and vomiting." On the day of admission, the patient's roommate reported that the patient was "sleeping too much and breathing really fast and deep."Available laboratory values are as follows: Serum glucose 490 mg/dL; pH 7.25; PaO_2 98 mm Hg; PCO_2 15 mm Hg; Bi-

carbonate 8.0 mEq/L. Which of the following interventions should the nurse perform first?

A. Administer the first infusion of antibiotics
B. Administer 20 units regular insulin via IV push
C. Administer 100 mL of bicarbonate solution via IV push
D. Administer 1000 mL of normal saline at 125 mL/hr

1-111. A nurse preceptor is working with an orientee who has just admitted a patient believed to have ventilator-associated pneumonia. In reviewing the various interventions that may be helpful in preventing this disorder, which should the preceptor emphasize as the most effective intervention for this purpose?

A. Locating the tip of a nasogastric feeding tube in the post-pyloric area
B. Maintaining the head of the bed elevated at 30 to 45 degrees
C. Suctioning the oropharynx and ET tube hourly
D. Using hyperalimentation instead of enteral feedings

1-112. The patient with the rhythm shown below is sleeping, and the automated BP during the rhythm records a blood pressure of 100/60 mm Hg. The nurse caring for the patient should perform which of the following actions?

A. Awaken the patient and obtain the BP with the patient awake
B. Continue to monitor the patient while asleep
C. Administer atropine 0.5 mg IV push
D. Place the patient on oxygen by nasal cannula at 2 L/min

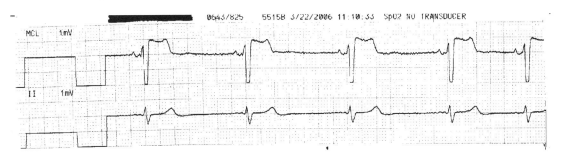

1-113. In order to improve resuscitation outcomes and reduce the incidence of multisystem organ failure for patients in shock, their serum lactate levels should be corrected in

    A. Less than 24 hours
    B. 24 to 48 hours
    C. 49 to 72 hours
    D. 73 to 96 hours

1-114. For a patient with an anterior wall MI, which of the following findings would the nurse be especially vigilant for?

    A. Sinus bradycardia with a rate of 40 BPM
    B. Hiccoughs and GI upset
    C. Signs and symptoms of heart failure
    D. JVD and peripheral edema

1-115. A patient is admitted to the ICU after a motor vehicle crash related to excessive consumption of alcohol. This is the patient's third accident in a year related to alcohol consumption and his first involving driving without a license. As the nurse enters the room, the patient is awake, oriented, and lying quietly. How should the nurse approach this patient?

    A. Enter the room but avoid talking about the most recent incident
    B. Discuss nonthreatening topics such as weather to engage in conversation
    C. Provide nonjudgmental encouragement aimed at reducing or ceasing alcohol consumption
    D. Ask the patient if he would like to talk about what happened

1-116. One hour after percutaneous coronary intervention (PCI) with stent placement, a patient with a Fem-o-stop in place complains of back and groin pain. Vital signs include BP 100/70 mm Hg, HR 112 BPM, and RR 20/min. There is no visible bleeding. The nurse caring for this patient would anticipate which of the following orders?

    A. Obtain a 12-lead ECG
    B. Administer morphine 2 mg IV for pain
    C. Obtain a serum hemoglobin and hematocrit
    D. No orders would be expected

1-117. A young woman is admitted to the unit after having ingested an unknown amount of amphetamines, barbiturates, and alcohol. She has three children who are currently with their grandparents and states that she has been out of work for over a month. The most effective approach for the nurse to provide for this patient's needs would be to

    A. Contact the patient's family to ensure the children are being cared for
    B. Arrange for a social worker to conduct a comprehensive assessment of needs
    C. Document that the patient is unemployed and may not be capable of providing for the children
    D. Refer to Alcoholics Anonymous for drug and alcohol rehabilitation

1-118. When the nurse provides discharge teaching for a patient recovering from an acute exacerbation of chronic obstructive pulmonary disease (COPD), which of the following should be emphasized as the best indicator for the patient to use to closely monitor this disease process?

    A. Peak flow measurements
    B. Pulse oximetry readings
    C. Changes in the amount or quality of sputum
    D. Experiences of dyspnea or breathlessness

1-119. A patient admitted to the ICU with exacerbation of heart failure and atrial fibrillation is currently receiving warfarin with therapeutic INR levels and diuretic therapy. The nurse recognizes that this patient is at highest risk for which of the following preventable complications?

    A. Stroke
    B. Exercise intolerance
    C. Falling
    D. Pulmonary edema

1-120. When providing postoperative care for coronary artery bypass surgery patients, the nurse needs to be especially vigilant to assess the patient for which problem that is associated with infection, impaired wound healing, and poor recovery?

    A. Pain
    B. Loss of control

C. Depression

D. Anemia

1-121. Which of the following medications prevents early complications and mortality associated with acute myocardial infarction after administration of thrombolytic therapy?

A. Calcium channel blockers

B. Magnesium sulfate

C. Lidocaine

D. Beta blockers

1-122. In a patient with cirrhosis and ascites who develops fever and generalized abdominal pain, the nurse needs to assess for additional evidence of

A. Acute appendicitis

B. Spontaneous bacterial peritonitis

C. Small bowel obstruction

D. Acute pancreatitis

1-123. A patient has had an indwelling pericardial catheter in place for 3 days. Which of the following findings is the most reliable indicator that this catheter may now be removed?

A. Absence of pericardial drainage for 3 hours

B. Absence of symptoms of pericardial tamponade

C. Normal cardiac silhouette on chest x-ray

D. Bedside echocardiography demonstrates absence of pericardial effusion

1-124. An immigrant from Haiti who has been in the United States for about 13 months is admitted with a diagnosis of metabolic syndrome. He has elevated blood pressure, blood glucose, and BMI. During the admission history, the nurse asks the patient what medications he is currently taking, and he replies that he takes an herbal substance known as "Kong." The nurse asks what Kong is for, and he replies "My wife can tell you more about it." Noting this patient's cultural background, his nurse is aware that in the Haitian culture

A. The family is matriarchcal, so the wife needs to answer some of these questions

B. Kong is an herbal substance widely used by young men

C. Kong is usually purchased at local grocery stores by women

D. The family is patriarchal, and questions of this nature are not considered appropriate for women to ask

1-125. A patient has survived a severe traumatic brain injury with a basilar skull fracture but has now developed an elevated temperature. Although the nurse's plan for managing fever in this patient population will be multifactorial, the most important aspect will center on identifying

A. Deep vein thrombosis, a frequently neglected complication of immobility

B. Meningitis, a potential complication of basilar skill fractures

C. Hypothalamic dysfunction or "storming," a potentially lethal febrile syndrome after head trauma

D. Foreign bodies still embedded in the skull base, a common source of infection

1-126. Laboratory values for a patient with acute gastric hemorrhage and hypotension are as follows: HCT 30%; Platelets 50,000/mm^3; INR 1.3. In addition to administering a fluid bolus of 250 mL normal saline, the nurse anticipates administration of which of the following?

A. One unit of packed red blood cells

B. 6 units/300 mL of platelets

C. Fresh frozen plasma 4 units/250 mL

D. 50 mL of salt poor albumin/25% albumin

1-127. Patients with pelvic fractures are at high risk for a number of potential complications. In order to optimize the pelvic fracture patient's potential for recovery, which member of the health care team should the nurse consult within the first 24 hours?

A. Psychiatrist

B. Nutritionist

C. Occupational therapist

D. Physical therapist

1-128. All of the following signs and symptoms were identified in a newly admitted patient with a history of severe asthma. Of these clinical findings, which poses the most significant concern to the nurse who suspects this patient may develop acute respiratory failure?

A. Inability to readily speak a three-word sentence
B. Wheezing audible without a stethoscope
C. Respiratory rate of 38/min
D. Inaudible breath sounds by auscultation

1-129. The nurse is providing education related to prevention of complications to a patient with liver failure and his family. Which of the following is the best explanation of why immunosuppression is a major concern for a patient with liver failure?

A. "You will be more susceptible to infection because of the medicines you take."
B. "You have been experiencing malnutrition for a long time because of your substance abuse."
C. "Because your liver does not process proteins properly, you no longer produce enough immune globulin to fight infection."
D. "Because your liver is impaired, you will not have sufficient stores of fat soluble vitamins and B_{12} to protect against infection."

1-130. A patient who sustained traumatic brain injury in an assault 4 hours ago is admitted directly to the ICU from the emergency department. He is endotracheally intubated and mechanically ventilated. The nurse's admission neurological examination findings are as follows: no response to voice or touch; when the patient's trapezius muscle is pinched, his eyes do not open, though he flexes his right arm and extends his left arm. This patient's total Glasgow Coma Scale score is

A. 6
B. 5
C. 3
D. 2

1-131. A 38-year-old man admitted to the ICU has been on hemodialysis for the past 6 months

and was found to be noncompliant with his diet and fluid restrictions. His labwork shows K+ 6.2 mEq/L, BUN 39, and creatinine 3.6 mg/dL, and he complains of severe fatigue and weakness. What is the best course of action for the nurse to take to understand this patient's noncompliance?

A. Consult a nutritionist for dietary education
B. Discuss his condition with his spouse
C. Tell the patient that his nonadherence increases the risk of a stroke
D. Ask the patient if he is interested in being placed on a transplant list

1-132. Which of the following is an absolute contraindication to the administration of thrombolytic agents in the patient with acute myocardial infarction?

A. Blood pressure 210/110 mm Hg
B. Transient ischemic attack (TIA) 3 days prior
C. Ischemic stroke 2 years prior
D. Age 75 years

1-133. A chronic renal failure patient with a right arm arteriovenous fistula complains of pain, numbness, and tingling of the right hand. Nursing management of the patient's symptoms would include

A. Elevating the arm on two pillows
B. Applying warm compresses to the arm
C. Keeping the arm flexed at 90 degrees
D. Placing the arm in a sling

1-134. A nurse is precepting a new ICU nurse who is assigned to a recent postoperative abdominal surgical patient. The patient has bladder pressure measurements ordered. The new nurse has a measurement of 15 mm Hg but states that she does not understand how to interpret the results. As a preceptor for this new nurse, which of the following points would represent a good starting place for instruction?

A. Pressures between 15 and 30 mm Hg may be normal after abdominal surgery
B. Pressures between 0 and 15 mm Hg may be normal after abdominal surgery
C. Bladder pressures are not always accurate, so an average of three measures is needed

D. Bladder pressures should only be done after the foley is clamped for 30 minutes

1-135. A patient with dilated cardiomyopathy secondary to myocardial infarction would benefit most from which of the following?

A. Administration of ACE inhibitors
B. Administration of diuretics
C. Coronary artery bypass surgery
D. Insertion of a permanent pacemaker

1-136. A patient who underwent a roux-en-y gastric bypass 7 days ago is now exhibiting fever >38.6° C, chills, tachycardia, nausea, malaise, and yellow-green drainage from the Jackson-Pratt drain. An increase in which of the following laboratory values would support the nurse's suspicion that this patient has developed a complication associated with this surgical procedure?

A. White blood cell count
B. Potassium
C. Platelets
D. Lipase

1-137. A patient is recovering from a complicated case of Klebsiella pneumonia. His morning assessment reveals diminished breath sounds at the right base, temperature 40° C, HR 120/min, BP 90/40 mm Hg, RR 30/min, and SO$_2$ 95% on 40% face mask. His chest x-ray reveals a right lower lobe fluid collection. The nurse should anticipate which of the following interventions?

A. Broncho-alveolar lavage (BAL) with a quantitative sputum culture
B. Stat hematocrit and chest tube insertion
C. Thoracentesis and antibiotic administration
D. Aggressive bronchopulmonary hygiene with right lower lobe chest physiotherapy

1-138. A patient is readmitted 2 years after surgical repair of an ASD with pulmonary hypertension. Which of the following complications is most likely responsible for this patient's hospitalization?

A. First degree heart block
B. Second degree heart block, Type 1

C. Second degree heart block, Type 2
D. Complete heart block

1-139. Long-term alcohol dependency often leads to a thiamine deficiency. In caring for a patient with a known history of alcohol abuse, which of the following would the nurse recognize as evidence that the patient has Korsakoff syndrome?

A. Gait disturbances
B. Paralysis of the eye muscles
C. Retrograde and anterograde amnesia
D. Nystagmus

1-140. An older woman is diagnosed with normo-progressive hydrocephalus and receives a ventricular shunt. During the postoperative period, she has a parietal stroke that leaves her with some blurred vision and expressive aphasia, which have impeded her recovery and caused her considerable frustration and anger. Her husband tells the nurse that he knows that she understands him, but he is distressed to see her get so upset every time she attempts to respond to his statements. He wonders if some type of activity would help his wife cope better. With which member of the health care team should the nurse consult for this problem?

A. Occupational therapist
B. Psychiatric social worker
C. Physical therapist
D. Speech therapist

1-141. A patient with inferior wall myocardial infarction and sinus bradycardia abruptly develops atrial fibrillation. Which of the following should the nurse anticipate administering?

A. Amiodarone
B. Diltiazem
C. Digoxin
D. Synchronized cardioversion

1-142. A middle-aged person is found unresponsive at a bus stop and is transported to the emergency department. The patient's capillary blood glucose measures 40 mg/dL and remains below normal limits after an initial IV push administration of 50 mL of 50%

dextrose solution. What orders would the nurse expect to receive next for this obtunded patient?

A. Administer a serving of orange juice
B. Begin an infusion of 10% dextrose intravenously
C. Administer 1 mg glucagon intravenously
D. Administer 10 units insulin glargine subcutaneously

1-143. The behaviors of health care providers can influence end-of-life decisions made by patients and their families. Which of the following nursing behaviors is usually most helpful at this time?

A. Acting as an arbitrator between family members
B. Requesting that only one person be the spokesperson
C. Avoiding the use of words such as death, dying, and suffering
D. Consulting clergy for support

1-144. The patient experiencing renal transplantation has been having an unremarkable recovery over the previous 5 days. Which of the following findings would the nurse need to report to the physician immediately?

A. Abdominal discomfort and bladder distention
B. Increasing urinary output with decreasing serum creatinine
C. Right upper quadrant tenderness with elevated serum bilirubin
D. Elevated serum glucose and decreasing level of conciousness

1-145. While observing a newly admitted patient with blunt force trauma to the left flank area, the critical care nurse notes that the patient's urine is dark and tea-colored. In planning care for this patient, which assessment finding indicates the achievement of patient management goals?

A. Urine pH of 7.20
B. Serum sodium of 152 mEq/L
C. Urine output of 100 mL/hr
D. Serum pH of 7.37

1-146. A patient admitted with the diagnosis of acute coronary syndrome is in the intensive care unit on oxygen 2 L/min by nasal cannula and unfractionated heparin per protocol. The patient complains of upper abdominal pain, which is described as discomfort 1 out of 10. The most appropriate initial intervention for the critical care nurse to perform would be to

A. Obtain serum troponin
B. Insert a nasogastric tube
C. Administer 1/150 nitroglycerin sublingual
D. Obtain a 12-lead ECG

1-147. When caring for a trauma patient with a hemothorax and chest tube, the nurse notes that the patient continues to drain 150 mL/hr of blood in the chest tube collection chamber. Which of the following findings would the critical care nurse be most concerned about with this patient?

A. Fluctuation or tidaling in the water-seal chamber
B. Discomfort at the chest tube insertion site
C. Sudden decrease or absence of drainage
D. Intermittent bubbling in the water-seal chamber

1-148. A 78-year-old woman with a severe cough treated with an over-the-counter cough medicine is admitted to the ICU with melana and pneumonia. On physical examination, the nurse finds that her abdomen is flat and nontender with hypoactive bowel sounds. Vital signs are BP 112/76 mm Hg, pulse 102 beats/min, respirations 15 breaths/min. Since her admission to the unit 2 days ago, the patient's stool has been normal in color and consistency. The nurse anticipates that the explanation for the patient's melana is

A. Hemorrhoidal bleeding
B. Gastric irritation from the cough medicine
C. Rupture of a diverticula
D. Slowly healing peptic ulcer

1-149. The nurse's neurological assessment reveals that her patient exhibits the following clinical findings: contralateral face, arm, and leg paralysis with sensory deficits; loss of half of the field of vision; ipsilateral Horner's syndrome; and aphasia. This set of neurologic findings indicates the need to plan and manage care tailored to a patient with stroke involving which of the following vessels?

A. Right middle cerebral artery
B. Right vertebral artery
C. Left anterior cerebral artery
D. Left internal carotid artery

1-150. An 80-kg patient diagnosed with acute respiratory distress syndrome is on mechanical ventilation with the following settings: continuous mandatory ventilation (CMV), tidal volume 400 mL, rate 12/min, PEEP 15 cm H_2O. Arterial blood gases on these settings are pH 7.28, PaO_2 75 mm Hg, $PaCO_2$ 62 mm Hg. Which of the following interventions is warranted at this time?

A. Increase the respiratory rate to decrease the $PaCO_2$
B. Increase the tidal volume to increase the PaO_2
C. Administer sodium bicarbonate to decrease the pH
D. Continue to monitor the patient on these ventilator settings

1-1. **(B)** Clinical signs of acute pulmonary edema include tachycardia, tachypnea, inspiratory crackles, and rhonchi with chest x-ray findings of Kerley B lines and peribronchial hilar enlargement. Enlargement of the cardiac silhouette reflects left ventricular enlargement owing to left ventricular failure. Pericardial tamponade (Option A) would be associated with an enlarged cardiac silhouette and widened mediastinum from blood accumulation in the pericardial space, but it is not associated with adventitious breath sounds. Pneumonia would be associated with adventitious breath sounds, but consolidation would be present on the chest x-ray. Right ventricular failure would be associated with clear lung fields and breath sounds.

References: Bixby, M. Turn back the tide of cardiogenic pulmonary edema. *Nursing 2005,* 35, 56-60, 2005.
Ware, L. B., Matthay, M. A. Acute pulmonary edema. *New Engl J Med,* 353, 2788-2796, 2005.

1-2. **(C)** The nurse should intervene when informed consent for a research study has not been correctly provided. The nurse recognizes that informed consent in human subjects has not occurred with this patient. Informed consent must include the description and purpose of the research, procedures that are experimental, foreseeable risks, how confidentiality will be maintained, and a clear understanding that the subject can withdraw at any time. Option A is incorrect because it will delay correcting the problem. Option B is incorrect because the investigator may not be readily available and informed consent should be corrected immediately. Option D is incorrect because, regardless of being a volunteer or paid employee, whoever is enrolling a subject in a study must ensure informed consent.

References: Arford, P. H. Working with human research protections. *J Nurs Scholarship,* 36(3), 265-271, 2004.
Molter, N. Professional caring and ethical practice. In J. G. Alspach (ed.). *Core Curriculum for Critical Care Nursing,* 6th ed. St. Louis, Elsevier, 2006, pp 1-44.
Stannard, D., Hardin, S. R. Advocacy and moral agency. In S. R. Hardin, K. Kaplow (eds.) *Synergy for Clinical Excellence.* Sudbury, Jones & Bartlett, 2005, pp 63-8.

1-3. **(C)** The administration of oxygen therapy is key to relieving the hypoxia associated with a pulmonary embolism. If there is severe cardiopulmonary compromise, intubation and mechanical ventilation will be necessary. Reassessment in 1 hour would neglect the need to significantly improve this patient's cardiopulmonary status, particularly with signs of possible cerebral hypoxia, tachypnea, tachycardia, and declining cardiac output. In a pulmonary embolism, early identification and intervention are key. The initiation of sequential compression devices is preventive, and at this stage it is more important to initiate supportive therapy and improve oxygenation. Thrombolytic therapy would represent a secondary line of treatment that would be used only in patients where cardiac failure is profound.

References: Chulay, M. Respiratory system. In M. Chulay, S. Burns (eds.). *AACN Essentials of Critical Care Nursing*. New York, McGraw-Hill, 2006, p 264.

Ellstrom, K. Pulmonary system. In J. G. Alspach (ed.). *Core Curriculum for Critical Care Nursing*, 6th ed. St. Louis, Elsevier, 2006, p 145.

1-4. **(C)** Since this patient received thrombolytics and subsequently had the groin accessed for PCI, this patient is at great risk for hematoma at the groin insertion site. Hourly inspection of the site to determine if a hematoma is present or expanding is essential to recognize and prevent permanent injury from this complication. The patient was alert and able to give consent to the physician, so an intracranial hemorrhage did not occur from the thrombolytics. Retroperitoneal bleeding would be suspected if signs of hypotension not associated with other obvious sources of bleeding were present. Gray Turner's sign (flank bruising) is seen in retroperitoneal bleeding, but it is a relatively late sign. Bowel sounds are not anticipated early in the postoperative course and are a nonspecific indicator of GI bleeding. The NG tube aspirate would be a better indicator of GI bleeding.

Reference: Woods, S. L., Froelicher, E. S., Motzer, S. U., Bridges, E. J. *Cardiac Nursing*, 5th ed. Philadelphia, Lippincott Williams & Wilkins, 2005.

1-5. **(B)** The purpose of the primary and secondary trauma survey is to provide a consistent method of caring for individuals with multiple injuries and to keep the team focused on care priorities. The primary survey involves a continuous process of assessment, intervention, and reevaluation. Potentially life-threatening injuries can be identified during the primary survey and appropriate interventions instituted. The components of the primary trauma survey are A—airway, B—breathing, C—circulation, D—disability (neurological deficits), and E—exposure and environmental control. Components of the secondary survey are F—full set of vital signs, facilitation of family presence, and five interventions (cardiac monitoring,

nasogastric/orogastric tube, urinary catheter, laboratory tests, and pulse oximetry); G—give comfort measures; H—history and head-to-toe examination; and I—inspect the posterior surfaces.

Reference: Newberry, L., Criddle, L. M. (eds.). *Sheehy's Manual of Emergency Care*, 6th ed. St. Louis, Elsevier, 2005, pp 601-605.

1-6. **(D)** Data suggest that leads III and V_3 should be used to perform ST segment monitoring in patients with acute coronary artery syndrome. Lead II (Option A) is useful for general cardiac monitoring, but it is not especially helpful for ST segment monitoring. Leads V_6 (Option B) and I (Option C) are helpful together for distinguishing ventricular aberration but not for ST segment monitoring.

Reference: AACN Practice Alert. ST Segment Monitoring. Available at www.aacn.org//AACN/practiceAlert.nsf/Files/ECG%20ST%20Segment/ Retrieved on July 1, 2006.

1-7. **(B)** Phenylephrine (Neosynephrine) is a potent vasoconstrictor which may cause bradycardia because it has no beta 1 or beta 2 activity. Dopamine, epinephrine and norepinephrine (Levophed) have strong beta 1 activity and increase the heart rate.

Reference: Chulay, M., Burns, S. M. *AACN Essentials of Critical Care Nursing*. New York, McGraw-Hill, 2006.

1-8. **(D)** Lung protective ventilation decreases pulmonary pressures by decreasing tidal volumes and preventing volutrauma. The patient's oxygenation is only minimally adequate and needs to be closely followed with the changes in tidal volume. Pressure support is not indicated with the clinical findings described. Although the patient is acidotic, increasing the ventilatory rate will not lessen the pressures, and lung protective strategies may include permissive hypercapnea.

References: Alspach, J. G. (ed.). *Core Curriculum for Critical Care Nursing*, 6th ed. St. Louis, Elsevier, 2006.

Petrucci, N., Iacovelli, W. Ventilation with lower tidal volumes versus traditional tidal volumes in adults for ALI and ARDS. *Cochrane Database Systematic Review*, 2004(2), CD003844.

1-9. **(C)** Common injuries resulting from blunt

abdominal trauma can include injury to the liver, spleen, mesenteric vessels, pancreas, or kidneys. In a nonoperative approach to blunt abdominal trauma, observation and monitoring include serial hematocrits to evaluate for intra-abdominal bleeding. The platelet count does not fluctuate unless there is a disease process (cirrhosis, leukemia) or significant blood loss. If there is significant blood loss, the platelet count is reduced along with total blood volume. Platelet levels are not good indicators for acute blood loss as they must be hand-counted and may be influenced by medications and volume resuscitation. Protime (prothrombin time) is a monitor of coagulation status. The level can be prolonged without active bleeding. This is not an accurate measure of intra-abdominal bleeding. Mean corpuscular volume measures the average volume or size of a single RBC and is used in classifying anemias. It is not a good measure of intravascular blood volume in acute bleeding situations.

References: Eckert, K. L. Penetrating and blunt abdominal trauma. *Crit Care Nurse Q,* 28(1), 41-59, 2005.

Pagana, K. D., Pagana, T. *Mosby's Manual of Diagnostic and Laboratory Tests,* 2nd ed. St. Louis, Elsevier, 2002.

1-10. **(C)** The patient may have initially presented with the large nonreactive pupil and ptosis. A little bit of detective work through reviewing the patient's medical record can help the nurse distinguish whether the examination findings are old or new. Since the examination is otherwise nonfocal and the GCS is 15, no acute change in her condition is apparent, so Option A, notifying the neurosurgeon is not indicated at this time. The findings are likely relatively old and do not warrant Option B, rushing the patient to the OR or CT scanner. The patient's level of consciousness has not diminished, so Option D, intubation, is not indicated.

Reference: Alspach, J. G. (ed.). *Core Curriculum for Critical Care Nursing,* 6th ed. Philadelphia, Elsevier, 2006, pp 481-483.

1-11. **(D)** The patient should be immediately disconnected from the circuit and machine because these findings suggest that the patient is experiencing a diaylzer or hemofilter reaction. Signs of this reaction include hypotension, pruritis, back pain, angioedema, and/or anaphylaxis. Once removed from the treatment, the patient is reassessed, and the symptoms are managed. At this time, administration of a fluid bolus may be used to manage hypotension. Assessment for bleeding at the access site is done routinely and with episodes of hypotension. The administration of diphenhydramine may occur if the patient continues to have pruritis, provided the patient is not hypotensive.

References: ANNA. *Continuous Renal Replacement Therapy.* Pitman, NJ, American Nephrology Nurses Association, 2005, pp 1-12.

Lough, M. E. Renal disorders and therapeutic management. In L. D. Urden, K. M. Stacy, M. E. Lough (eds.). *Thelan's Critical Care Nursing: Diagnosis and Management,* (5th ed.). St. Louis, Elsevier, 2006, pp 813-846.

Stark, J. L. The renal system. In J. G. Alspach (ed.). *Core Curriculum for Critical Care Nursing,* 6th ed. St. Louis, Elsevier, 2006, pp 525-607.

1-12. **(A)** The 12-lead ECG represents a narrow complex tachycardia. Immediate interventions for this stable tachycardia with an acceptable blood pressure include having the patient perform vagal maneuvers to slow conduction from the SA node to the AV node. If this is ineffective in slowing or terminating the tachycardia, the next intervention would be to administer adenosine. Adenosine causes transient block in AV node conduction, which may cause asystole. If the patient is stable, administration of a medication that may cause asystole is contraindicated. Diltiazem is indicated for rate control in atrial fibrillation with a rapid ventricular rate. Synchronized cardioversion is indicated for unstable supraventricular tachycardias.

Reference: Field, J. M., Hazinski, M. F., Gilmore, D. (eds.). *Handbook of Emergency Cardiovascular Care for Healthcare Providers.* Dallas, American Heart Association, 2006.

1-13. **(D)** Two large-bore IV lines should be immediately inserted to enable fluid administration and vasopressor support. Laboratory studies for type and crossmatch should be obtained for anticipated blood replacement. Surgery should not be delayed to complete a pericardiocentesis. Labetolol administration is contraindicated in hypotension. Norepinephrine administration is contraindicated in hypovolemia and will increase the force of contraction, which may cause the dissection to rupture.

Reference: Stone, C. K., Humphries, R. L. *Current Emergency Diagnosis and Treatment* (5ᵗʰ ed.). New York, McGraw-Hill, 2004.

1-14. **(A)** Individuals with ICDs often fear that the device will shock them. These patients do not report concerns about being awakend by the device or about the device being triggered by exertion, nor do they experience depression owing to dependence on the ICD.

Reference: Dunbar, S. Psychosocial issues of patients with implantable cardioverter defibrillators. *Am J Crit Care,* 14(4), 294-303, 2005.

1-15. **(D)** The patient has likely suffered an aspiration. Cultures will need to be completed to determine the causative organism(s), and pulmonary hygiene will assist in clearing the lobar pneumonia. Administration of broad-spectrum antibiotics should await completion of the cultures. Bronchoalveolar lavage does not reach the distal airways, so it is not likely to help this patient. Steroid therapy is not indicated for this condition.

References: Ellstrom, K. The pulmonary system. In J. G. Alspach (ed.). *Core Curriculum for Critical Care Nursing,* 6ᵗʰ ed. Philadelphia, Elsevier, 2006.

Marik, P. E. Aspiration, pneumonitis and pneumonia. In M. P. Fink, E. Abraham, J. L. Vincent, P. M. Kochanek (eds.). *Textbook of Critical Care,* 5ᵗʰ ed. Philadelphia, Elsevier, 2005.

1-16. **(C)** At this point, the nurse should focus on educating the patient and family regarding the benefits of treatment options available with early intervention. This patient delayed hospitalization and therefore missed an opportunity to received needed therapy that might have averted the acute MI. Unless the patient will be taking thrombolytics, additional instruction related to their use is not indicated. There is no indication that the patient's delay was owing to any inability to reach a telephone, so Option B is not warranted. Admonishing the patient may resemble scolding, blaming, or scare tactics, and it does not represent an appropriate means of enabling an adult to improve his or her self-care.

Reference: Banks, A. D., Dracup, K. Factors associated with prolonged prehospital delay of African Americans with acute myocardial infarction. *Am J Crit Care*, 15(2), 149-157, 2006.

1-17. **(D)** MODS is characterized by the presence of progressive physiologic dysfunction of two or more organ systems after an acute threat to systemic homeostasis. SIRS is characterized by a generalized systemic inflammation in organs remote from an initial insult. Septic shock is sepsis-induced shock with hypotension despite adequate fluid resuscitation, along with the presence of perfusion abnormalities. Bacteremia is the presence of viable bacteria in the blood.

References: Alspach, J. G. (ed.). *Core Curriculum for Critical Care Nursing,* 6ᵗʰ ed. St. Louis, Elsevier, 2006, pp 753-754.

Urden, L. D., Stacy, K. M., Lough, M. E. *Thelan's Critical Care Nursing, Diagnosis and Management,* 5ᵗʰ ed. St. Louis, Elsevier, 2006, p 1023.

1-18. **(A)** The persistent air leak could suggest a bronchopleural fistula or other pulmonary parenchymal pathology. If the leak worsens, the patient could start losing tidal volume into the leak, which would be demonstrated by a discrepancy in his inspiratory and expiratory tidal volumes as well as adverse effects on his ABGs (Option A). The scenario does not suggest that this is an acute change, so STAT diagnostic tests are not warranted (Option B). Tracheal deviation is a late sign of a tension pneumothorax, which is unlikely as long as the chest tube drainage system is functioning properly (Option C). Placing the chest tube to water seal could place the patient at risk for accumulating a tension pneumothorax (Option D).

Reference: Lois, M., Noppen, M. Bronchopleural fistulas: An overview of the problem with special attention to endoscopic management. *Chest,* 128, 3955-3965, 2005.

1-19. **(A)** A patient complaint of shoulder pain during peritoneal dialysis can result from the presence of air in the infusion tubing. To prevent this problem, the critical care nurse should ensure that all air is primed out of the infusion tubing. Once the problem has occurred, the nurse needs to drain the effluent with the patient in the knee-chest position. The knee-chest position facilitates the movement of air to the lower abdomen where it may be expelled. Changing the patient to the right side-lying position will not move the air to the lower abdomen and is usually done to manage fluid obstruction. Failure to warm the infusion will cause severe abdominal cramping and hypothermia. Increasing the dwell time will affect the amount of fluid removed from the peritoneal capillaries; however, the increase is not proportional due to osmotic equilibrium.

References: Lough, M.E.: Renal disorders and therapeutic management. In L. D. Urden, K. M. Stacy, M. E. Lough (eds.). *Thelan's Critical Care Nursing: Diagnosis and Management,* 5th ed. St. Louis, Elsevier, 2006, pp 813-846.

Mitchell, J. K. Renal disorders and therapeutic management. In L. D. Urden, K. M. Stacy, M. E. Lough (eds.). *Priorities in Critical Care Nursing,* 4th ed. St. Louis, Elsevier, 2005, pp 333-356.

Stark, J. L. The renal system. In J. G. Alspach (ed.). *Core Curriculum for Critical Care Nursing,* 6th ed. St. Louis, Elsevier, 2006, pp 525-607.

1-20. **(B)** Diabetes insipidus may develop after trauma to the central nervous system. Criteria for this malady include urinary output of more than 500 mL/hr for 2 consecutive hours and low specific gravity. Failure to control diabetes insipidus may result in drastic shifts of fluids and electrolytes, which may evoke seizures, ventricular ectopy, circulatory collapse, and, eventually, death. Increases in abdominal girth measurement would be useful for detection of abdominal bleeding but cannot account for this patient's increased urine output. An elevated capillary glucose measurement may lead to polyuria; however, this is not as ominous a situation as a decrease in specific gravity, and polyuria will subside with treatment of hyperglycemia. The potassium level will change with polyuria, but discovering the source of the polyuria and treating the cause will limit the potential alteration in electrolyte balance.

References: Newberry, L., Criddle, L. *Sheehy's Manual of Emergency Care,* 6th ed. Philadelphia, Elsevier, 2006, pp 433-434.

Urden, L. D., Stacy, K. M., Lough, M. E. *Thelan's Critical Care Nursing: Diagnosis and Management,* 5th ed. St. Louis, Elsevier, 2006, pp 952-953.

1-21. **(C)** The normal BNP is less than 100 pg/mL. Levels greater than 500 pg/mL are consistent with heart failure. A CPK-MB level of 5% and troponin level of 0.3 ng/mL do not support a diagnosis of acute myocardial infarction. Tricuspid valve insufficiency generally results in peripheral edema. ECG signs of pericarditis include diffuse ST segment elevation rather than depression.

Reference: Mueller, C., Frana, B., Rodriguez, D., et al. Emergency diagnosis of congestive heart failure: impact of signs and symptoms. *Can J Cardiol,* 21, 2005, 921-924.

1-22. **(A)** Heparin-induced thrombocytopenia is the result of an antigen/antibody response to the drug heparin. The ELISA test establishes the presence of the antigen for heparin-induced thrombocytopenia, and a platelet count of 30% to 50% of baseline is the key indicator of this condition. While international normalized ratio and partial thromboplastin time would help in understanding the degree of anticoagulation that has occurred with routine use of coumadin and heparin, respectively, they are not specific to heparin-induced thrombocytopenia. The complete blood count may be decreased for many different reasons, whereas the differential white count would not provide information needed to diagnose this autoimmune situation. Comparison of arterial with mixed venous gases provides information about gas exchange and oxygen use and would not be helpful in making this decision.

References: Francis, J. L., Drexler, A. J. Striking back at heparin induced thrombocytopenia. *Nursing,* 36(5), 2006, pp S12-S15.

Urden, L. D., Stacy, K. M., Lough, M. E. *Thelan's Critical Care Nursing: Diagnosis and Management,* 5th ed. St. Louis, Elsevier, 2006, pp 1136-1139.

1-23. **(A)** The patient needs to understand the possible causes for development of pancreatitis. If the patient's history does not include alcoholism, other possible etiologies associated with pancreatitis include gallstones and diet. Options B, C, and D are of a lesser concern for a diagnosis of pancreatitis. Option B does not apply because the patient scenario did not mention weight loss, and in any case that finding is not true for all patients with pancreatitis. Determining food preferences (Option C) will become important if the pancreatitis is related to gallstones. Option D is inappropriate because nothing in the scenario suggests that the patient's prognosis is poor or terminal.

Reference: Radovich, P. The gastrointestinal system. In J. G. Alspach (ed.). *Core Curriculum for Critical Care Nursing*, 6th ed. St. Louis, Elsevier, 2006, pp 725-729.

1-24. **(C)** Increased pulmonary capillary pressure (as measured by the PCWP) causes fluid to move out of the pulmonary capillaries into the pulmonary extravascular tissues and alveoli. Increased right atrial pressures cause fluid to accumulate in the venous system proximal to the lungs in the extremities. Decreased cardiac output may be a symptom of pulmonary edema related to redistribution of blood volume into lung tissue. Increased systemic blood pressure may precipitate pulmonary edema, but only when lymphatic drainage is insufficient to compensate for fluid accumulation in lung tissue.

Reference: Baird, M. S., Keen, J. H., Swearingen, P. L. *Manual of Critical Care Nursing*, 5th ed. St. Louis, Elsevier, 2005.

1-25. **(D)** In either pulmonary or fat embolism to the pulmonary vasculature, reduced preload results from obstruction to pulmonary blood flow, increased pulmonary resistance, and reduction in cardiac output (CO). The hypotension associated with a fall in CO then triggers release of catecholamines, prostaglandins, serotonin, and histamine, which attempt to restore CO by raising systemic vascular resistance via peripheral vasoconstriction. Increased afterload, then, occurs as a compensatory response to the development of hypotension. The right heart dysfunction, rather than intravascular volume, elevates CVP. Cardiomyopathy may be due to viral infections, coronary heart disease, congenital heart defects, vitamin deficiency, or alcoholism, but this patient does not show any risk factors for cardiomyopathy.

References: Koran, Z., Howard, P. K. Respiratory emergencies. In *Sheehy's Emergency Nursing Principles and Practice,* 5th ed. St. Louis, Elsevier, p 442.

Lessig, M. L. Cardiovascular system. In J. G. Alspach (ed.). *Core Curriculum for Critical Care Nursing,* 6th ed. St. Louis, Elsevier, 2006, p 362.

1-26. **(A)** During endovascular repair of AAA, fluoroscopy is used to determine that the position of the endograft is appropriate and does not occlude the renal artery. Blood losses are generally minimal with the endovascular approach unless retroperitoneal or endoleak bleeding is present. Fluoroscopic evidence of renal artery patency negates occlusion as a cause of diminished urine output. Absence of signs of bleeding such as tachycardia, hypotension, and delayed capillary refill indicate that hypovolemia and bleeding are not the cause of the decreased urinary output.

Reference: Hall, S. W. Endovascular repair of abdominal aortic aneurysm. *AORN J, 77,* 630-642, 2003.

1-27. **(D)** Dumping syndrome is a set of postprandial vasomotor and GI symptoms that occurs in some patients who have had gastric surgery or vagotomy that alters upper GI anatomy and neurologic innervation. When a volume of simple carbohydrates is consumed, accelerated gastric emptying causes hyperosmolar contents to be rapidly moved into the upper small intestine, causing bowel distention, abdominal fullness, and intestinal hypermotility that lead to osmotic fluid shifts from the intravascular compartment into the gut lumen, creating relative intravascular volume contraction and hemoconcentration. Compensatory changes lead to release of vasoactive GI hormones, which produce peripheral and splanchnic vasodilation and vasomotor symptoms such as tachycardia, weakness, fainting, dizziness, palpitations, diaphoresis, cramping, diarrhea, and reactive hypoglycemia. An acute MI may cause diaphoresis, nausea, and vomiting, but would usually produce chest pain and ECG changes, which this patient does not exhibit. Pulmonary embolism can occur suddenly in a postsurgical patient, but this patient lacks common risk factors such as prolonged immobility and has experienced no chest pain or hemoptysis. Symptoms of hyperglycemia are polyuria, polydypsia, and blurred vision. This patient does not exhibit any of these symptoms.

References: Elliot, K. Nutritional considerations after bariatric surgery. *Crit Care Nurse Q, 26,* 132-128, 2003.

Ukleja, A. Dumping syndrome. *Practical Gastroenterology*, 29(2), 32, 34-46, 2006.

1-28. **(A)** Advocating for the patient in this scenario means contacting the appropriate agency for filing a report to start an investigation into the care of this older woman. The nurse recognized a finding that clearly constitutes evidence of neglect and failure by a caregiver to adequately meet the physical, social, or emotional needs of a dependent older person. Option B is an action that a nurse would take with any notable assessment finding and would not advocate for this patient's protection. Options C and D will delay getting an investigation of this incident started.

References: Fulmer, T., Paveza, G., Abraham, I., Fairchild, S. Elder neglect assessment in the emergency department. *J Emerg Nurs,* 216(5), 436-443, 2000.

Hoban, S., Kearney, K. Elder abuse and neglect. *Am J Nurs,* 100(11), 49-50, 2000.

Molter, N. Professional caring and ethical practice. In J.G. Alspach (ed.). *Core Curriculum for Critical Care Nursing,* 6th ed. St. Louis, Elsevier, 2006, pp 1-44.

1-29. **(B)** Nitroglycerin is not harmful to the fetus and reduces blood pressure by vasodilation and afterload reduction. Sodium nitroprussode (Nipride) is rarely used in the treatment of pre-eclampsia due to the risk of thiocyanate toxicity in the fetus. ACE inhibitors such as captopril should not be administered in the antepartum period as they have been shown to potentiate fetal abnormalities. Phentolamine (Regitine) is an alpha adrenergic blocker indicated in the treatment of acute hypertension related to cocaine or catecholamine stimulating conditions such as pheochromocytoma.

Reference: Poole, J. H., Spreen, D. T. Acute pulmonary edema. *J Perinat Neonat Nurs,* 19, 316-331, 2005.

1-30. **(A)** The peak inspiratory pressure reflects airway resistance and compliance of lung tissue. The decrease in peak inspiratory pressure indicates that less pressure is necessary to deliver tidal volume and signifies improvement in compliance or distensibility of lung tissue. The decrease in $PaCO_2$ is not specific and may be related to the patient's respiratory rate rather than to any improvement. The increase in PaO_2 is minimal and may be related to factors such as suctioning, position change, or other laboratory factors.

An increase in respiratory rate may be related to patient agitation, activity, or decrease in sedation.

Reference: Wiegand, D. J., Carlson, K. K. (eds.). *AACN Procedure Manual for Critical Care,* 5th ed. St. Louis, Elsevier, 2005.

1-31. **(A)** One of the most common sites of origin for bacteremia and sepsis is the respiratory tract. For patients who are intubated for an extended period of time (greater than 24 hr), the incidence of VAP increases significantly. Aspiration of oral and/or gastric fluids and colonization of the mouth are presumed to be precursors to the development of VAP. Patients in the supine position have an increased incidence of aspiration. Elevating the HOB to an angle of 30 to 45 degrees decreases that incidence. Oral care should be given every 2 to 4 hr for optimal outcomes; if care is delayed more than 4 hr, these benefits are lost. Research has shown that there is no increase in the incidence of VAP associated with prolonged use of ventilator circuits; as a result, frequent changes of the circuit are not warranted. Saliva serves a protective function for the oral mucosa. Mechanical ventilation causes drying of the oral mucosa, affecting salivary flow and contributing to mucositis and gram-negative colonization. Mouth moisturizer should be applied with each cleansing.

References: Lynn-McHale Wiegand, D. J., Carlson, K. K. (eds.). *AACN Procedure Manual for Critical Care,* 5th ed. St. Louis, Elsevier, 2005, pp 28-33.

Urden, L. D., Stacy, K. M., Lough, M. E. *Thelan's Critical Care Nursing, Diagnosis, and Management,* 5th ed. St. Louis, Elsevier, 2006, pp 674-676.

1-32. **(B)** Hypertension after coronary artery bypass graft surgery should be treated promptly to prevent stress on graft sites and decrease bleeding. The nitroglycerin infusion should be increased to enhance vasodilation and decrease the blood pressure. Although the PAD and RAP are borderline low, the urine output indicates that the patient is not hypovolemic at this point, so a fluid bolus is not yet indicated. Increasing the pacing rate will increase the cardiac output, but CO of 3.5 L/min is acceptable immediately after surgery and does not require treatment. Beta-blocking medications are generally avoided in the early postoperative cardiac surgery period because of their negative inotropic effects during the period when myocardial stunning may be present.

Reference: Woods, S. L., Froelicher, E. S., Motzer, S. U., Bridges, E. J. *Cardiac Nursing,* 5th ed. Philadelphia, Lippincott Williams & Wilkins, 2005.

1-33. **(D)** In a patient with longstanding asthma, respiratory acidosis and hypercarbia are signs of worsening gas exchange and a diminishing respiratory effort. These are generally considered ominous signs, so expeditious intubation is the best answer (Option D). Anti-inflammatory agents such as steroids and leukotriene inhibitors (Options A and B) are administered in concert with the bronchodilator therapy but should be added prior to the development of hypercarbia. Inhaled nitric oxide (Option C) via an endotracheal tube is used for the treatment of ARDS and pulmonary hypertension.

References: Corbridge T., Corbridge S. J. Severe asthma exacerbation. In M. P. Fink, E. Abraham, J. L. Vincent, P. M. Kochanek (eds.). *Textbook of Critical Care,* 5th ed. Philadelphia, Elsevier, 2005.

Ellstrom. K. The pulmonary system. In J. G. Alspach (ed.). *Core Curriculum for Critical Care Nursing,* 6th ed. Philadelphia, Elsevier, 2006.

1-34. **(C)** This question illustrates the nurse's competency for System Thinking. Options A and B would diminish VAP incidence within the hospital, but not to the extent afforded by Option C, which, by implementing a vaccination program for all patients age 65 years and older who come to the facility, clearly has the farthest-reaching impact. DVT prophylaxis has not been associated with decreasing VAP. When choosing an intervention to improve outcomes, wide-reaching solutions should be considered over those with more limited impact.

References: Houghton, D. HAI prevention: the power is in your hands. *Nurs Manage,* 37, S1-S7, 2006.

Molter, N. Professional caring and ethical practice. In J. G. Alspach (ed.). *Core Curriculum for Critical Care Nursing,* 6th ed. St. Louis, Elsevier, 2006, pp 1-44.

Tablan, O., Anderson, L., Besser, R., et al. Guidelines for preventing healthcare associated pneumonia, 2003: Recommendations of CDC and the healthcare infection control practices advisory committee. *Morb Mortal Wkly Rep,* 53(RR3), 1-36, 2004.

1-35. **(C)** Before administering interventions such as medications or food, the nurse should assess the patient. In this case, the capillary glucose level should be assessed, as restlessness and irritability are classic signs of hypoglycemia, and this patient has an insulin drip. Except as part of the nurse's admission appraisal, there is no indication apparent for auscultating breath sounds. Administration of an anxiolytic medication without first determining whether that medication is warranted could potentially be detrimental to a patient who needed glucose. Because irritability may also indicate hypoxemia, this would be an appropriate second area in which to assess this patient. While providing milk and crackers for this patient will help to alleviate hypoglycemia over a long period of time, a person experiencing hypoglycemia initially needs a rapidly absorbed source of glucose after the assessment is completed.

References: Newberry, L., Criddle, L. *Sheehy's Manual of Emergency Care,* 6th ed. Philadelphia, Elsevier, 2006, pp 428-432.

Urden, L. D., Stacy, K. M., Lough, M. E. *Thelan's Critical Care Nursing: Diagnosis and Management,* 5th ed. Philadelphia, Elsevier, 2006, p 926.

1-36. **(A)** Allowing the patient to have things that make him or her feel more at home helps to reduce anxiety. Cats tend to carry many pathogens, owing to their bathing habits and litter box use, that could become opportunistic for this patient. School-aged children spend a large part of their days in a confined area with 20 to 30 other people, sharing many communicable diseases, and they may not be well-served by adult-sized masks, gowns, and gloves (used as barrier devices), so they pose potential sources of pathogens to the patient. Fresh foods may improve a patient's appetite and enhance a sense of well-being, but they carry the risk of transmitting bacteria and viruses from the fields in which they were grown, so commercially canned foods are preferable.

References: Newberry, L., Criddle, L. *Sheehy's Manual of Emergency Care,* 6th ed. Philadelphia, Elsevier, 2006, pp 419-421.

Urden, L. D., Stacy, K. M., Lough, M. E. (eds.). *Thelan's Critical Care Nursing: Diagnosis and Management,* 5th ed. Philadelphia, Elsevier, 2006, pp 75-77.

1-37. **(C)** Unstable tachycardia should be treated with immediate synchronized cardioversion. Stable ventricular tachycardia, stable tachycardias of uncertain etiology and atrial fibrillation with Wolff-Parkinson-White syndrome may be treated with amiodarone. Stable supraventricular tachycardia may be treated with adenosine. Defibrillation is indicated for unstable ventricular tachycardia or ventricular fibrillation.

Reference: Field, J. M., Hazinski, M. F., Gilmore, D. (eds.). *Handbook of Emergency Cardiovascular Care for Healthcare Providers.* Dallas, American Heart Association, 2006.

1-38. **(A)** Using evidence-based protocols, policies, standards, and guidelines to improve patient care reflects the use of clinical inquiry. Option A indicates that the nurse needs to conduct a literature search for evidence-based practice for patients at high risk for SRMD and that the nurse's practice should be protocol-driven. Although Option B (use of proton pump inhibitors) would be useful as an intervention for SRMD, not every patient needs to be placed on a PPI, and prevention of SRMD is preferred over allowing the condition to develop. Option C turns the problem over to a medical committee, where nurse input may not be included in development of the protocol. Option D adds needless delay to address the issue.

References: Molter, N. Professional caring and ethical practice. In J. G. Alspach (ed.). *Core Curriculum for Critical Care Nursing*, 6th ed. St. Louis, Elsevier, 2006, pp 1-44.

Spirt, M. J., Stanley, S. Update on stress ulcer prophylaxis in critically ill patients. *Crit Care Nurse*, 26(1), 18-29, 2006.

1-39. **(A)** Paradoxical pulse, a variation in pulse or blood pressure with respiration, is a sign of pericardial tamponade or hypovolemia. Pericardial tamponade may occur after PCI owing to coronary artery dissection or perforation of the myocardium. Coronary artery spasm causes signs of myocardial ischemia such as chest pain and ECG changes but does not affect blood pressure. Dysrhythmias such as atrial fibrillation and premature ventricular contractions may cause irregularities in pulse pressure, but do not cause paradoxical pulse. Vasovagal reactions cause decreased blood pressure and bradycardia.

Reference: Woods, S. L., Froelicher, E. S., Motzer, S. U., Bridges, E. J. *Cardiac Nursing,* 5th ed. Philadelphia, Lippincott Williams & Wilkins, 2005.

1-40. **(B)** Morbid obesity contributes to immobility, one of the risk factors for deep vein thrombosis (DVT) and pulmonary embolism. Sudden onset of dyspnea and chest pain indicate an acute condition such as pneumothorax, aspiration or pulmonary embolus. The chest x-ray findings of an enlarged, or prominent pulmonary artery suggest that pulmonary obstruction is due to pulmonary embolism. There is no radiologic evidence of pneumothorax. Acute MI would be indicated by ST segment elevation. Aspiration pneumonia would not likely have acute onset unless the aspirate was large in volume (which would be demonstrated on x-ray) or acid in pH.

Reference: Sole, M. L., Klein, D. G., Moseley, M. J. *Introduction to Critical Care Nursing*, 4th ed. St. Louis, Elsevier, 2005.

1-41. **(C)** The patient is experiencing hyperphosphatemia and requires the administration of aluminum hydroxide. Calcium and phosphorus are regulated at the renal level by parathyroid hormone (PTH). PTH facilitates calcium reabsorption and phosphorus excretion in people with normal renal function. Patients with chronic renal failure require medications that bind with phosphorus (e.g., aluminum hydroxide) so that phosphorus can be excreted via the stool. As the serum phosphorus level decreases, blood calcium levels increase. Administration of a potassium supplement will not correct the patient's hyperphosphatemia. Supplementing the patient with oral phosphates will worsen the problem. Sodium bicarbonate administration will not address the hyperphosphatemia.

References: Hinkle, C. Renal system. In Chulay, M., Burns, S. M. (eds.). *AACN Essentials of Critical Care Nursing.* New York, McGraw-Hill, 2006, pp 341-355.

Lough, M. E. Renal disorders and therapeutic management. In L. D. Urden, K. M. Stacy, M. E. Lough (eds). *Thelan's Critical Care Nursing: Diagnosis and Management,* 5th ed. St. Louis, Elsevier, 2006, pp 813-846.

Stark, J. L. The renal system. In J. G. Alspach (eds.). *Core Curriculum for Critical Care Nursing,* 6th ed. St. Louis, Elsevier, 2006, pp 525-607.

1-42. **(B)** Inferior wall MI is caused by occlusion of the right coronary artery, which also supplies the right ventricle. ST segment elevation is present in II, III, and aVF indicating inferior wall MI. In right ventricular MI, the right ventricle fails and requires higher volume to produce adequate cardiac filling and output, causing hypotension after administration of nitroglycerin. Although some drop in BP is expected after nitroglycerin administration, hypotension to this extent would not be anticipated in the supine position and, if hypersensitivity to nitroglycerin was the source, hypotension would likely have been accompanied by other findings such as nausea and vomiting. Papillary muscle rupture causes signs of left ventricular failure; symptoms would diminish after administration of nitroglycerin due to decreased afterload. Rupture of the ventricular free wall would cause symptoms of pericardial tamponade and shock.

Reference: Woods, S. L., Froelicher, E. S., Motzer, S. U., Bridges, E. J. *Cardiac Nursing,* 5th ed. Philadelphia, Lippincott Williams & Wilkins, 2005.

1-43. **(B)** The best reply is to provide the patient with an instructional rationale for holding fluids until it is safe for them to drink again. Option A is incorrect because the patient may be able to swallow and still not have a gag reflex. Option C ignores the patient's request and lacks any instructional value. Option D is incorrect because lunch cannot be given without verification that the patient has intact and fully functioning reflexes (gag, cough, etc.) and can safely ingest fluids and the assigned diet.

Reference: Zuckerman, G. R., Lotsoff, D. S. Upper and lower gastrointestinal bleeding: principles of diagnosis and management. In R. S. Irvin, J. M. Rippe, H. Goodgeart (eds.). *Irwin & Rippe's Intensive Care Medicine,* 5th ed. Philadelphia, Lippincott Williams & Wilkins, 2003, pp 1089-1092.

1-44. **(C)** Studies have found that routine ventilator circuit changes do little to prevent the development of VAP. As a result, the Centers for Disease Control and Prevention (CDC) no longer calls for routine changes of the ventilator circuit (tubing, exhalation valve, and attached humidifier) but instead recommends changing these components only when the equipment is visibly soiled or malfunctioning. In a related recommendation, the CDC recommends draining and discarding condensate that collects in the ventilator tubing and not allowing it to drain back toward the patient.

Reference: Chulay, M. VAP prevention: the latest guidelines. RNweb. Posted March 1, 2005. Accessed at http://rnweb.com/rnweb/article/articleDetail.jsp?id=149672 (November 7, 2006).

1-45. **(B)** A pacemaker magnet placed over the ICD generator will disable the ICD and prevent further inappropriate discharge. Trancutaneous pacing is indicated for symptomatic bradycardia. Medication administration will not prevent inappropriate shock delivery. Diltiazem will control the rate and amiodarone might convert the atrial fibrillation to sinus rhythm.

References: Aviles, J. M., Aviles, R. J. Advances in cardiac biomarkers. *Emerg Med Clin North Am,* 23, 954-975, 2005.

Woods, S. L., Froelicher, E. S., Motzer, S. U., Bridges, E. J. *Cardiac Nursing,* 5th ed. Philadelphia, Lippincott Williams & Wilkins, 2005.

1-46. **(C)** Exogenous corticosteroid administration frequently results in a hyperglycemic state related to inhibition of gluconeogenesis and increased insulin resistance. Untreated, the serum glucose gradually climbs, but the presence of exogenous insulin prevents the development of diabetic ketoacidosis. In response to polyuria, the patient becomes hyperosmolar. Diabetes insipidus would cause hyperosmolarity but would not result in a serum glucose of 624 mg/dL. In Type 1 diabetes with such a high serum glucose, ketoacidosis would have been evidenced in the laboratory work. While the patient may develop polycythemia vera after years of poor oxygenation, that condition would not produce this serum glucose value.

References: Newberry, L., Criddle, L. *Sheehy's Manual of Emergency Care,* 6th ed. Philadelphia, Elsevier, 2006, pp 431-433.

Urden, L. D., Stacy, K. M., Lough, M. *Thelan's Critical Care Nursing: Diagnosis and Management,* 5th ed. Philadelphia, Elsevier, 2006.

1-47. **(A)** The normal ejection fraction is 50-75%. Patients with diastolic dysfunction often have decreased early diastolic filling time and preserved ejection fraction. The left ventricular ejection time is reduced due to diminished left ventricular end-diastolic volume. Beta-blocking agents prolong the diastolic filling time, resulting in improved left ventricular contraction and decreased diastolic pressure.

Reference: Colonna, P., Pinto, F. J., Soreno, M., et al. The emerging role of echocardiography in the screening of patients at risk of heart failure. *Am J Cardiol,* 96, 42L-51L, 2005.

1-48. **(B)** Researching the current ICD registries in use, the typical complications monitored, and the type of reporting required by the FDA should be the nurse's initial step in designing a program to monitor ICDs in the facility. When asked to develop a new program, current strategies should be researched to identify best practices. Option A would most likely provide information on that vendor's ICD but not other vendors' devices, and any vendor information would need to be considered for potential bias. Option C overlooks considering the complexity of the device and may therefore neglect appraisal of important features. Option D fails to demonstrate any competency in clinical inquiry.

References: Maisel, W. H. Pacemaker and ICD generator reliability: meta-analysis of device registries. *J Am Med Assoc,* 295(16), 1929-1934, 2006.

Molter, N. Professional caring and ethical practice. In J. G. Alspach (ed.). *Core Curriculum for Critical Care Nursing,* 6th ed. St. Louis, Elsevier, 2006, pp 1-44.

1-49. **(B)** Large-bore IV insertion is a priority in this patient so that initiation of fluid resuscitation can begin to ensure maintenance of a MAP of 60 mm Hg. The monitoring of coagulation studies will be of importance if there is prolonged bleeding or after the administration of blood products. These values adjust to reflect the patient's condition over time. An upright KUB will assist in the determination if there is free air in the abdomen; however, stabilization of the patient's circulatory status is the initial focus for the nurse. Monitoring fluid balance and renal function is an ongoing intervention for this patient. It will be important to replace fluid losses and maintain intravascular volume, but this aspect of care is not the most immediate need of the patient.

References: Krumberger, J., Parrish, C. R., Krenitsky, J. Gastrointestinal system. In M. Chulay, S. Burns (eds.). *AACN Essentials of Critical Care Nursing.* New York, McGraw-Hill, 2006, p 320.

Radovich, P. Gastrointestinal system. In J. G. Alspach (ed.). *Core Curriculum for Critical Care Nursing,* 6th ed. St. Louis, Elsevier, 2006, p 732.

1-50. **(C)** The most appropriate action for the nurse to take would be to inform the patient of the spouse's concerns and determine what his current wishes are. A trial period, or a trial period with time limitations, may be an option that the patient is willing to consider. An open atmosphere for both the patient and his spouse to express their desires and concerns should be encouraged. Although it is correct that the DPA is not in effect until the patient is no longer able to make decisions, informing the spouse of this fact may make the spouse feel that the nurse is not willing to listen to the spouse's concerns. A dyspneic patient is not likely to be able to carry on a discussion of this nature, and expectations that the patient would be physically able to discuss an emotional topic such as end-of-life decisions with his spouse are unrealistic under these circumstances.

Reference: Baird, M. S., Keen, J. H., Swearingen, D. L. *Manual of Critical Care Nursing: Nursing Interventions and Collaborative Management.* St. Louis, Elsevier, 2005.

1-51. **(A)** Coronary artery spasm is common after coronary atherectomy. Treatment with intravenous nitroglycerin and fluids maintains coronary artery dilation and prevents spasm. Calcium channel blockers lower blood pressure through vasodilation, but do not prevent coronary artery spasm. Heparin and glycoprotein IIb/IIIa inhibitors prevent new clot formation and aid in promoting thrombus dissolution but do not affect coronary spasm.

Reference: Woods, S. L., Froelicher, E. S., Motzer, S. U., Bridges, E. J. *Cardiac Nursing,* 5th ed. Philadelphia, Lippincott Williams & Wilkins, 2005.

1-52. **(A)** After surviving aneurysmal subarachnoid hemorrhage, patients are primarily at risk for developing any or all of the following three problems: (1) rebleed of the aneurysm if unsecured, (2) hydrocephalus owing to problems with reabsorption of CSF, or (3) vasospasm. Blood in the subarachnoid space can block reabsorption of CSF by the arachnoid villi. This is a type of communicating hydrocephalus. A thrombus (Option B) could potentially cause an obstruction of CSF flow; however, hydrocephalus after SAH is generally communicating rather than obstructive in nature. Mass effect (Option C) can block CSF flow but would more likely be associated with a brain tumor than with SAH. This patient population is at risk of developing vasospasm (Option D), which can result in further stroke, but vasospasm directly affects blood flow, not CSF flow.

References: Bader, M. K., Littlejohns, L. R. (eds.). *AANN Core Curriculum for Neuroscience Nursing,* 4th ed. St. Louis, Elsevier, 2004.

Greenberg, M. S. (ed.). *Handbook of Neurosurgery,* 6th ed. New York, Thieme Medical Publishers, 2006.

Hickey, J. V. (ed.). *The Clinical Practice of Neurological and Neurosurgical Nursing,* 5th ed. Philadelphia, Lippincott Williams & Wilkins, 2002.

1-53. **(C)** Decreased urine output may be the first indication that early compensatory mechanisms to prevent shock are occurring. Activation of the sympathetic nervous system causes vasoconstriction, which decreases renal blood flow. When renal blood flow decreases, renin and angiotensin are released and produce vasoconstriction, which increases capillary refill time. Hypotension and tachycardia are later signs seen in a more advanced stage of shock.

Reference: Lewis, S. M., Heitkemper, M. M., Dirksen, S. R. *Medical-Surgical Nursing: Assessment and Management of Clinical Problems*, 6th ed. St. Louis, Elsevier, 2004.

1-54. **(B)** Administration of oxygen is the first priority in this emergent situation. Although this patient likely has a pneumothorax, the physician will confirm that finding with a chest x-ray unless the patient is acutely decompensating. The patient may have pain, but administration of narcotics may decrease his respiratory drive and worsen hypoxia. Older patients with rib fractures often require 24 to 48 hours of observation in the ICU, but treatment of hypoxia takes priority at this time.

References: Alspach, J. G. (ed.). *Core Curriculum for Critical Care Nursing,* 6th ed. Philadelphia, Elsevier, 2006.

McQuillan, K. A., Von Rueden, K., Hartsock, R., et al. (eds.). *Trauma Nursing,* 3rd ed. Philadelphia, Elsevier, 2002.

1-55. **(A)** Clinical inquiry is demonstrated when the nurse uses evidence-based information to make changes in nursing practice. Implementing a change in practice requires first identifying the key stakeholders for the change in order to introduce the proposed change. Research utilization and experiential knowledge can be applied to improve patient outcomes when others are part of the change process. Numerous studies have demonstrated the safety and accuracy of drawing blood from peripheral venous access devices (VADs) for aPTTs. The intended change has already been identified. Option C is incorrect because one does not implement a change without getting input from key stakeholders. Option D is incorrect because evaluation would not be performed until after the change had been implemented.

References: Molter, N. Professional caring and ethical practice. In J. G. Alspach (ed.). *Core Curriculum for Critical Care Nursing,* 6th ed. St. Louis, Elsevier, 2006, pp 1-44.

Prue-Owen, K. K. Use of peripheral venous access devices for obtaining blood samples for measurement of activated partial thromboplastin time. *Crit Care Nurse,* 26(1), 30-38, 2006.

1-56. **(C)** In pericardial tamponade, the patient becomes hypotensive due to inadequate cardiac filling. Right and left heart pressures equalize and the patient may develop jugular venous distension and tachycardia. Beck's triad is the classic presentation for cardiac tamponade and includes decreased systolic blood pressure, increased CVP/JVP and muffled heart tones. Tachycardia may not be present in the early postoperative period of the open heart surgery patient due to myocardial stunning. Chest tube output is not a reliable indicator of whether pericardial tamponade is present because chest tube output may be decreased due to clot formation. No evidence of MI was presented in the case described.

Reference: Woods, S. L., Froelicher, E. S., Motzer, S. U., Bridges, E. J. *Cardiac Nursing* (5th ed.). Philadelphia, Lippincott Williams & Wilkins, 2005.

1-57. **(C)** Several recreational drugs and stimulants are associated with development of rhabdomyolysis, particularly agents that either mimic or stimulate the sympathetic nervous system. The appearance of discolored urine is indicative of large amounts of myoglobin in the urine and is often the initial clinical finding in rhabdomyolysis. The goal of treatment for rhabdomyolysis is to prevent renal failure. This is achieved by maintaining a urine output >150 mL/hr with intravascular volume expansion using isotonic crystalloid and diuretics. Myoglobin is a dark red protein responsible for supplying oxygen to the myocytes. The breakdown of myoglobin produces a pigment-induced nephropathy with subsequent sloughing of the tubular epithelium. This exfoliate, together with large myoglobin molecules, results in the formation of brown casts that obstruct renal tubules. Low urinary pH facilitates the formation of casts and also promotes the dissociation of myoglobin molecules into cytotoxic components. The addition of sodium bicarbonate to IV solutions alkalinizes urine to prevent dissociation of myoglobin into its nephrotoxic components. The goal for urinary pH is to maintain >6.0. The purpose of insertion of an indwelling catheter and hemodynamic monitoring is to guide the bedside nurse in management and evaluation of the patients' response to fluid administration and diuretic therapy, not to prevent renal failure.

  Reference: Criddle, L. M. Rhabdomyolysis. Pathophysiology, recognition and management: *Crit Care Nurse,* 23(6), 14-32, 2003.

1-58. **(B)** SPECT perfusion imaging is the most helpful in diagnosing myocardial ischemia in a patient with left bundle branch block. LBBB may mask ST and T wave abnormalities, making it difficult to determine if ischemia is present. Perfusion defects are demonstrated during SPECT studies. Those which appear during exercise and disappear during rest indicate ischemia. MRI is useful in demonstrating structural defects of the heart, aorta, and pericardium, but not the coronary arteries. MR angiography (MRA) may be useful to determine if coronary grafts are patent.

  Reference: Woods, S. L., Froelicher, E. S., Motzer, S. U., Bridges, E. J. *Cardiac Nursing,* 5th ed. Philadelphia, Lippincott Williams & Wilkins, 2005.

1-59. **(D)** The nurse in this situation should promote patient-centered decision making that honors the rights and interests of the patient even when the patient's choice is not what the nurse would chose. The patient has the right to have his reports of pain believed. Options A, B, and C do not involve the patient in the decision-making process. Giving the NTG before giving the morphine may be viewed by the patient as the nurse's not listening to his needs. Option B is incorrect because administering the morphine assumes that this is the drug the patient wants. Making the patient wait 30 minutes may imply to the patient that the nurse does not believe he is having pain and that his pain needs are not being met.

  References: Molter, N. Professional caring and ethical practice. In J. G. Alspach (ed.). *Core Curriculum for Critical Care Nursing*, 6th ed. St. Louis, Elsevier, 2006, pp 24, 36.

  Stannard, D. Hardin S. R. Advocacy and moral agency. In S. R. Hardin, K. Kaplow (eds.). *Synergy for Clinical Excellence*. Sudbury, Jones & Bartlett, 2005, pp 63-68.

1-60. **(A)** The optimal ventilation strategy for this patient includes use of low tidal volumes, minimizing potential barotrauma, and carefully monitoring respiratory rates. Patients in status asthmaticus are at great risk for air trapping and developing auto-PEEP due to airway constriction. As a result, high tidal volumes and high PEEP place the patient at risk for barotrauma (Options B, C, D).

  References: Corbridge, T., Corbridge, S. J. Severe asthma exacerbation. In M. P. Fink, E. Abraham, J. L. Vincent, P. M. Kochanek (eds.). *Textbook of Critical Care,* 5th ed. Philadelphia, Elsevier, 2005.

  Ellstrom, K. The pulmonary system. In J. G. Alspach (ed.). *Core Curriculum for Critical Care Nursing,* 6th ed. St. Louis, Elsevier, 2006.

1-61. **(A)** Revasularization may result in the release of products of anaerobic metabolism, lactic acid and potassium, into circulation. Acidosis and potassium imbalance place the patient at increased risk of dysrhythmias. Elevated CPK levels are expected after revascularization due to skeletal muscle ischemia. Graft occlusion may occur if hypotension or coagulopathy occur. Pulmonary embolus is a risk of surgery, but is usually associated with venous thrombus. Heart failure is a complication of fluids administered during surgery and the effects of anesthetics, but is not indicated by an elevated potassium and metabolic acidosis.

Reference: Fahey, V. A. *Vascular Nursing*, 4ᵗʰ ed. St. Louis, Elsevier, 2004.

1-62. **(D)** The first three questions provide important information related to this patient's medical history, but only Option D poses a question that may solicit a belief or value rather than a fact.

References: Hardin, S. R. Response to diversity. In S. R. Hardin, R. Kaplow (eds.). *Synergy for Clinical Excellence*. Sudbury, Jones & Bartlett, 2005, pp 91-96.

Molter, N. Professional caring and ethical practice. In J. G. Alspach (ed.). *Core Curriculum for Critical Care Nursing*, 6ᵗʰ ed. St. Louis, Elsevier, 2006, pp 1-44.

1-63. **(A)** COPD is an umbrella term for a variety of pathologies such as emphysema and chronic bronchitis. Patients typically have components of both diseases, so they often benefit from carefully monitored increases in FiO_2. While ABGs should be drawn to guide care of this patient, they should not be the sole determinant for clinical interventions. Manipulations of oxygen should be done with careful monitoring of the patient's clinical response; however, hypoxia is a greater concern for this patient than respiratory drive. Hypoxemic vasoconstriction is a compensatory process that maximizes V/Q matching in this patient population. It does not create a diffusion defect.

Reference: Calverley, P. Chronic obstructive pulmonary diseases. In M. P. Fink, E. Abraham, J. L. Vincent, P. M. Kochanek (eds.). *Textbook of Critical Care*, 5ᵗʰ ed. Philadelphia, Elsevier, 2005.

1-64. **(D)** The initial therapy would be calcium chloride 1000 mg in 1000 mL NS (calcium gluconate might also be considered) because the patient is manifesting signs of hypocalcemia. In acute pancreatitis, calcium precipitates in the pancreas. Signs of hypocalcemia include positive Chvostek's and Trousseau's signs, tetany, seizures, respiratory arrest, bronchospasm, stridor, wheezing, paralytic ileus, and diarrhea.

Magnesium sulfate would be used to manage hypomagnesemia. Plicamycin is used to treat hypercalcemia and vasopressin is used for hyperosmolar disorders.

References: Hinkle, C. Renal system. In M. Chulay, S. M. Burns (eds.). *AACN Essentials of Critical Care Nursing*. New York, McGraw-Hill, 2006, pp 341-355.

Lough, M. E. Renal disorders and therapeutic management. In L. D. Urden, K. M. Stacy, M. E. Lough (eds.). *Thelan's Critical Care Nursing: Diagnosis and Management,* 5ᵗʰ ed. St. Louis, Elsevier, 2006, pp 813-846.

Stark, J. L. The renal system. In J. G. Alspach (ed.). *Core Curriculum for Critical Care Nursing*, 6ᵗʰ ed. St. Louis, 2006, Elsevier, pp 525-607.

1-65. **(B)** The causes of erosive gastritis include drugs (especially NSAIDs), alcohol, and acute stress. When viewed with an endoscope, superficial erosions are seen that do not penetrate into the deeper layers of the stomach. They are frequently accompanied by some degree of hemorrhage. When gastritis is diffuse, the amount of blood loss can be extensive. A pulmonary embolism usually occurs in the setting of deep vein thrombosis. This patient has not been immobilized for a significant period of time. The signs and symptoms of a pulmonary embolism include acute chest pain, cough, and hemoptysis, which this patient is not exhibiting. Intracranial hypertension presents with widening pulse pressure and bradycardia, findings inconsistent with this patient's presentation. Dehydration owing to alcohol abuse may contribute to this patient's overall hydration status. Dehydration does not usually result in gastrointestinal bleeding.

Reference: Radovich, P. The gastrointestinal system. In J. G. Alspach (ed.). *Core Curriculum for Critical Care Nursing,* 6ᵗʰ ed. St. Louis, Elsevier, 2006, p 729.

1-66. **(C)** Thiocyanate toxicity generally occurs when sodium nitroprusside is used for longer than 48 hours. Thiocyanate is a metabolite of sodium nitroprusside and causes oxygen to bind to hemoglobin, preventing its release to tissues; as a result, SpO_2 is not a reliable indicator of tissue oxygenation. Early symptoms include mental status changes and delirium. Stroke may present as altered mental status, but it is unlikely if the patient is receiving appropriate blood pressure reduction therapy. Myocardial infarction is also unlikely owing to the vasodilatory effects of sodium nitroprusside and lack of chest pain complaints. Encephalopathy would have been evident earlier in the treatment of hypertensive crisis if blood pressure reduction was too rapid for cerebral autoregulation to be maintained.

Reference: Chulay, M., Burns, S. M. *AACN Essentials of Critical Care Nursing.* New York, McGraw-Hill, 2006.

1-67. **(C)** In septic shock, HR increases in response to stimulation of the sympathetic nervous system baroreceptors and release of epinephrine and norepinephrine by the adrenal gland. Mixed venous oxygen saturation (SVO_2) reflects the balance between O_2 delivery and O_2 consumption. A normal SVO_2 is 60% to 80%. Several factors can increase the SVO_2—increase in oxygen saturation and/or increase in cardiac output. In the patient with septic shock, a *decrease* in oxygen consumption occurs at the cellular level owing to a reduced ability of the cells to use the oxygen and inadequate tissue perfusion related to vasoconstriction. The oxygen is not extracted from the blood at the tissue level, resulting in an abnormally elevated SVO_2.

The patient's temperature is elevated in response to pyrogens released from invading microorganisms, immune mediator activation, and increased metabolic activity. Urine output declines because of decreased perfusion to the kidneys. Dilation of the arterial system causes SVR to fall, thereby reducing left ventricular afterload. If the patient is euvolemic, these compensatory changes help to produce a normal to high CO. Dilation of the venous system leads to a decrease in venous return to the heart, which results in decreased preload as evidenced by a decreased RAP. Ventilation and perfusion mismatching occurs in the lungs as a result of pulmonary vasoconstriction and the presence of pulmonary microemboli. Hypoxemia occurs, and the RR increases to compensate for the lack of oxygen.

Reference: Urden, L. D., Stacy, K. M., Lough, M. E. *Thelan's Critical Care Nursing: Diagnosis and Management,* 5th ed. St. Louis, Elsevier, 2006, pp 1026-1027.

1-68. **(B)** The best approach to establishing a comprehensive program of oral care should begin with forming a multidisciplinary team that can review supporting scientific literature and develop a policy or protocol, provide hospital wide education, and measure outcomes of the intervention. Option A is incorrect because placing kits at the bedside does not ensure their use. Merely obtaining staff input does not designate any accountability for the project as Option B does. Option D is of very limited help because the nature of those oral care orders needs to coincide with a best-practices approach to care before outcomes could be expected to improve.

Reference: Cutler, C. J., Davis, N. Improving oral care in patients receiving mechanical ventilation, *Am J Crit Care,* 14(5), 389-394, 2005.

1-69. **(B)** The patient's blood pressure is adequate to give the beta blocker, but because of worsening symptoms of heart failure, a reduced dose is warranted. Abrupt discontinuation of beta blocker therapy can cause rebound hypertension and tachycardia. Tachycardia will worsen heart failure, as it increases oxygen consumption and reduces ventricular filling time. Additional doses of beta blockers may worsen symptoms. ACE inhibitor therapy reduces afterload and decreases sodium retention. ACE inhibitors have a mild diuretic effect and may be added to current therapy, but additional doses are not warranted to treat worsening symptoms.

Reference: Woods, S. L., Froelicher, E. S., Motzer, S. U., Bridges, E. J. *Cardiac Nursing,* 5th ed. Philadelphia, Lippincott Williams & Wilkins, 2005.

1-70. **(B)** Noninvasive ventilatory techniques (CPAP, BiPAP) are routinely used for COPD patients with moderate respiratory failure. NIV therapies improve respiratory mechanics by allowing the patient to take larger tidal volumes and preventing fatigue of respiratory muscles, which often precipitates a need for intubation. NIV is not an option for every patient, however, including those with significant cardiovascular compromise, arrhythmias with hypotension, or impaired consciousness (except O_2 induced) and those with significant risk of aspiration. Heavy sedation is contraindicated with NIV as this therapy requires that the patient be able to spontaneously ventilate and be sufficiently conscious to protect their airway. NIV reduces work of breathing in patients with COPD. Use of masks versus nasal pillows is a matter of patient preference and is not required for COPD patients.

Reference: Calverley, P. Chronic obstructive pulmonary diseases. In M. P. Fink, E. Abraham, J. L. Vincent, P. M. Kochanek (eds.). *Textbook of Critical Care,* 5th ed. Philadelphia, Elsevier, 2005.

1-71. **(B)** Breakdown of fat cells produces ketone bodies, which are acids. An increase in metabolic acids results in an increase of urinary output in an attempt to decrease serum glucose, diminish the concentration of acids, and rebalance electrolyte levels. The patient may have faithfully adhered to his routine of managing his type 1 diabetes, yet developed ketoacidosis when emotional or physical stress, such as a viral illness led to increased release of cortisol. The next most likely cause of ketoacidosis would be inadequate insulin in relation to caloric intake. Type 2 diabetes, not type 1, has been found to have a genetic predisposition. Type 1 is currently believed to be autoimmune in origin. Increased levels of activity would result in hypoglycemia rather than hyperglycemia and ketoacidosis.

References: Newberry, L., Criddle, L. *Sheehy's Manual of Emergency Care,* 6th ed. Philadelphia, Elsevier, 2006, pp 428-431.
Urden, L. D., Stacy, K. M., and Lough, M. E. *Thelan's Critical Care Nursing: Diagnosis and Management,* 5th ed. Philadelphia, Elsevier, 2006, p 943.

1-72. **(C)** This patient needs continued fluid resuscitation with crystalloids such as Ringer's lactate or normal saline. Continued administration of crystalloid will enable renal excretion of excess hydrogen ions and resolve acidosis. Administration of sodium bicarbonate may induce alkalosis and prevent oxygen release to tissues. The hematocrit is greater than 28% so transfusion is not indicated. Endotracheal intubation is not indicated with a PaO_2 of 80 mm Hg.

Reference: Kelly, D. Hypovolemic shock. *Crit Care Nurs Q,* 28, 2-19, 2005.

1-73. **(C)** Stabilization of the airway with endotracheal intubation is warranted given the patient's increasing respiratory distress. In patients with severe respiratory distress, increasing the FIO_2 is appropriate; however, it would be increased to 100% at least until airway intubation is completed. There is no radiologic evidence of a pneumothorax, so placement of a chest tube would not be appropriate, and there is no indication that a repeat chest x-ray is warranted at this time. Once intubation has been completed, the chest x-ray can be repeated to confirm correct placement of the endotracheal tube.

References: Ellstrom, K. Pulmonary system. In J. G. Alspach (ed.). *Core Curriculum for Critical Care Nursing,* 6th ed. St. Louis, Elsevier, 2006, p 148.
Yamamoto, L., Schroeder, C., Morely, D., Beiveau, C. Thoracic trauma: the deadly dozen. *Crit Care Nurs Q* (28)1, 22-40, 2005.

1-74. **(D)** Controlling a dying patient's pain minimizes any suffering, a common fear related to end-of-life concerns. Option A is incorrect because there is no evidence that any particular staffing pattern will assure a "good death." Option B is incorrect because unrestricted visiting may be exhausting and undesired for the patient. Encouraging hope when there is none represents a barrier to providing a good death.

Reference: Beckstrand, R. L., Callister, L. C., Kirchhoff, K. T. Providing a "good death": critical care nurses suggestions for improving end of life care. *Am J Crit Care,* 15(1), 38-46, 2006.

1-75. **(A)** Aortic regurgitation may be caused by congenital or degenerative cardiac disease or by endocarditis. Symptoms of aortic regurgitation include systolic ejection murmur, bounding or water-hammer peripheral pulses, head bobbing with each heart beat, dyspnea, syncope, and signs of left ventricular failure. Mitral valve stenosis may cause symptoms of right heart failure, atrial fibrillation, jugular venous distention (JVD), and a diastolic murmur. Tricuspid regurgitation causes a high-pitched holosystolic murmur and symptoms of right heart failure. Signs of pericardial effusion include jugular venous distention (JVD), tachycardia, and symptoms of decreased cardiac output. The ECG in pericardial effusion would typically demonstrate low voltage and tachycardia.

Reference: Bekeredjian, R., Grayburn, P. A. Valvular heart disease, aortic regurgitation. *Circulation,* 11, 125-134, 2005.

1-76. **(C)** All of the options are possible reasons for seizures, but substance withdrawal is the most likely choice among these possibilities. Hypoxia (Option A) is less likely because the patient just started this activity of clenching on his endotracheal tube. Delirium tremens (Option B) is another possibility, but DTs usually occur 48 to 72 hours after cessation of alcohol intake. The patient received seizure prophylaxis for post-traumatic seizures (Option D), so while this is possible, it is a less likely cause.

References: Alspach, J. G. (ed.). *Core Curriculum for Critical Care Nursing,* 6th ed. Philadelphia, Elsevier, 2006.

Bader M. K., Littlejohns, L. R. (eds.). *AANN Core Curriculum for Neuroscience Nursing,* 4th ed. St. Louis, Elsevier, 2004.

1-77. **(B)** Absorption describes the extent and rate of substance removal from outside the body to the bloodstream. Factors affecting absorption include the route and the bioavailability of the particular substance. Clearance is the measurement of the body's ability to eliminate a substance from blood or plasma over time. Distribution is the way in which a substance disseminates throughout the body. Chelation describes one means by which toxic minerals, metals, or chemical substances may be removed from the body via chemical bonding with a chelating agent for elimination in urine and feces.

References: Alspach, J. G. (ed.). *Core Curriculum for Critical Care Nursing,* 6th ed. St. Louis, Elsevier, 2006, p 826.

Newberry, L., Criddle, L. M. (ed.). *Sheehy's Manual of Emergency Care,* 6th ed. St. Louis, Elsevier, 2005, pp 463-464.

1-78. **(A)** Since the medications and transcutaneous pacemaker are equally accessible, the initial intervention should be to initiate transcutaneous pacing. Atropine IV, dopamine or epinephrine infusions may be administered for symptomatic bradycardia if there would be a delay in initiating pacing.

Reference: Field, J. M., Hazinski, M. F., Gilmore, D. (eds.). *Handbook of Emergency Cardiovascular Care for Healthcare Providers.* Dallas, American Heart Association, 2006.

1-79. **(B)** Among the groups listed, only Anglo-American families are typically organized around the nuclear family. All of the other listed options (Asians, African Americans, and Native Americans) reflect cultures where the common family unit is an extended family.

References: Sole, M. L., Klein, D. G., Mosley, M. J. *Introduction to Critical Care Nursing,* 4th ed. St. Louis, Elsevier, 2005.

1-80. **(C)** Classic symptoms of cardiac tamponade include Beck's triad: hypotension, jugular venous distension and distant heart tones. Breath sounds are equal bilaterally, so pneumothorax requiring chest tube insertion or needle thoracostomy is not suspected. The SpO_2 is adequate so intubation is not indicated.

Reference: Sole, M. L., Klein, D. G., Moseley, M. J. (eds.). *Introduction to Critical Care Nursing*, 4th ed. St. Louis, Elsevier, 2005.

1-81. **(D)** The absence of breath sounds over all of the right lung fields strongly suggests a pneumothorax. If there is no penetrating trauma creating a sucking chest wound, these findings are significant for a tension pneumothorax. If the tension pneumothorax enlarges without relief, the patient can go into cardiopulmonary collapse within minutes. Inspiratory wheezing is indicative of narrowed airways; when wheezing clears with coughing, it indicates an intermittent and reversible concern. If the patient were receiving large volumes of IV fluids, frequent auscultation would be warranted. Decreased breath sounds in the bases or over the right lung fields may indicate areas of atelectasis, a collapsed lobe, or a hemothorax. Although these may be significant complications, they are not immediately life-threatening.

References: Ellstrom, K. Pulmonary system. Core Curriculum for Critical Care Nursing, 6th ed. St. Louis, Elsevier, 2006, p 149.

Yamamoto, L. Schroeder, C., Morely, D., Beiveau, C. Thoracic trauma: The deadly dozen. *Crit Care Nurse Q,* (28)1, 22-40, 2005.

1-82. **(D)** Fifty percent of patients with cirrhosis develop esophageal varicies. Variceal hemorrhage accounts for one third of deaths in patients with cirrhosis. The veins of the esophagus represent a high-flow but low-pressure system. When there is increased resistance to blood flow within the liver, the pressure within this system increases, resulting in portal hypertension and the development of esophageal varicies. The varicies are prone to rupture if they are not eliminated by endoscopy or if the pressure is not reduced by a beta blocker. While portal hypertension can increase the risk of right-sided heart failure, heart failure does not cause gastrointestinal bleeding. In cirrhosis, shunting and vasodilatation occur with elevated pressure in the venous portal system, but circulating blood volume does not increase. Normal liver tissues are not fibrotic. Damage to the liver causes hepatocyte necrosis, collapse of the healthy tissue, and replacement with fibrotic tissue. It is not until the liver becomes cirrhotic that portal hypertension leads to a risk of hemorrhage.

References: Elta, G. H. Approach to the patient with gross gastrointestinal bleeding. In T Yamada (ed.). *Textbook of Gastroenterology,* 4th ed. Philadelphia, Lippincott Williams & Wilkins, 2003.

Krumberger, J. M. How to manage an acute upper GI bleed. *RN,* 68(3), pp 34-39, 2005.

1-83. **(A)** Right bundle branch block is demonstrated by an rSR′ pattern in leads V_1 or V_2 (the right chest leads), a slurred S wave in V_5 and V_6 and a QRS duration of greater than 0.12 seconds. LBBB would be demonstrated by a deep S wave in the right chest leads and a QRS greater than 0.12 seconds in leads V_5 and V_6. The heart rate is 100 BPM in this ECG so it does not qualify as tachycardia. There is ST segment depression in the anterior leads (V_2-V_5), which does not signify acute MI. Acute anterior wall MI would be demonstrated by ST segment elevation or Q waves in the anterior leads.

Reference: Woods, S. L., Froelicher, E. S., Motzer, S. U., Bridges, E. J. *Cardiac Nursing,* 5th ed. Philadelphia, Lippincott Williams & Wilkins, 2005.

1-84. **(A)** Postoperative care basics are universal and include optimizing airway, breathing, circulation, pain management, wound care, and intake and output. In the neurosurgical patient, those universals also need to incorporate monitoring and optimizing cerebral perfusion and blood flow. Brain, blood, and CSF are the contents of the cranium. If

blood flow—either arterial inflow or venous outflow—is altered, cerebral perfusion may be compromised. If jugular venous outflow is obstructed, cerebral blood volume increases. That volume directly corresponds to pressure, particularly since the cranium is fixed in size and cannot accommodate varying volumes or pressures. Not only would this affect intracranial pressure, but it may also influence postoperative bleeding. Generally, the nurse would not try to decrease CPP (Option B). The usual goal CPP in monitored patients with intracranial processes is 60–70 mm Hg. Positioning of a postoperative patient does not affect CSF flow (Option C) within the central nervous system. No physiologic benefits derive from immobilizing the surgical site or the head (Option D).

Reference: Bader, M. K., Littlejohns L. R. (eds.). *AANN Core Curriculum for Neuroscience Nursing,* 4th ed. Elsevier, St. Louis, 2004.

1-85. **(C)** Sudden onset of back pain and neurological changes such as syncope are classic findings in aortic dissection. BP differences and facial edema may be the initial indicators that a thoracic aortic aneurysm is present. Pressure differences greater than 20 mm Hg between the left and right arm may indicate the presence of an aortic aneurysm, but do not signal that dissection is occurring unless they are accompanied by other findings. A pulsatile abdominal mass associated with a bruit is a sign that an abdominal aortic aneurysm is present, and may be found on routine abdominal examination. These findings may be difficult to appreciate in the obese patient. Hypertension and renal insufficiency are frequently found in patients with abdominal aortic aneurysm owing to decreased renal blood flow.

References: Beese-Bjurstrom, S. Hidden danger aortic aneurysms and dissection. *Nursing 2004,* 34, 36-41, 2004.

Jones, L. E. Endovascular stent grafting and thoracic aortic aneurysms. *J Cardiovasc Nurs,* 20, 376-384, 2005.

1-86. **(C)** Bronchodilators, oxygen, mucolytic agents, antibiotics, and glucocortocoids are all commonly employed to treat acute exacerbations of COPD. Although viral infections are a frequent cause of these exacerbations, antiviral therapy is not routinely administered to COPD patients. Inhaled prostacycline is an option for maximizing V/Q matching in patients with ARDS, and its intravenous administration is a common treatment for pulmonary hypertension, but it is not used in COPD. A recent review of evidence related to the efficacy of antibiotics in this patient population supports use of antibiotics for patients with COPD exacerbations who are moderately or severely ill with increased cough and colored sputum. Cholinergic agents would not be used in patients with COPD since they would intensify airway bronchoconstriction; COPD patients receive anticholinergic agents, which antagonize acetylcholine, thereby leading to bronchodilation.

Reference: Ram, F. S. F., Rodgriquez-Roisin, R., Grandos-Navarette, A., et al. Antibiotics for exacerbation of chronic obstructive pulmonary disease. *Cochrane Database of Systematic Reviews,* 2006 (2) CD004403.

1-87. **(A)** Percutaneous coronary intervention would eliminate the cause of the dysrhythmia, which is right coronary artery (RCA) occlusion. The RCA supplies the sinus node in most people, and patients with RCA occlusion and IWMI typically have bradycardia. ECG changes associated with RCA occlusion are ST segment elevation in leads II, III, and aVF. Temporary pacing and atropine will only temporarily treat the bradycardia associated with IWMI.

Reference: Woods, S. L., Froelicher, E. S., Motzer, S. U., Bridges, E. J. *Cardiac Nursing,* 5th ed. Philadelphia, Lippincott Williams & Wilkins, 2005.

1-88. **(C)** This question illustrates the nurse's competency for systems thinking. Systems thinking is displayed as the nurse makes a connection between insertion of an ICD, its malfunction, regulatory requirements related to the incident, and impact on the facility. FDA regulations require manufacturers and hospitals to report all pacemaker and ICD malfunctions, especially those that result in death or surgery. Failure to communicate this device problem may lead to underreporting of their potential defects. Between 1990 and 2002, the average rate of ICD device malfunction was 20.7 per 1000 new implants. Option A reflects an expanded concern that includes effects on the facility but does not approach the still wider repercussions of this scenario on the safety of numerous patients with ICDs. Providing emotional support to the family is an obvious and immediate concern but neglects recognition of the system effects of this incident. There is no evidence that indicates staff need instruction regarding ICD malfunctions, so that option is inappropriate at this time.

References: Molter, N. Professional caring and ethical practice. In J. G. Alspach (ed.). *Core Curriculum for Critical Care Nursing,* 6th ed. Elsevier, St. Louis, 2006, pp 1-44.
Wilkoff, B. L. Pacemaker and ICD malfunction-an incomplete picture. *J Am Med Assoc,* 295(16), 1944-1946, 2006.

1-89. **(B)** Administration of fluid (crystalloid) would be the most appropriate and *immediate* treatment at this time. The patient is hemodynamically compromised with hypotension and tachycardia. With the patient's history of nausea, vomiting, and diarrhea, intravascular volume deficit is the rationale for the patient's hemodynamic status. Inotropic support would be detrimental to this patient until volume resuscitation is provided. The patient is anemic and will need a blood transfusion, but it will require time to prepare the packed RBCs; therefore, this is not considered an *immediate* treatment. β-blocker therapy to decrease the heart rate is not indicated for this patient in the presence of hypotension, since the tachycardia is likely a compensatory change for hypovolemia.

Reference: Dellinger, R. P., Carlet, J. M., Masur, H., et al. Surviving Sepsis Campaign guidelines for management of severe sepsis and septic shock. *Crit Care Med,* 32(3), 858-873, 2004.

1-90. **(A)** Therapeutic goals for the patient in cardiogenic shock include achieving a mean arterial pressure (MAP) sufficient to ensure central and peripheral perfusion. A MAP of 60 mm Hg will provide cerebral perfusion. Elevated systemic vascular resistance increases left ventricular work and the potential for decreased end organ perfusion. A heart rate nearing normal further indicates that myocardial work has decreased and oxygenation potentially improved.

Reference: Baird, M. S., Keen, J. H., Swearingen, D. L. *Manual of Critical Care Nursing: Nursing Interventions and Collaborative Management.* St. Louis, Elsevier, 2005.

1-91. **(A)** The patient should have autonomy in deciding how the information will be shared and with whom. Option B completely avoids providing the patient with the information. Suggesting the chaplain's presence shrouds the reply in an undue, ominous tone that is inappropriate. Option D is inappropriate as it reflects a biased reply related to how the information should be conveyed.

Reference: Forest, K., Simpson, S. A., Wilson, B. J., et al. To tell or not to tell: barriers and facilitators in family communication about genetic risk. *Clin Genet*, 64, 317-326, 2003.

1-92. **(B)** More than 50% of COPD exacerbations are related to bacterial or viral infections. Patients with COPD typically experience considerable sputum production, but these secretions do not become inspissated in this disorder. Airway inflammation and sputum production typically occur as a result of the exacerbation, rather than as its cause.

References: Calverly P. M. Chronic obstructive pulmonary disease. In Fink, M. P., Abraham, E., Vincent, J. L., Kochanek, P. M. (eds.). *Textbook of Critical Care,* 5th ed. Philadelphia, Elsevier, 2005.

Ellstrom, K. The pulmonary system. In J. G. Alspach (ed.). *Core Curriculum for Critical Care Nursing,* 6th ed. St. Louis, Elsevier, 2006.

1-93. **(B)** Hypotension and a low PCWP require volume replacement. Surgical blood loss that causes such a dramatic decrease in PCWP requires blood replacement. Packed cells would replenish intravascular blood volume. Normal saline bolus would be a temporary volume replacement and may enter the extravascular space in several hours. Vasoconstricting agents such as dopamine and vasopressin should be withheld until volume status is corrected.

Reference: Baird, M. S., Keen, J. H., Swearingen, P. L. *Manual of Critical Care Nursing.* St. Louis, 2005, Elsevier.

1-94. **(C)** The patient is in acute renal failure. Given that the patient is fluid overloaded and hemodynamically unstable, continuous renal replacement therapy is the treatment modality of choice. Administering fluid boluses to a patient who is in the oliguric phase of ATN will worsen the fluid overload. Hemodialysis requires the patient to be hemodynamically stable. Peritoneal dialysis is not an option owing to the patient's having recently undergone abdominal surgery.

References: ANNA. *Continuous Renal Replacement Therapy.* Pitman, NJ, American Nephrology Nurses Association, 2005, pp 1-12.

Hinkle, C. Renal system. In M. Chulay, S. M. Burns (eds.). *AACN Essentials of Critical Care Nursing.* New York, McGraw-Hill, 2006, pp 341-355.

Lough, M. E. Renal disorders and therapeutic management. In L. D. Urden, K. M. Stacy, M. E. Lough (eds.). *Thelan's Critical Care Nursing: Diagnosis and Management,* 5th ed. St. Louis, Elsevier, 2006, pp 813-846.

Stark, J. L. The renal system. In J. G. Alspach (ed.). *Core Curriculum for Critical Care Nursing*, 6th ed. St. Louis, Elsevier, 2006, pp 525-607.

1-95. **(A)** Weight gain is an early and reliable sign of fluid retention and potentially worsening heart failure, so these patients require instruction regarding daily weights and reinforcement that an increase in weight should be reported to health care providers to prevent a hospital readmission. Option B is incorrect in that not all heart failure patients have anemia. The literature reports that approximately 30% will experience fatigue and/or anemia. Option C is incorrect even though compliance with appointments might help to ensure early identification of problems by the health care provider. Fluid restriction is important and may eventually prevent a readmission; however, immediate intervention is needed when the patient identifies a weight gain.

Reference: Hoyt, R. E., Bowling, L. S: Reducing admissions for congestive heart failure. *Am Fam Phys*, 63(3), 1593-1598, 2001.

1-96. **(B)** Symptoms of pericardial tamponade include hypotension, narrowed pulse pressure, JVD, and pulsus paradoxus. Tamponade may also cause pulsus paradoxus owing to cardiac compression and decreased stroke volume. Hypovolemia may cause tachycardia, hypotension, and decreased stroke volume, but it is not associated with JVD or a friction rub. Tension pneumothorax may cause hypotension and tachycardia but would be associated with severe dyspnea. Superior vena cava syndrome would cause enlargement of neck veins, edema of the face, shortness of breath, and altered mental status.

Reference: Woods, S. L., Froelicher, E. S., Motzer, S. U., Bridges, E. J. *Cardiac Nursing,* 5th ed. Philadelphia, Lippincott Williams & Wilkins, 2005.

1-97. **(A)** The protracted vomiting and abdominal fluid sequestration associated with acute pancreatitis may result in significant electrolyte imbalances, especially those of calcium, magnesium, and potassium. If severe hypocalcemia occurs, the QT intervals lengthen on the ECG, and seizures may occur. Cullen's sign, a bluish discoloration of the periumbilical skin typically associated with subcutaneous intraperitoneal hemorrhage, may or may not be observed in patients with acute pancreatitis, and measurements of abdominal girth are not typically warranted. Although pain control is essential for patients with acute pancreatitis, fluids would not be restricted in patients with vomiting and diarrhea. These patients would be expected to have diminished bowel sounds owing to fluid sequestration. Although vascular stasis and coagulopathies may eventually arise, peripheral pulses are not typically compromised.

Reference: Whitcomb, D. C. Acute pancreatitis. *N Engl J Med,* 354, 2142-2150, 2006.

1-98. **(A)** The first nursing action is discontinuation of the tube feeding to remove the threat of aspiration and its associated complications such as aspiration pneumonia. Metoclopramide should be given after the tube feeding is stopped in order to promote gastrointestinal motility and stomach emptying, further diminishing the chance of aspiration of tube feedings. Checking feeding tube or endotracheal tube placement may be helpful to determine whether dislodgment of either tube is causing the aspiration rather than a reopening of the fistula, though auscultation of air through a feed tube is often unreliable for assessing such dislodgment. Other diagnostic studies such as bronchoscopy or endoscopy are indicated prior to continuing or resuming feedings.

References: Alspach, J. G. (ed.). *Core Curriculum for Critical Care Nursing,* 6th ed. St. Louis, Elsevier, 2006.

McQuillan, K. A., Whalen, E., Flynn Makic M. B. (eds.). *Trauma Nursing,* 3rd ed. St. Louis, Elsevier, 2002.

1-99. **(C)** Sinus rhythm at a rate of less than 100 beats/min indicates that the workload on the left ventricle has decreased effectively, and oxygenation has improved. The heart rate would be elevated if hypoxia was present. Because respiratory effort may cause exhaustion, a slow respiratory rate may indicate fatigue and impending respiratory failure. The amount of diuresis is not a specific indicator that pulmonary fluid overload has resolved. Systolic blood pressure is influenced by multiple factors, including catecholamine release, blood volume, and vasodilation, making it a nonspecific indicator for resolution of pulmonary edema.

Reference: Albert, N. M., Eastwood, C. A., Edwards, M. L. Evidence based practice for acute decompensated heart failure. *Crit Care Nurs,* 24, 14-31, 2004.

1-100. **(C)** The response to cytokine release during sepsis results in (1) systemic vasodilation with decreased afterload ($\downarrow$ SVR) and hypotension; (2) increased capillary permeability with decreased preload ($\downarrow$ CVP), third-spacing, and interstitial edema; (3) relative hypovolemia; and (4) decreased tissue oxygen extraction ($\uparrow$ SVO$_2$). The hemodynamic values in Option A are consistent with a patient in cardiogenic shock. The elevated SVR reflects the sympathetic nervous system response of vasoconstriction. The CVP is elevated owing to pump dysfunction. The SVO$_2$ is decreased owing to low cardiac output. Option B illustrates a patient with loss of vascular tone as seen in spinal cord injury. The patient has adequate preload and normal oxygen extraction at the tissue level. Option D describes a patient with hypovolemic shock. Again, the SVR is elevated as a compensatory response to low pressure with vasoconstriction. The low preload ($\downarrow$ CVP) is consistent with decreased circulating volume. The SVO$_2$ is decreased in relation to the low preload with resultant low cardiac output.

Reference: Alspach, J. G. (ed.). *Core Curriculum for Critical Care Nursing,* 6th ed. St. Louis, Elsevier, 2006, pp 756-763.

1-101. **(A)** Chest tube output greater than 200 mL for 2 consecutive hours indicates a need to return to the operating room to determine if there is a correctable source of bleeding. Low MAP requires pharmacologic support and increasing the rate of dopamine infusion, changing therapy to norepinephrine (Levophed), and fluid bolus to increase blood pressure. Low cardiac output may indicate a need for vasopressor support, fluid administration, increased pacing rate, or cardiac assist with IABP. Elevated PCWP should be treated with vasodilators or possible IABP support to decrease afterload.

Reference: Whitlock, R., Crowther, M. A., Ng, H. J. Bleeding in cardiac surgery, its prevention and treatment, an evidence-based review. *Crit Care Clin,* 21, 589-610, 2005.

1-102. **(C)** The patient must be repositioned because effective chest compressions need to be delivered with the patient in a supine position. Instructing the new nurse on use of the *2006 Guidelines for Cardiopulmonary Resuscitation and Emergency Cardiovascular Care* from the AHA provides current information on correct patient placement from an authoritative source and clarifies that the Trendelenburg position should not be used. Option A is incorrect because in order for chest compressions to be effective, the patient must first be positioned for optimal compression. Option B is a good response but not the best response. The nurse should begin CPR immediately, and then the preceptor can initiate the unit's code blue response. Option D is important, but suction should already be available at an ICU patient's bedside.

Reference: Bridges, N., Jarquin-Valdivia, A. A. Use of the Trendelenburg position as the resuscitation position: to T or not to T? *Am J Crit Care,* 14(5), 364-368, 2005.

1-103. **(C)** In hypertrophic cardiomyopathy, obstruction is decreased when afterload is increased and when preload is decreased; as a result, treatment aims toward increasing afterload and/or increasing preload. Nitroglycerin decreases both preload and afterload, so when it is administered to patients with hypertrophic cardiomyopathy, both of these effects worsen the obstruction and intensify symptoms. Since hypertrophic cardiomyopathy is associated with diastolic dysfunction, medications (such as beta blockers and calcium channel blockers) that slow the heart rate allow increased diastolic filling, which increases preload and promotes myocardial stretch with more efficient emptying of the ventricle. Amiodarone may be used in the treatment of hypertrophic cardiomyopathy to treat atrial or ventricular dysrhythmias.

Reference: Bruce, J. Getting to the heart of cardiomyopathies. *Nursing 2005,* 35, 44-47, 2005.

1-104. **(C)** Regardless of the factors contributing to the development of disseminated intravascular coagulopathy, the definitive treatment is to eliminate the potential causes of this malady. Until this has been accomplished, the patient's situation will continue to deteriorate. Use of heparin may or may not be useful for the patient experiencing DIC, depending on the factors related to the etiology. Subcutaneous administration of any medication may lead to prolonged bleeding from the injection site and should be avoided, especially because the impairment of circulation would limit absorption. While supportive care is necessary, unless the cause of the DIC is addressed, the patient will not survive.

References: Schilling McCann, J. A. *Professional Guide to Pathophysiology.* Philadelphia, Lippincott Williams & Wilkins, 2003, pp 442-444.

Urden, L. D., Stacy, K. M., Lough, M. E. *Thelan's Critical Care Nursing: Diagnosis and Management,* 5th ed. St. Louis, Elsevier, 2006, pp 1131-1134.

1-105. **(B)** Although septic shock is usually associated with vasodilation caused by the release of proinflammatory cytokines and prostaglandins, not all blood vessels dilate. The arterioles in the microcirculation remain vasoconstricted, leading to a maldistribution of blood flow and subsequent inadequate tissue perfusion. Inadequate tissue perfusion is evaluated by tissue oxygen indices, which include oxygen delivery (DO_2) and consumption (VO_2). Normal oxygen delivery is approximately 1000 mL/min, while normal oxygen consumption is estimated at 250 mL/min. In septic shock, the absolute intravascular volume may be normal, but because of acute vasodilation, a relative hypovolemia occurs. Myocardial depression can occur in patients with septic shock and is characterized by reversible biventricular dilation, decreased ejection fraction, altered myocardial compliance, and decreased contractile response to fluid resuscitation and catecholamines. It is caused primarily by myocardial depressant factors released as a result of sepsis and not by altered coronary perfusion or global ischemia. The patient's hemodynamic values indicate the patient has not received adequate volume resuscitation.

Reference: Bridges, E. J., Dukes, M. S. Cardiovascular aspects of septic shock: pathophysiology, monitoring, and treatment. *Crit Care Nurse,* 25(2), 14-42, 2005.

1-106. **(C)** An emergent tracheotomy will provide immediate access to and maintenance of a patent airway so the patient can be ventilated and enable management of the pulmonary trauma that has resulted in the subcutaneous emphysema. The rapid onset of airway obstruction suggests that the obstruction is located in the upper airways, so oral intubation will be ineffective to solve the problem. A fiberoptic bronchoscopy can only be used after the airway has been secured. There is no indication that cardiac compressions for initiation of cardiopulmonary resuscitation are warranted, as the patient has not lost pulses.

References: Ellstrom, K. Pulmonary system. In J. G. Alspach (ed.). *Core Curriculum for Critical Care Nursing,* 6th ed. St. Louis, Elsevier, 2006, p 149.

Yamamoto, L., Schroeder, C., Morely, D., Beiveau, C. Thoracic trauma: the deadly dozen. *Crit Care Nurse Q,* 28(1), 22-40, 2005.

1-107. **(B)** Risk factors for intracerebral hemorrhage (ICH) include low weight (<70 kg), hypertension, advanced age (>70 yr), and thrombolytic therapy. Coagulopathies must be reversed as soon as possible. Warfarin should be reversed with vitamin K (three 10 mg IV doses) and fresh frozen plasma to normalize prothrombin time. Factor IX concentrate can be used along with vitamin K. IV bolus dosing of recombinant factor VIIa can be administered within the first 3 to 4 hours after symptom onset or in patients at risk of additional bleeding, such as

those with warfarin-related coagulopathies. It may limit hematoma enlargement and reduce morbidity and mortality after ICH. Surgery (Option A) for evacuation of a large deep hemispheric clot has been found ineffective in reducing mortality or disability. CT scan is appropriate for diagnostic evaluation in this case. MRI (Option C) may be considered in cases where the clot morphology, location, or presentation is inconsistent with typical ICH. However, this patient does not present with any atypical findings. Epsilon-aminocaproic acid (EACA) (Option D) is indicated in patients who recently received a thrombolytic and are deteriorating. EACA can enhance hemostasis when fibrinolysis contributes to bleeding, but it can also cause excessive thrombosis and is generally not indicated in this scenario.

References: Hickey J. V. (Ed). *The Clinical Practice of Neurological & Neurosurgical Nursing,* 5th ed. Philadelphia, Lippincott Williams & Wilkins, 2002.

Wijdicks, E. F. M. *The Clinical Practice of Critical Care Neurology.* New York, Oxford University Press, 2003.

1-108. **(B)** Identifying and locating resources that the patient's wife could use would help relieve the heavy burden of the husband's care. There is no basis for involving the ethics committee in this situation. Option C has a somewhat judgmental tone and is at odds with the wife's stated feelings and perspective on the situation. Option D may be supportive to some extent, but fails to address the issues of greatest concern at the moment.

Reference: Molter, N. Professional caring and ethical practice. In J. G. Alspach (ed.). *Core Curriculum for Critical Care Nursing,* 6th ed. St. Louis, Elsevier, 2006, pp 1-44.

1-109. **(D)** Renal insufficiency as demonstrated by elevated creatinine should be reported to the cardiologist as adjustments in the amount or type of contrast used for the catheterization may be necessary. Premedication with fenoldopam or acetylcysteine and hydration may be ordered to prevent nephrotoxicity from the contrast agent. Heparin will be continued during catheterization and will be discontinued prior to sheath removal. A serum troponin level of 0.2 ng/dL is not indicative of myocardial ischemia. The potassium level is within normal limits. Contrast media frequently cause diuresis, which may decrease the serum potassium.

Reference: Woods, S. L., Froelicher, E. S., Motzer, S. U., Bridges, E. J. *Cardiac Nursing,* 5th ed. Philadelphia, Lippincott Williams & Wilkins, 2005.

1-110. **(B)** Administration of insulin will begin to correct the patient's acid-base imbalances. This initial bolus should be followed up with an IV drip of regular insulin, which is fast acting and will stop the formation of ketone bodies, thereby correcting metabolic acidosis. Administration of antibiotics may not be an appropriate intervention, as there is no indication the patient is febrile or producing purulent sputum or urine. The patient is compensating for his metabolic acidosis through an increase in the depth and rate of respirations, and bicarbonate level will likely return to a normal level as the cause of the metabolic acidosis is corrected. Normal saline is important for its hydrating effects; however, this rate of infusion would be inadequate to replace fluids lost over a 4-day period.

References: Newberry, L., Criddle, L. *Sheehy's Manual of Emergency Care,* 6th ed. Philadelphia, Elsevier, 2006, pp 426-431.

Urden, L. D., Stacy, K. M., Lough, M. E. *Thelan's Critical Care Nursing: Diagnosis and Management,* 5th ed. St. Louis, Elsevier, 2006, pp 934-937.

1-111. **(B)** Elevation of the head of the bed 30 to 45 degrees has been shown to decrease the rate and risk of aspiration and hospital-acquired pneumonia. Feeding tube placement does not decrease the risk of aspiration. No matter where the tip of a feeding tube is placed, residuals increase the risk of aspiration. In order to prevent tissue trauma and unwarranted oxygen desaturation, patients should be only suctioned when clinically indicated by the presence of secretions. Enteral feedings appropriately delivered have been shown to decrease mortality and morbidity when compared with hyperalimentation.

Reference: Isakow, W., Kollef, M. H. Preventing ventilator associated pneumonia: an evidence based approach of modifiable risk factors. *Sem Resp Crit Care Med,* 27, 5-17, 2006.

1-112. **(B)** The patient's rhythm strip indicates first degree AV block with bradycardia and the automated blood pressure is adequate, therefore no immediate interventions are necessary. Bradycardia is common in healthy persons during sleep. If the automated blood pressure was below 90 mm Hg systolic, the nurse may awaken the patient to determine if symptomatic bradycardia is present. If the patient had low blood pressure or symptoms of decreased perfusion such as altered mental status, administration of atropine would be warranted. Administration of oxygen is indicated for symptomatic bradycardia.

Reference: Woods, S. L., Froelicher, E. S., Motzer, S. U., Bridges, E. J. *Cardiac Nursing,* 5th ed. Philadelphia, Lippincott Williams & Wilkins, 2005.

1-113. **(A)** The body uses oxygen to generate high-energy phosphates via cellular metabolism. If oxygen delivery is not sufficient to meet cellular demands—as seen during periods of shock—the body must rely on anaerobic metabolism. The end product of anaerobic metabolism is lactate. Serum lactate can be used as an alternative parameter to measure the adequacy of oxygen delivery. Although initial serum lactate levels do not differ significantly between survivors and nonsurvivors, survival rates are highest in patients whose serum lactate levels return to normal within the first 24 hours. Thereafter, the longer it takes for lactate levels to clear, the higher the incidence of organ failure and mortality.

Reference: Boswell, S. A., Scalea, T. M. Sublingual capnometry: an alternative to gastric tonometry for the management of shock resuscitation. *Adv Pract Acute Crit Care,* 14(2), 176-184, 2003.

1-114. **(C)** The anterior wall is synonymous with the left ventricle. Acute myocardial infarction of the left ventricle is associated with left ventricular failure and signs of heart failure. Occlusion of the right coronary artery is associated with SA and AV block and bradycardia. Hiccoughs and GI upset are also common with inferior wall MI. Right ventricular MI may cause right ventricular failure and related signs such as JVD and peripheral edema.

Reference: Diepenbrock, N. H. *Quick Reference to Critical Care,* 2nd ed. Philadelphia, Lippincott Williams & Wilkins, 2004.

1-115. **(C)** Option C is the best because hospitalized patients are often highly motivated to change their lifestyles to improve their health, so hospitals are appropriate sites for prevention. Option A does not facilitate communication. Options B and D avoid discussing an obvious and potentially life-threatening behavior problem.

> **References:** Hardin, S. R. Caring practices. In S. R. Hardin, R. Kaplow (eds.). *Synergy for Clinical Excellence*. Sudbury, Jones & Bartlett, 2005, pp 69-74.
> Willaing, I., Ladelund, S. Nurse counseling of patients with an overconsumption of alcohol. *J Nurs Scholarship*, 37(1), 30-35, 2005.

1-116. **(C)** Signs of retroperitoneal bleeding after PCI include back and groin pain. This condition may be seen when access is difficult due to obesity and the iliac artery is punctured anteriorly and posteriorly during sheath insertion. The serum hemoglobin and hematocrit would decrease with blood loss into the peritoneal space. The 12-lead ECG would not show changes related to bleeding other than tachycardia, or sometimes bradycardia. Morphine administration would relieve pain, but would not stop bleeding.

> **Reference:** Woods, S. L., Froelicher, E. S., Motzer, S. U., Bridges, E. J. *Cardiac Nursing,* 5th ed. Philadelphia, Lippincott Williams & Wilkins, 2005.

1-117. **(B)** This client requires referral to a social worker or psychiatric clinical nurse specialist who can conduct a comprehensive assessment of this patient's needs related to child care issues, financial and employment issues, and drug rehabilitation. Option A is not an immediate concern since the children are being cared for. Although the patient's employment status is a relevant point to document, the patient's competence to care for her children depends on numerous factors and cannot be assumed without further assessment. Referrals for drug and alcohol rehabilitation can be arranged by the social worker or CNS.

> **Reference:** Sommer, M. S., Bolten, P. L. Multisystem. In J. G. Alspach (ed.). *Core Curriculum for Critical Care Nursing*, 6th ed. St. Louis, Elsevier, 2006, p 841.

1-118. **(A)** COPD is primarily a disease of pulmonary mechanics and is best monitored by measuring ease of expiratory flow, which can be done using serial peak flow measurements. Hypoxia is usually a later sign during an exacerbation. Excessive mucous production is a common problem in COPD and exacerbations may be caused by infectious processes, but this will not track respiratory function. Patient reports of dyspnea are multifactorial and are not necessarily associated with an exacerbation.

> **References:** Calverly, P. M. Chronic obstructive pulmonary disease. In M. P. Fink, E. Abraham, J. L. Vincent, P. M. Kochanek (eds.). *Textbook of Critical Care,* 5th ed. Philadelphia, Elsevier, 2005.
> Ellstrom, K. The pulmonary system. In J. G. Alspach (ed.). *Core Curriculum for Critical Care Nursing,* 6th ed. St. Louis, Elsevier, 2006.

1-119. **(C)** The patient is at highest risk of falling due to diuretic use. Concomitant use of anticoagulants places the patient at higher risk of bleeding complications at points of fall contact. Hematomas and cerebral bleeds will prolong this patient's hospital stay. The risk of stroke is decreased owing to anticoagulants, and if therapeutic levels are maintained, that risk is potentially preventable. While the patient is in the acute phase of care, exercise expectations are restricted to patient abilities and may be restricted to sitting in a chair. It is anticipated that treatment with diuretics will prevent the occurrence of pulmonary edema.

> **Reference:** Woods, S. L., Froelicher, E. S., Motzer, S. U., Bridges, E. J. *Cardiac Nursing,* 5th ed. Philadelphia, Lippincott Williams & Wilkins, 2005.

1-120. **(C)** Following CABG surgery, patient depression is associated with a high incidence of adverse outcomes. Early identification (within the first 48 hours) of a postoperative CABG patient experiencing depression enables prompt intervention to improve the patient's psychological health. Option A is incorrect because postoperative pain is associated with virtually all types of surgery, is readily identified, and does not, in itself, lead to these complications. Option B is incorrect as a loss of control is not associated with poor outcomes in CABG patients. Option D is incorrect as anemia can be readily identified and corrected with blood products.

References: Doering, L. V., Moser, D. K., Lemankiewicz, W., et al: Depression, healing and recovery from coronary artery bypass surgery. *Am J Crit Care*, 14(4), 316-324, 2005.

Hardin, S. R. Caring practices. In S. R. Hardin, R. Kaplow (eds.). *Synergy for Clinical Excellence*. Sudbury, Jones & Bartlett, 2005, pp 69-74.

1-121. **(D)** Beta blocking medications decrease the incidence of myocardial reinfarction as well as the incidence of ventricular and supraventricular dysrhythmias, reduce myocardial remodeling, and prevent sympathetic stress on the myocardium, making beta blockers useful in reducing mortality in acute MI. Calcium channel blocking agents do not prevent ventricular dysrhythmias and have not been shown to reduce mortality in acute MI. Magnesium prophylaxis does not reduce development of ventricular dysrhythmias in the setting of acute MI after thrombolytic therapy. Lidocaine decreases ventricular dysrhythmias, but side effects such as bradycardia, paresthesias, and altered mental status, which persist after the reperfusion dysrhythmias, make it a poor treatment choice.

Reference: International Liaison Committee on Resuscitation. Part 5: acute coronary syndromes. *Resuscitation,* 67, 249-369, 2005.

1-122. **(B)** Spontaneous bacterial peritonitis is the infection of ascites fluid and is a common complication of decompensated cirrhosis. This should be suspected when a patient with cirrhosis and ascites also develops fever, abdominal pain, or deterioration in mental status. Although these clinical findings may be subtle, spontaneous bacterial peritonitis may precipitate septic shock, renal failure, and liver failure. Acute appendicitis typically manifests as a vague midline abdominal pain accompanied by nausea, vomiting, and lack of appetite that slowly migrates to the right lower quadrant over 24 hours. A small bowel obstruction presents with nausea, vomiting, and severe cramping abdominal pain that often comes in waves at intervals every 5 to 15 minutes but does not include fever. Acute pancreatitis will present with severe upper abdominal pain, nausea, vomiting, and fever.

References: Sargent, D. The management and nursing care of cirrhotic ascites. *Br J Nurse,* 15(4), 212-219, 2006.

Yamada, T. *Handbook of Gastroenterology,* 2nd ed. Philadelphia, Lippincott Williams & Wilkins, 2005.

1-123. **(D)** Echocardiography best determines the absence of pericardial effusion and tamponade. While the pericardial catheter is in place and functioning properly, the patient should demonstrate absence of symptoms of pericardial effusion and tamponade. A lack of drainage may signal catheter obstruction and does not necessarily indicate that pericardial effusion has resolved. Approximately 250 mL of pericardial fluid is necessary for the effusion to be visualized on chest x-ray as an enlarged cardiac silhouette or water-bottle shape.

Reference: Wiegand, D. J., Carlson, D. J. (eds.). *AACN Procedure Manual for Critical Care*, 5th ed. St. Louis, Elsevier, 2005.

1-124. **(A)** In Haitian culture, the family is matriarchcal. The wife is instrumental in decision making and overseeing major decisions. Kong is not widely used in the Haitian culture and is not a product for young men. Kong is used to increase virility and is not sold at local grocery stores. Haitian culture is matriarchal rather than patriarchal.

References: Colin, J. M., Paperwalla, G. Haitian-Americans,1998, retrieved April 20, 2006, from http://www-unix.oit.umass.edu/~efhayes/haitian.htm

Desrosiers, A., St. Fleurose, S. Treating Haitian patients: key cultural aspects. *Am J Psychotherapy*, 56(4), 508-521, 2002.

1-125. **(B)** Meningitis is a potential complication of basilar skull fracture, and an elevated temperature is a key examination finding. Deep vein thrombosis (Option A) may present with an elevated white count and/or elevated temperature. Screening would include venous duplex of the extremities. However, infectious sources are a more likely cause of fever. Hypothalamic dysfunction or "storming" (Option C) characteristically presents with hypertension, tachycardia, and fever. The scenario presented does not include all of these key features. While a retained foreign body (Option D) may eventually result in infection, the scenario described suggests a more common and likely source of infection for this patient.

References: Alspach, J. G. (ed.). *Core Curriculum for Critical Care Nursing,* 6th ed. St. Louis, Elsevier, 2006.

Bader, M. K., Littlejohns, L. R. (eds.). *AANN Core Curriculum for Neuroscience Nursing*, 4th ed. St. Louis, Elsevier, 2004.

1-126. **(B)** The nurse would anticipate administration of platelets to decrease bleeding in this patient. The normal platelet count is 250,000 to 500,000/mm³. Packed RBCs are not indicated unless the hematocrit falls below 28%. Fresh frozen plasma would be indicated to replace clotting factors if the INR was greater than 1.5. Salt poor albumin is used to replace volume in patients with low albumin or extravascular fluid overload.

Reference: Baird, M. S., Keen, J. H., Swearingen, P. L. *Manual of Critical Care Nursing*. St. Louis, Elsevier, 2005.

1-127. **(B)** Patients with pelvic fractures require prompt and effective nutritional support to optimize recovery. A specialist should evaluate nutritional needs and begin feeding within 24 hours of admission. Nutrition is key to ensuring adequate healing. Option A is not warranted unless the patient has an underlying psychiatric problem that needs to be addressed. Neither Option C nor Option D is required at this point in the patient's care.

Reference: Frakes, M. A., Evans, T. Major pelvic fractures. *Crit Care Nurse*, 24(2), 18-32, 2004.

1-128. **(D)** A "silent chest" represented by inaudible breath sounds on auscultation is the most ominous sign of acute respiratory failure in the asthmatic patient because it reflects significantly diminished ventilation or movement of air into and out of the lungs. Poor ventilation may be due to respiratory muscle fatigue or bronchoconstriction. Wheezing indicates bronchoconstriction but also reflects the patient's ability to move sufficient air to produce the wheezing sounds. Although sentence length is a general indicator of severity of shortness of breath, it is not an indicator of respiratory failure. Tachypnea may lead to respiratory failure if its prolonged duration results in respiratory muscle fatigue.

Reference: Sole, M. L., Klein, D. G., Moseley, M. J. *Introduction to Critical Care Nursing*, 4th ed. St. Louis, Elsevier, 2005.

1-129. **(C)** When the liver loses its ability to break down and conjugate new proteins, immune globulins are produced in progressively smaller quantities. The pathophysiology of liver failure, not the patient's medications, is the cause of the patient's immune compromise. Adhering to the medication regimen will increase the patient's ability to ward off infection as laboratory values become more normal. Long-term malnutrition and impaired uptake of nutrients are not the primary reason for decreased immunity. While it is true that fewer fat-soluble vitamins and vitamin B-12 are stored, this is not the primary reason for immune compromise.

References: Pagana, K. D., Pagana, T. J. *Mosby's Manual of Diagnostic and Laboratory Tests,* 3rd ed. St. Louis, Elsevier, 2006, pp 324-329.

Urden L. D., Stacy K. M., Lough, M. E. (eds.). *Thelan's Critical Care Nursing: Diagnosis and Management,* 5th ed. St. Louis, Elsevier, 2006, pp 854, 1112-1113.

1-130. **(B)** The highest Glasgow Coma Scale (GCS) score a patient can receive is 15, and the lowest is 3. For the eye score, the patient receives one point because his eyes do not open (even to noxious stimuli). His verbal score is 1 since he is intubated (although given his motor response, he is unlikely to make any better response). He flexes his right upper extremity (motor score of 3) and extends his left upper extremity (motor score of 2) to noxious stimuli. As the best motor score is used to calculate a patient's GCS score, his total GCS score is 5 (Eye = 1, Verbal = 1, Motor = 3).

References: Alspach, J. G. (ed.). *Core Curriculum for Critical Care Nursing,* 6th ed. St. Louis, Elsevier, 2006, p 418

Jennett, B., Teasdale, G. Assessment of coma and impaired consciousness. A practical scale. *Lancet*, 2(7872), 81-84, 1974.

Teasdale, G., Jennett, B. Assessment and prognosis of coma after head injury. *Acta Neurochir*, 34, 45-55, 1976.

1-131. **(A)** Research shows that many (over 70%) patients have difficulty following the dietary and fluid restrictions necessary while on hemodialysis, especially younger male patients. The best response is to have a nutritionist determine the need for additional education regarding renal diet and fluid restriction and provide any supplementation warranted. The nutritionist needs to design a dietary plan and work with the patient (and, if patient wishes, with his spouse or other family members who assist with food shopping and cooking) to identify food selection and short-term goals. Option B would be implemented only at the patient's request. Option C may be a true statement, but attempts to improve compliance based on induced fear are not supported in the literature. Option D is a discussion he should have with his nephrologist and does not afford an immediate solution to his problem of diet and fluid protocol nonadherence.

Reference: Kugler, C., Vlaminck, H., Haverich, A., Maes, B. Nonadherence with diet and fluid restrictions among adults having hemodialysis. *J Nurs Scholarship*, 37(1), 25-29, 2005.

1-132. **(A)** Uncontrolled hypertension is an absolute contraindication to the administration of thrombolytics. Blood pressure may be reduced with beta blockers or vasodilators to enable administration of thrombolytics to reduce the risk of intracerebral bleeding. Although TIA may increase the risk of stroke, it does not necessarily indicate that a thrombus is present, and the risk of intracerebral bleed should be weighed against the benefit of thrombolytic administration. History of stroke is a relative contraindication to administration of thrombolytics. Remote stroke should not prevent administration of thrombolytics because intracerebral clots should be absorbed over time through normal processes. Age is also a relative contraindication. If percutaneous intervention (PCI) is available within 90 minutes for an elderly patient with acute myocardial infarction, PCI would be a better alternative. If PCI is not available, the patient should receive thrombolytic therapy.

Reference: Baird, M. S., Keen, J. H., Swearingen, D. L. *Manual of Critical Care Nursing: Nursing Interventions and Collaborative Management.* St. Louis, Elsevier, 2005.

1-133. **(B)** The patient is experiencing vascular steal syndrome. This syndrome occurs when blood is shunted away from tissues, causing tissue hypoperfusion. The incidence of vascular steal syndrome is higher in patients with grafts and/or upper arm accesses, in diabetics, and in the elderly; the incidence in-creases in extremities with previous access procedures. Management of the patient's symptoms includes comfort measures such as applying warm compresses and administering ordered analgesics that improve vascular supply to the hand. All other options would reduce blood flow and further exacerbate the patient's symptoms.

References: Lough, M. E. Renal disorders and therapeutic management. In L. D. Urden, K. M. Stacy, M. E. Lough (eds.). *Thelan's Critical Care Nursing: Diagnosis and Management,* 5th ed. St. Louis, Elsevier, 2006, pp 813-846.

Mitchell, J. K. Renal disorders and therapeutic management. In L. D. Urden, K. M. Stacy, M. E. Lough (eds.). *Priorities in Critical Care Nursing,* 4th ed. St. Louis, Elsevier, 2005, pp 333-356.

1-134. **(B)** Option B is the correct reply not only because it is factually correct, but also because the easiest way to begin learning about a procedure such as this is by recognizing what constitutes a "normal" finding. Option A is factually incorrect. Both Option C and Option D are incorrect because these activities are not included in the procedures related to measuring bladder pressures.

Reference: Gallagher, J. J. Ask the expert. *Crit Care Nurse*, 26(1), 67-70, 2006.

1-135. **(C)** If cardiomyopathy is due to myocardial ischemia, the most definitive treatment is to restore coronary circulation by either percutaneous coronary intervention or coronary bypass surgery. ACE inhibitors can decrease pulmonary congestion and prevent ventricular remodeling, but they do not afford definitive benefit. Likewise, diuretics only temporarily relieve symptoms such as pulmonary congestion. Permanent pacing could be used to treat dysrhythmias or improve cardiac output caused by lack of AV synchrony.

Reference: Haworth, K., Mayer, B. H., Munden, J., et al (eds.). *Critical Care Nursing Made Incredibly Easy.* Philadelphia, Lippincott Williams & Wilkins, 2004.

1-136. **(A)** Enteric leakage from anastomotic sites is a complication of the roux-en-y gastric bypass. In addition to an elevated WBC count, patients may have subtle signs of infection or have signs of sepsis and hemodynamic instability. In most cases of infection, the WBC count is elevated and the platelet count remains unchanged. Potassium levels usually are reduced in patients with increased gastrointestinal drainage. Platelet counts are elevated in patients with hematological disorders or in those who have undergone a splenectomy, neither of which pertain to this patient. Lipase is elevated in pancreatic disorders. This patient does not exhibit clinical evidence of pancreatic dysfunction.

Reference: Marshall, J. S., Srivastava, A., Gupta, S. K., et al. Roux-en-y gastric bypass leak complications. *Arch Surg,* 138, 520-524, 2003.

1-137. **(C)** Gram-negative pneumonia and persistent immunocompromise are both risk factors for developing a lung abscess or parapneumonic effusion. This patient's clinical and diagnostic test findings are consistent with those associated with these conditions and warrant manual thoracic drainage and antibiotic administration. Results from a BAL would not reflect a process in the pleural space. Option B identifies interventions for hemothorax, a condition not evidenced in this patient's clinical presentation. Bronchial hygiene interventions will not affect an intrapleural process.

Reference: Schiza, S., Siafakas, N. M. Clinical presentation and management of empyema, lung abscess and pleural effusion. *Curr Opin Pulm Med,* 12, 205-211, 2006.

1-138. **(D)** The patient has most likely developed complete heart block from scar formation subsequent to surgical repair of the atrial septal defect (ASD). Prior to the patient's surgery, the left to right atrial shunt associated with ASD caused pulmonary hypertension, which resulted in right ventricular and right atrial enlargement; RA and RV enlargement, in turn, may precipitate development of right bundle branch block (complete or incomplete) and delayed conduction from the SA to AV node evidenced by a prolonged PR interval. As a result, first and second degree AV block, Type 1, could have existed preoperatively with progression to complete AV block occurring gradually with scar tissue formation postoperatively.

Reference: Cheever, K. H. An overview of pulmonary artery hypertension: risks, pathogenesis, clinical manifestations and management. *J Cardiovasc Nurs,* 20, 108-116, 2005.

1-139. **(C)** Korsakoff syndrome is characterized by retrograde and anterograde amnesia, decreased spontaneity, decreased initiative, and confabulation (filling in memory gaps with distorted facts). Gait disturbances, paralysis of the eye muscles, and nystagmus are clinical manifestations of Wernicke's encephalopathy. Both conditions are the result of chronic alcohol ingestion and a thiamine deficiency. Thiamine plays a key role in glucose metabolism. The major organ systems that are affected by a thiamine deficiency are those that depend on energy from metabolism of carbohydrates: the peripheral nerves, heart and brain. Other symptoms of thiamine deficiency include peripheral neuropathy with myelin degeneration, hypertension, and cardiomyopathy.

Reference: McKinley, M. G. Alcohol withdrawal syndrome. Overlooked and mismanaged? *Crit Care Nurse* 25(3), 40-49, 2005.

1-140. **(D)** The immediate need of this patient is to alleviate her frustration by consulting a speech therapist who can assist the patient in regaining and improving her speech expression. Progress in that area will, in turn, help to alleviate the patient's vexation with her current limitations. Nothing in the scenario described supports this patient's need for either occupational or physical therapy. Although the patient's responses of anger and frustration might suggest the need for a psychiatric social worker, these are perfectly normal early behavioral responses to the patient's current physical challenges.

Reference: McQuillan, K. A., Belden, J. M. The neurologic system. In J. G. Alspach (ed.). *Core Curriculum for Critical Care Nursing,* 6th ed. St. Louis, Elsevier, 2006, pp 489-500.

1-141. **(D)** Immediate treatment with cardioversion is appropriate to treat atrial fibrillation in this patient. Inferior wall infarction decreases perfusion to the right atrium and may result in SA node ischemia and atrial dysrhythmias. Atrial fibrillation decreases cardiac output and may further compromise coronary perfusion. Although amiodarone, diltiazem, and digoxin are all possible antiarrhythmic agents that may be used to treat atrial fibrillation, the time it takes for these pharmacologic interventions to circulate and take effect may allow detrimental effects of myocardial ischemia to occur.

Reference: Woods, S. L., Froelicher, E. S., Motzer, S. U., Bridges, E. J. *Cardiac Nursing,* 5th ed. Philadelphia, Lippincott Williams & Wilkins, 2005.

1-142. **(B)** A continuous infusion of 10% dextrose is less irritating to the peripheral veins than repeated doses of 50% dextrose and will allow correction of fluid and electrolyte imbalances to occur at a slower and more steady pace, helping to avoid seizure or dysrhythmia activity. Because the patient has a diminished level of consciousness, it would not be safe to administer any form of glucose as an oral fluid. After beginning the 10% dextrose infusion, glucagon may be administered intramuscularly, not intravenously. While glargine insulin produces a steady control of glucose, this patient is in an acute phase and reduction of glucose would not be desirable at this time.

References: Newberry, L., Criddle, L. *Sheehy's Manual of Emergency Care,* 6th ed. Philadelphia, Elsevier, 2006, pp 428-432.
Urden, L. D., Stacy, K. M., Lough, M. E. *Thelan's Critical Care Nursing: Diagnosis and Management,* 5th ed. St. Louis, Elsevier, 2006, p 926.

1-143. **(A)** Acting as an arbitrator between family members is the most helpful behavior for families. Though often used by nurses, Option B is incorrect because all family members should be involved in understanding options at the end of life. Option C is incorrect because the use of terms such as death and dying is realistic and often helps the family understand the patient's prognosis. Option D should be pursued only when the family requests clergy support.

References: Hardin, S. R. Caring practices. In S. R. Hardin, R. Kaplow (eds.). *Synergy for Clinical Excellence.* Sudbury, Jones & Bartlett, 2005, pp 69-74.
Thelen, M. End-of-life decision making in intensive care. *Crit Care Nurse,* 25(6), 28-37, 2005.

1-144. **(A)** Abdominal discomfort and bladder distention indicate urinary tract obstruction, which could progress to renal transplant graft failure. An increase in urinary output and decreasing serum creatinine indicate improved renal function. Right upper quadrant tenderness and elevation of liver enzymes and bilirubin are indicative of rejection of a transplanted liver. Elevation of serum glucose with symptoms of hyperglycemia are associated with pancreatic rejection and would appear days after signs and symptoms of renal rejection in the case of transplant of multiple organs.

References: Schell, H., Puntillo, K. A. *Critical Care Nursing Secrets,* 2nd ed. St. Louis, Elsevier, 2006, pp 587-589
Urden, L. D., Stacy, K. M., Lough, M. E. *Thelan's Critical Care Nursing: Diagnosis and Management,* 5th ed. St. Louis, Elsevier, 2006, pp 1114-1124.

1-145. **(D)** Dark, tea-colored urine suggests that the patient has myoglobinuria. Once myoglobinuria is diagnosed, treatment is aimed at preventing subsequent renal failure. Aggressive administration of IV fluids increases renal blood flow and decreases the concentration of nephrotoxic pigments. Continuous infusion of mannitol and sodium bicarbonate will alkalinize the urine and prevent myoglobin crystallization in the renal tubules. Nursing management is aimed at achieving fluid and electrolyte balance. The patient needs to be assessed for hypernatremia, hyperosmolality, and volume overload. Patient management goals include maintaining a serum pH less than 7.5, serum Na of 135 to 145 mEq/L, urine output greater than or equal to 200 mL/hr, and urine pH of 6.0 to 7.0.

References: Adams, K., Johnson, K. Trauma. In L. D. Urden, K. M. Stacy, M. E. Lough (eds.). *Thelan's Critical Care Nursing: Diagnosis and Management,* 5th ed. St. Louis, Elsevier, 2006, pp 969-1008.
Stark, J. L. The renal system. In J. G. Alspach (ed.). *Core Curriculum for Critical Care Nursing,* 6th ed. St. Louis, Elsevier, 2006, pp 525-607.

1-146. **(C)** Patients with inferior wall MI often complain of abdominal or gastrointestinal symptoms. A 12-lead ECG should be performed prior to administration of nitroglycerin in order to detect changes owing to ischemia. NG decompression should be attempted with caution in a patient on heparin. Troponin studies should be performed after the 12-lead ECG and nitroglycerin are administered.

Reference: Swap, C. J., Nagurney, J. T. Value and limitations of chest pain history in the evaluation of patients with suspected acute coronary syndromes. *J Am Med Assoc,* 29, 2623-2629, 2005.

1-147. **(C)** A sudden decrease or absence of chest drainage may indicate an obstruction in the chest tube caused by tube kinking or the presence of a blood clot or tissue debris. Tube obstruction can interfere with the re-expansion of the lung following hemothorax or pneumothorax and contribute to hemodynamic compromise. Fluctuation or tidaling in the water-seal chamber indicates a properly functioning chest tube. Discomfort at the chest tube insertion site can be relieved with analgesics. Intermittent bubbling in the water-seal chamber may occur when the system is initially placed to suction and may continue until the patient's lung is re-expanded.

> **Reference:** Lynn-McHale Wiegand, D. J., Carlson, K. K. (eds.). *AACN Procedure Manual for Critical Care,* 5th ed. St. Louis, Elsevier, 2005, pp 151-169.

1-148. **(B)** Some over-the-counter cough medications contain aspirin. This can cause gastric irritation resulting in a blood loss of 100-200 mL, which presents as melana. Since the patient has not been taking the cough medicine during the hospitalization, the cause of the irritation has been removed. Hemorrhoidal bleeding presents as bright red blood on the outside of the stool, sometimes coloring the toilet water light pink. A ruptured diverticula would present with crampy abdominal pain and bright red bleeding. A healing peptic ulcer would not have any bleeding associated with it.

> **References:** Beers, M. H., Porter, R. S., Jones, T. V. Gastrointestinal bleeding. In *The Merck Manual of Diagnosis and Therapy,* 18th ed. New York, Wiley, 2006, pp 241-245.
> Krumberger, J., Parrish, C. R., Krenitsky, J. Gastrointestinal system. In M. Chulay, S. Burns (eds.). *AACN Essentials of Critical Care Nursing.* New York, McGraw-Hill, 2006, p 318.

1-149. **(D)** In most people, the dominant internal carotid artery is on the left, so a stroke involving that artery would be expected to produce the clinical picture described. A right middle cerebral artery (Option A) stroke would produce left-sided motor or sensory loss (greater in arm than leg), left-sided motor loss in lower face, left-sided visual field loss, and aphasia. A right vertebral artery (Option B) stroke would likely cause right facial weakness and numbness, facial and eye pain, clumsiness, ataxia, vertigo, nystagmus, hiccups, dysphagia, and dysarthria. Left anterior cerebral artery (Option C) stroke would typically result in confusion, personality changes, perseveration, incontinence, and right-sided motor or sensory loss (greater in leg than arm).

> **Reference:** Alspach, J. G. (ed.). *Core Curriculum for Critical Care Nursing,* 6th ed. St. Louis, Elsevier, 2006, pp 491-492.

1-150. **(D)** The most appropriate nursing action is to continue to monitor the patient on the current ventilator settings. Permissive hypercapnea is used in ARDS to prevent volutrauma from large tidal volumes and high PEEP levels. The use of tidal volumes from 5-8 mL/kg decreases the risk of volutrauma in noncompliant lung tissue. Increased respiratory rates increase patient energy use and may also increase the risk of alveolar damage owing to air trapping. Therapy goals in ARDS include maintaining the pH greater than 7.20. If the pH decreases below 7.20, sodium bicarbonate may be used to raise the pH.

> **Reference:** Sole, M. L., Klein, D. G., Moseley, M. J. *Introduction to Critical Care Nursing*, 4th ed. St. Louis, Elsevier, 2005.

2 Core Review Test 2

2-1. A patient with ARDS has a PaO_2 of 60% on mechanical ventilation with an FiO_2 of 80% and 20 cm H_2O of PEEP. Physical assessment findings include patient is unresponsive to pain, respiratory rate at ventilator setting of 12/min, temperature 101.6° F (38.6° C), BP 88/64 mm Hg, HR 112/min. Urine output is 20 mL for 2 hours. Chest x-ray shows complete opacification on left lung as well as right lower and middle lobes with radiolucence in right middle lobe. Which of the following immediate interventions should the nurse now anticipate?

   A. Insertion of a chest tube to relieve pneumothorax
   B. Administration of furosemide (Lasix) 40 mg intravenous to stimulate diuresis
   C. Administration of norepinephrine (Levophed) to support systolic BP
   D. Obtaining a sputum culture prior to precede initiation of antibiotics

2-2. A patient has been in the ICU for 5 days with maximal medical management after a large left-sided (dominant) middle cerebral artery ischemic stroke. Since admission, the patient has not improved from a Glasgow Coma Scale score of three. Pupils are equally nonreactive, and the neurologist is at the bedside to evaluate the patient for brain death. Which of the following neurologic deficits would the nurse correctly interpret as supporting a determination of brain death?

   A. Loss of vascular tone
   B. Loss of response to barbiturate infusion
   C. Loss of spinal reflex arc response
   D. Loss of spontaneous respiratory effort

2-3. A 77-year-old man is admitted for dysrhythmias and chest pain after 4 days of frequent vomiting. His workup for myocardial infarction is negative, and his nurse suspects that the patient's clinical problems may be related to electrolyte deficiencies. Which of the following sets of clinical findings would support the nurse's contention?

   A. Hyperglycemia, peaked T waves, diarrhea
   B. Hypoglycemia, headache, tremors, disorientation
   C. Headache, nausea, muscle weakness, orthostatic hypotension
   D. Jaundice, water retention and swelling, cramps

2-4. A patient is admitted to the CCU following a motor vehicle crash with a diagnosis of thoracic trauma with a flail chest. Assessment of this patient's chest reveals "paradoxical chest wall motion," which refers to the unstable, injured segment moving

A. Outward during inspiration, inward during expiration
B. Outward during inspiration, outward during expiration
C. Inward during inspiration, outward during expiration
D. Inward during inspiration, inward during expiration

2-5. A patient complains of chest pain, and a 12-lead ECG is performed that demonstrates sinus rhythm with ST segment depression of 2 mm and T wave inversion in leads V_5 and V_6. These ECG findings are consistent with

A. Subendocardial ischemia of the lateral wall
B. Transmural infarct of the lateral wall
C. Subendocardial ischemia of the anterior wall
D. Transmural infarct of the anterior wall

2-6. Which of the following patient descriptions suggests a late complication of renal injury?

A. Blunt trauma to the flank region with absent bowel sounds
B. A gunshot wound to the flank region with a WBC count of 16,000/mm³
C. A laceration of the right ureter with a serum creatinine of 6.0 mg/dL
D. A stab wound to the left flank with a BP of 186/90 mm Hg

2-7. The nurse is providing patient teaching while administering immunosuppressive therapy to an organ transplant recipient. Which of the following statements indicates that the patient has a correct understanding of their planned immunosuppressive regimen?

A. "If I miss a dose of my immunosuppressive medication, I can just double the dose the next time to make up for it."
B. "I will need to have levels of my immunosuppressive medications monitored each week by the laboratory."
C. "In order to reduce the chance of stomach ulcers, I will take my immunosuppressive medication with chocolate milk."
D. "My blood pressure will increase when I take my immunosuppressive medication, but this is normal."

2-8. A 62-year-old patient recently admitted with new onset of heart failure appears distressed regarding her health condition. During the admission assessment, the nurse should determine how this patient has viewed past successes in life as well as her health and satisfaction with life because considering these issues can

A. Encourage patients to adapt to new challenges
B. Explain their current health problems
C. Enable patients to view their life within context
D. Help patients confront their own mortality

2-9. During a code blue incident in an outpatient clinic, the patient was found to be hypoglycemic. Resuscitative efforts were successful after 50 mL of 50% dextrose were administered. When should the patient's capillary glucose measurement be repeated?

A. 10 minutes after the patient's cardiac rhythm and pulse are restored.
B. 15 minutes after the dose of 50% dextrose was administered
C. Upon admission to the ICU
D. 30 minutes after the last capillary glucose measurement

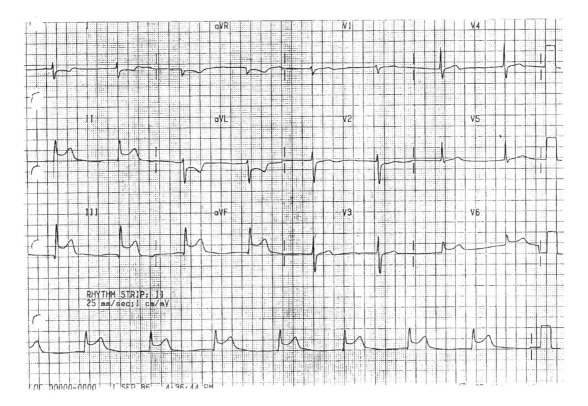

2-10. The most appropriate action for the nurse obtaining the ECG above would be to

   A. Obtain a right side ECG
   B. Obtain a second ECG in 30 minutes
   C. Institute transcutaneous pacing at a rate of 60
   D. Administer atropine 0.5 mg IV

2-11. A patient has a central venous catheter, which was placed emergently during a code. Which of the following is indicated to help reduce the incidence of a catheter-related bloodstream infection?

   A. Use chlorhexidine gluconate solution for site care
   B. Change the intravenous tubing with crystalloid therapy every 48 hours
   C. Replace the transducer, flush device, flush solution, and tubing every 48 hours
   D. Collaborate with the physician to re-place the catheter within 72 hours

2-12. Recommendations for monitoring patients thought to have carbon monoxide poison-ing include obtaining carboxyhemoglobin levels and ABG samples to evaluate the SaO$_2$. In this patient population, the primary reason why pulse oximetry measurements (SpO$_2$) are considered unreliable and inac-curate for monitoring SaO$_2$ is because the

   A. SpO$_2$ is often spurious in hemodynami-cally unstable patients
   B. Cherry-red skin color changes associ-ated with this disorder invalidate oxim-etry measurements
   C. Patient must receive 100% oxygen
   D. SpO$_2$ does not specifically reflect the percentage of hemoglobin saturated with oxygen

2-13. Treatment for pulmonary artery hyperten-sion with a mean pulmonary artery pressure of 30 mm Hg and signs of right heart failure including tricuspid regurgitation murmur consists of administration of oxygen and

   A. Phlebotomy to maintain hematocrit at 48%
   B. Fluid bolus to increase right ventricular output
   C. Epoprostenol (Flolan) to dilate pulmo-nary arteries
   D. Inotropic agents to increase right ven-tricular contractility

2-14. A morbidly obese patient is admitted to the unit following a laparoscopic cholecystectomy. The nurse knows that this patient is at risk for developing a hospital-associated pneumonia because

- A. His body habitus causes him to hypoventilate, leading to atelectasis
- B. Elevated intra-abdominal pressures related to morbid obesity predispose to aspiration
- C. All patients with cholecystitis are at risk for developing pneumonia
- D. Morbidly obese individuals have altered neutrophil activity

2-15. A patient is in the critical care unit following emergent right hemicolectomy for a penetrating shotgun wound. Clinical findings include pulse 145 beats/min, temperature 102° F, abdominal distention, hypoactive bowel sounds, BP had been 140/86 mm Hg but is now 108/80 mm Hg, and extremities very warm to touch with bounding pulses. The physician orders rapid fluid administration, blood cultures, and antibiotics. What clinical finding would the nurse look for in this patient as evidence of an optimal clinical response to rapid IV fluid administration?

- A. Central venous pressure of 4 mm Hg
- B. Lactate level less than 4 mmol/L
- C. Urine output of 25 mL/hr
- D. Cool, dry skin

2-16. Which of the following medications is administered to prevent sudden death associated with dilated cardiomyopathy?

- A. Warfarin to prevent clot formation
- B. Calcium channel blockers to control tachycardia
- C. Nitrates to improve coronary artery perfusion
- D. Digoxin to reduce atrial dysrhythmias and improve contractility

2-17. A patient is admitted with pallor, shortness of breath, dyspnea on exertion, syncope, and chest pain related to right ventricular ischemia. He has a loud S_2 in the pulmonic area, a right ventricular heave, and a pulmonary flow murmur. He is diagnosed with pulmonary hypertension and is to be started on treprostinil sodium (Remodulin®). Which of the following topics should the nurse be prepared to discuss with the patient regarding treprostinil administration?

- A. Operation of a programmable pump
- B. Potential for pelvic bleeding
- C. Need to take the medication with food
- D. The use of wireless technology

2-18. A 54-year-old end-stage renal disease (ESRD) patient is admitted to the ICU after falling down three flights of stairs. The patient's BP is 200/116 mm Hg, HR is 118/min, and RR is 32/min. The patient complains of fatigue, headache, lightheadedness, and palpitations; laboratory work reveals hemoglobin 7.6 g/dL, hematocrit 22.8%. The patient is currently receiving 3000 units of Epoetin Alfa (Epogen, Procrit) three times per week. Which of the following interventions is the most warranted at this time?

- A. Transfuse with one unit of packed red blood cells
- B. Increase Epoetin Alfa by 1000 units
- C. Transfuse with two units of packed red blood cells
- D. Decrease Epoetin Alfa by 500 units

2-19. A patient who has had chest pain intermittently for 16 hours, unrelieved by aspirin and nitroglycerin, is admitted to the ICU. A 12-lead ECG shows ST segment elevation in leads II, III, and aVF. Which of the following interventions would most benefit this patient?

- A. Administration of thrombolytic therapy such as streptokinase or TNK
- B. Transfer to a hospital able to perform open heart surgery
- C. Administration of heparin and G IIb/IIIa inhibitor
- D. Immediate transfer to the cardiac catheterization suite for percutaneous coronary intervention

2-20. When the health care team plans care for a patient with sepsis, coordination of laboratory studies with fluid and pharmaceutical therapies becomes especially important. Which of the following collaborations is consistent with current recommendations for optimal management of the patient with sepsis?

A. Collaborate with the intensivist regarding administration of human recombinant activated protein C
B. Consult with the clinical pharmacologist regarding which vasopressor to administer to correct hypotension prior to fluid replacement
C. Collaborate with the physician to determine the best approach for maintaining blood glucose levels at <150 mg/dL
D. Perform a cortisol stimulation test and then consult with the pharmacist about initiating high-dose corticosteroids.

2-21. A patient is admitted to the ICU after a motor vehicle collision. The patient is currently alert and oriented but had experienced a transient loss of consciousness at the scene. The only significant injury is a linear left temporal skull fracture. Within 2 hours of admission, the patient's neurological status deteriorates. The nurse should now anticipate which of the following actions?

A. Cerebral angiography and coil embolization
B. Ventriculostomy and cerebrospinal fluid drainage
C. Osmotic diuretic and corticosteroid therapy
D. Burr holes and clot evacuation

2-22. A teenager who has received a heart transplant was recently admitted to the Intensive Care Unit with pyelonephritis, urinary frequency, and cloudy urine, which she has experienced for a number of weeks. Which of the following should the nurse relate to effectively address the patient's knowledge deficit and prevent delays in treatment of future infections?

A. "You need to restrict your physical activities to avoid complications."
B. "Avoid foods high in folic acid so your immunosuppressive therapy remains effective."
C. "Be sure to drink plenty of fluids to avoid becoming dehydrated."
D. "Report any unusual sensations you experience as they may be a sign of infection."

2-23. Three days after surgical repair of an abdominal aortic aneurysm, a morbidly obese patient continues to be mechanically ventilated. The patient required fiberoptic intubation preoperatively. Current ventilator settings include FiO_2 40%, TV 600 mL, SIMV rate 10/min. The patient over-breathes the ventilator during the day, but not at night. Daily chest x-rays show an enlarged heart and linear densities consistent with alveolar hypoventilation. Arterial blood gas values consistently demonstrate a PaO_2 over 80 mm Hg and $PaCO_2$ 40 mm Hg. Which of the following should the nurse anticipate as this patient's weaning strategy?

A. Change the mode of ventilation to pressure support
B. Place the patient on T-piece
C. Add CPAP to SIMV and decrease the FiO_2
D. Extubate the patient and initiate BiPAP

2-24. A postoperative patient who sustained multiple trauma from a motor vehicle crash is in the ICU. On multidisciplinary rounds, which of the following should the nurse suggest to help prevent deep vein thrombosis in this patient?

A. Pneumatic compression devices
B. Unfractionated heparin
C. Below-the-knee graded stockings
D. Low molecular weight heparin

2-25. A patient with a high output enterocutaneous fistula is NPO on hyperalimentation at a rate of 80 mL/hr. The patient is listless but responds to commands appropriately. Heart rate is 124/min sinus tachycardia, BP 88/50 mm Hg. Respiratory rate is 24/min on 40% face mask with an SpO_2 of 100%. Other assessment findings include 2+ edema in dependent areas and capillary refill time of 4 seconds. Admission laboratory values include hematocrit 30%, serum sodium 150 mEq/L, glucose 90 mg/dL, albumin 1.9 g/dL. The nurse anticipates immediate administration of which of the following?

A. One unit of packed red blood cells
B. 25 mL of dextrose 50%
C. A 250 mL normal saline bolus
D. 250 mL of 5% albumin

2-26. A patient presents with flu-like symptoms, lymphadenopathy, a diffuse erythematous rash, and severe muscle weakness. The nurse admits the patient for close monitoring and further diagnostic workup to identify the cause of these findings. The patient suddenly loses consciousness followed by a brief period of muscle rigidity and then rhythmic muscle jerking. The best immediate course of action for the nurse is to

A. Obtain a serum laboratory specimen for STAT identification of a disease-specific antigen or antibody causing this syndrome
B. Observe, record, and report all details of these clinical events to the physician as soon as these muscular movements have subsided
C. Administer benzodiazepine per standing order to stop the seizure activity
D. Quickly apply soft restraints to prevent injury

2-27. A patient of Chinese descent is in the ICU for aggressive fluid resuscitation. When nursing staff inform the physician that the patient appears to be experiencing hallucinations and delusional episodes and periodically is aggressive toward the staff, haloperidol (Haldol®) 2.5 mg intramuscularly is prescribed. The nurse caring for this patient should initially

A. Hold the order until volume repletion has occurred in case dehydration is the cause of these symptoms
B. Collaborate with the intensivist to determine the need for a loading dose of this medication
C. Question the dose as it might be too high for this patient
D. Check to determine if this patient has a deficiency of glucose-6-phosphate dehydrogenase (G6PD) enzyme

2-28. Which of the following medication regimens would be most appropriate to relieve chest pain in a patient with a diagnosis of myocarditis?

A. Nitroglycerin 1/150 grains sublingual
B. Furosemide 40 mg IV
C. Ibuprofen 800 mg PO
D. Morphine sulfate 2 mg IV

2-29. A patient presents to the emergency department with acute jaundice, elevated liver enzymes, and malaise. Throughout nursing assessment of this patient, a primary concern will be to determine whether this patient manifests clinical features associated with

A. Intractable hypotension
B. Early stages of esophageal bleeding
C. Development of systemic infection
D. Diminished level of consciousness

2-30. A patient complains of substernal pressure and becomes diaphoretic. A 12-lead ECG obtained during chest pain demonstrates tall, broad R waves and ST segment depression in leads V_1-V_2. These findings suggest that the nurse now needs to

A. Continue monitoring the patient for unstable angina
B. Assess the patient for fever and other signs of pericarditis
C. Examine the patient for findings related to posterior wall MI
D. Prepare the patient for possible cardioversion for septal MI

2-31. A 16-year-old female admitted with diabetic ketoacidosis has a serum glucose of 250 mg/dL and is asking to use the phone to call her friends to assure them that she is all right. Since her vital signs and other clinical parameters are stable, the nurse may allow the patient to use the phone in order to respond to the patient's needs for

A. Social support
B. Reducing anxiety
C. Overcoming boredom
D. Controlling her environment

2-32. A 30-weeks'-pregnant female is admitted to the ICU with heart failure owing to cardiomyopathy. The patient has a BP of 140/90 mm Hg, heart rate 116/min, sinus tachycardia, respiratory rate 28/min, labored with pulmonary rales. Anticipated treatment for this patient would include

A. Immediate C-section so that cardiomyopathy can be medically treated
B. Cautious use of diuretics and antihypertensives to prevent hypotension
C. Use of ACE inhibitors to reduce blood pressure and promote diuresis

D. Avoidance of beta blockers which may cause hypoglycemia in the fetus

2-33. A patient with chronic pulmonary disease is admitted to ICU with worsening dyspnea and pulmonary mechanics. The patient's medical history includes chronic bronchitis that requires home oxygen, anxiety, and a 5-kg weight loss over the last 4 weeks. In noting these findings, the critical care nurse will plan nursing care with the understanding that in this patient population, weight loss is typically associated with

A. Cor pulmonale
B. Increased mortality
C. Improved thoracic excursion
D. Dehydration

2-34. An orientee is caring for a patient 1 week post gastric bypass surgery. The patient has been unable to be weaned from mechanical ventilation. While reviewing the orientee's care of this patient, which of the following interventions would the nurse preceptor likely suggest adding to improve this patient's chances of survival?

A. Consult with the wound and ostomy nurse to assess early signs of wound infection
B. Collaborate with the dietitian to carefully assess for nutritional deficiencies
C. Collaborate with the physician to start a bowel regimen
D. Consult with pharmacy regarding initiation of low-molecular-weight heparin

2-35. During sheath removal after percutaneous coronary intervention (PCI), a patient's heart rate decreases to 40 beats/min, BP decreases to 80/50 mm Hg, and the patient complains of nausea. Appropriate treatment for this patient would include which of the following?

A. Continue to monitor the patient, anticipating the heart rate and BP will return to baseline within 5 minutes
B. Administer atropine 0.5 mg intravenously to treat vasovagal reaction
C. Administer prochlorperazine (Compazine) 10 mg IV to reduce nausea
D. Notify the MD immediately of potential retroperitoneal bleeding

2-36. A patient with a history of angina, hypercholesterolemia, and hypertension is admitted to the ICU for management of chest pain. Current medications include atenolol (Tenormin®) and hydrochlorothiazide. The patient also uses garlic pills for the hypercholesterolemia. Which of the following should be taught to the patient if invasive tests or procedures are required in the future?

A. "Be sure to take all of your medications with only a sip of water on the day of the procedure."
B. "Stop taking garlic if invasive procedures are likely."
C. "There is no added value in complementary therapies with the medication regimen you are taking, and those therapies are not FDA approved."
D. "Do not take atenolol the day of a procedure as the anesthesia might slow your heart rate as a side effect."

2-37. Treatment of right ventricular myocardial infarction includes administration of which of the following?

A. Diuretics
B. Intravenous fluid bolus
C. Morphine
D. Nitroglycerin

2-38. During the neurologic assessment of a patient who was the driver involved in a head-on collision, the critical care nurse finds no evidence of motor function or ability to sense pain or temperature below the nipple line. These neurologic findings suggest that this patient will require nursing management for

A. Anterior cord syndrome
B. Central cord syndrome
C. Brown-Sequard syndrome
D. Posterior cord syndrome

2-39. A patient is admitted after receiving several shocks in succession from his AICD. Device interrogation reveals that the shocks were delivered appropriately. What further assessments are warranted to identify this patient's problem?

A. 12-lead ECG with magnet in place to identify intrinsic cardiac rhythm

B. Chest x-ray to determine if lead fracture has occurred

C. Evaluation of serum electrolytes to identify source of dysrhythmia

D. Electrophysiology testing to determine the source of the dysrhythmia

2-40. A patient recuperating from a stroke continues to exhibit diminished level of consciousness and expressive aphasia and is being closely monitored for any difficulty coughing or swallowing. To detect the earliest clinical evidence of aspiration in this patient, which of the following should the nurse look for?

A. Increased $PaCO_2$

B. Chest x-ray demonstrating bilateral infiltrates

C. Tachypnea and tachycardia

D. Coughing and positive sputum cultures

2-41. The patient was admitted with a serum glucose level of 468 mg/dL. After 2 hours of therapy with 4 units/hr of regular Humulin in normal saline via the intravenous route, the patient's serum glucose is 400 mg/dL. Which of the following is the most appropriate nursing intervention at this time?

A. Document the laboratory results and continue to monitor

B. Increase the hourly insulin infusion dose by 2 units/hr

C. Begin administration of intravenous insulin at 8 units/hr and continue to monitor

D. Change from a regular insulin infusion to subcutaneous insulin glargine

2-42. A patient complains of chest pain. The 12-lead ECG performed prior to administering 1/150 grains of nitroglycerin appears below. Serum troponin is 0.1 ng/mL. The treatment plan for this patient would include which of the following?

A. Immediate percutaneous coronary intervention

B. Administration of thrombolytic therapy

C. Serial ECG and troponin levels

D. Administration of aspirin, heparin and ACE inhibitor

2-43. A nurse working the ICU night shift notes that over the past 6 months a number of patients with abdominal aortic aneurysm (AAA) repairs have experienced poor outcomes. The nurse approaches her nurse manager and asks if this trend has been noted by anyone else. The manager replies "No," and suggests that the nurse should

A. Start developing a list of patients admitted for AAA repairs and document the outcomes for each over the next 6 months

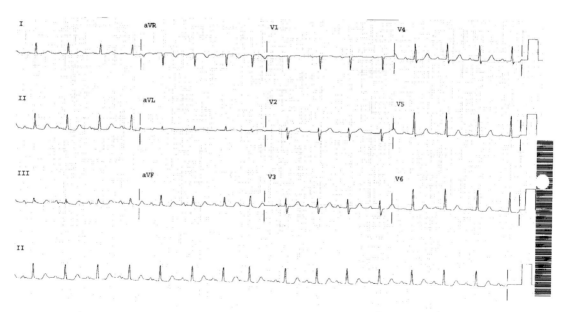

25 mm/sec 10.0 mm/mV

B. Conduct a chart audit of all the AAA repairs over the past 6 months
C. Talk to the thoracic surgeon about the observation
D. Present the concern at the next staff meeting

2-44. Which action should the nurse anticipate for a patient with supratentorial intracerebral hemorrhage?

A. Aggressive reduction of blood pressure
B. STAT completion of cerebral angiography
C. Correction of coagulopathy
D. Surgical evacuation of the clot

2-45. A patient undergoes a right posterolateral thoracotomy for repair of a membranous tracheal tear located 4 cm above the carina associated with pneumomediastinum and bilateral pneumothoraces. A few hours after the patient's return from surgery, a bronchoscopy is performed to clear secretions. Over the next few hours, it is important that the nurse monitors the chest drainage system to ensure

A. Bubbling in the water seal chamber
B. Adequate dependent loops in tubing
C. Positive pressure in the closed drainage system
D. Clamping of the chest tube

2-46. A patient in the critical care unit continues to exhibit signs and symptoms of hypoperfusion related to septic shock despite receiving adequate amounts of crystalloid and colloid for fluid resuscitation, so the physican now orders initiation of vasopressor therapy. Given the following patient information, which vasopressor agent would be the best choice for this patient? HR 110/min, sinus tachycardia; BP 80/40 mm Hg; ScVO$_2$ 60%; PAP 30/16 mm Hg; PCWP 14 mm Hg; CO 10.0 L/min; CI 5.2 L/min/cm^2; SVR 500 dynes/sec/cm^{-5}.

A. Dopamine
B Epinephrine
C. Norepinephrine
D. Vasopressin

2-47. A trauma patient will require massive transfusions of red blood cells and aggressive fluid resuscitation. Which of the following

nursing interventions will prevent the greatest number of complications for this patient?

A. Use of warmed blood components and intravenous fluids
B. Vigilant monitoring of laboratory values
C. Premedication with antihistamines and anti-inflammatory agents
D. Intramuscular administration of tetanus toxoid

2-48. A patient with a left ventricular assist device placed as a bridge to cardiac transplant is at greatest risk for which of the following complications?

A. Hemorrhage and stroke related to anticoagulation
B. Social isolation related to infection secondary to immunosuppression
C. Postoperative sepsis related to neutropenia
D. Transplant failure related to immunological sensitization

2-49. A patient is admitted to the ICU with a diagnosis of hypertensive urgency 2 weeks after roux-en-y gastric bypass surgery. The patient says, "I don't understand how my blood pressure can still be so high. I thought that operation was going to fix my blood pressure problems." The most appropriate nursing response is

A. "I will ask the nutritionist to review your preoperative nutrition counseling materials with you. It might be from the food you are eating."
B. "An adjustable band was placed around the upper part of your stomach to create a small pouch. The band is adjustable and can be tightened to allow feelings of being full longer. Your band may be a bit tight now, causing you stress."
C. "A leak is a common complication of your procedure and could potentially cause changes in blood pressure."
D. "Hypertensive patients taking antihypertensive medications have small blood pressure reductions after this surgery."

2-50. Upon turning a postoperative coronary artery bypass patient, the nurse observes 200 mL of bloody drainage in the chest tube drainage system. The nurse should perform which of the following?

    A. Autotransfuse the patient

    B. Aggressively strip the chest tube

    C. Obtain laboratory specimens for coagulation studies

    D. Continue to monitor the patient's chest tube drainage

2-51. Early goal-directed therapy for management of severe sepsis or septic shock involves maximizing cardiac preload, afterload, and contractility to balance oxygen delivery with demand. During the first 6 hours of resuscitation for sepsis-induced hypoperfusion, which of the following pairs of parameters represents desired target values?

    A. CVP: 12-15 mm Hg; $ScVO_2 \geq 60\%$

    B. CVP: 8-12 mm Hg; urine output ≥ 1 mL/kg/hr

    C. $ScVO_2 \geq 70\%$; MAP ≥ 65 mm Hg

    D. Urine output ≥ 0.5 mL/kg/hr; MAP ≥ 55 mm Hg

2-52. A patient with acute exacerbation of heart failure is receiving a continuous infusion of nesiritide (Natrecor) at 0.1 mcg/kg/min. Currently, the patient has the following vital signs: HR 116 beats/min, sinus tachycardia with atrial premature contractions, BP 78/48 mm Hg, RR 28/min, and SpO_2 90% on 40% BiPAP mask. Immediate interventions by the nurse would include which of the following?

    A. Discontinue the nesiritide (Natrecor) infusion

    B. Place the patient in a supine position

    C. Administer a 250 mL normal saline fluid bolus.

    D. Continue the nesiritide (Natrecor) infusion and administer 40 mg furosemide (Lasix) intravenously.

2-53. A 55-year-old patient is postoperatively admitted to the ICU following right lower lobectomy for adenocarcinoma. He is alert and oriented with stable vital signs, respiratory rate 25/min, and requires 4 L of oxygen via nasal cannula to maintain an O_2 satura-tion of 95%. During the night, his SaO_2 falls to 90%, his respiratory rate increases to 40, and he complains of increased pain in the right chest. His breath sounds are diminished to bilateral bases, but otherwise are clear. What are the most appropriate nursing actions?

    A. Place patient on a face mask at FiO_2 .40 and draw an ABG

    B. Administer pain medication and encourage the patient to cough and use the incentive spirometer

    C. Obtain an order for chest x-ray to evaluate for hemothorax and increase oxygen to 6 L/min

    D. Administer a sedative and encourage use of deep breathing and relaxation techniques

2-54. In acute pancreatitis, acute respiratory distress syndrome (ARDS) represents a common complication caused by the release of pancreatic enzymes into the circulation. Which of these other possible complications of pancreatitis can then complicate management of ARDS?

    A. Hypovolemia

    B. Fistula formation

    C. Pleural effusion

    D. Severe pain

2-55. After bedside insertion of a temporary transvenous pacemaker, a patient's BP drops to 96/78 mm Hg from 130/70 mm Hg and respiratory rate increases to 30/min, shallow with clear, equal breath sounds. JVD is visible. The heart rate is 70 beats/min 100% paced. The most likely cause of these findings is

    A. Hemothorax

    B. Pneumothorax

    C. Pericardial tamponade

    D. Pacemaker syndrome

2-56. A new graduate is being precepted and is caring for a patient with neurologic impairment. The patient is intubated and on blowby. The orientee inserts a nasogastric (NG) tube and is about to administer medication through the tube. When the preceptor asks how NG tube placement was verified, the orientee says that it was verified by auscultation of insufflated air at the gastric area. The preceptor's best initial response is to

A. Explain that observing for exhalation bubbles when the tube's hub is held under water is a more accurate method to verify tube placement

B. Verify the medication order before allowing the orientee to proceed

C. Observe the patient for the onset of respiratory symptoms (such as coughing, cyanosis, or dyspnea) for a few minutes before medication administration

D. Confirm placement with pH paper and discuss research studies that support use of this method

2-57. In planning the care of a patient in acute renal failure, the critical care nurse ascertains the patient is at risk for infection owing to

A. Excessive carbohydrate intake
B. Fluid overload
C. Protein-calorie malnourishment
D. Fluid restriction

2-58. A patient with end-stage heart failure is admitted to the intensive care unit minimally responsive with a heart rate 86 beats/min, BP 80/66 mm Hg, RR 26/min, on 60% Bi-PAP facemask. The patient has crackles at both bases. Home medications include furosemide, atenolol, potassium, and captopril (Capoten). Admitting labs include a serum albumin level of 2.0 g/dL, HCT 52%, BUN 62 mg/dL, and creatinine 3.0 mg/dL. The most appropriate initial treatment for this patient would be to

A. Initiate a dobutamine infusion
B. Initiate a norepinephrine (Levophed) infusion
C. Administer a 250 mL bolus of normal saline
D. Administer 40 mg of furosemide (Lasix) IV

2-59. The critical care nurse is aware that anxiety and depression are common psychological comorbidities for patients with COPD. Knowing that fact, which of the following should the nurse plan to provide for COPD patients?

A. Administering more benzodiazepines than for non-COPD patients

B. Restarting the patient's normal daily medications prior to discharge

C. Having a psychology consultation completed during their hospitalization

D. Continuing the patient's normal daily routines and practices

2-60. Which of the following statements is true regarding spirituality of patients in the ICU?

A. Spirituality issues should be addressed in the ICU after the patient has been stabilized

B. Addressing spirituality is best reserved for patients at end of life

C. Spirituality may impact understanding of illness in the ICU

D. Inquiring about spirituality preferences does nothing to alleviate the stress associated with an acute condition that requires ICU admission

2-61. Intra-aortic balloon counterpulsation is used to manage cardiogenic shock in order to increase

A. Coronary artery perfusion during systole
B. Myocardial oxygen supply
C. Left ventricular filling volume
D. Left ventricular systolic pressure

2-62. An older patient, who resides in a nursing home, is admitted to the ICU from the general medical floor with hypotension. The patient has been in the hospital for 10 days with an indwelling urinary catheter. The patient is confused and has been oliguric for the past 8 hours. The patient's vital signs on arrival are temperature 102° F; HR 100 beats/min sinus; RR 24/min; BP 76/42 mm Hg; SaO$_2$ 95% on 40% venti-mask. Despite several fluid boluses, the patient's hemodynamic status does not improve. The physician orders the administration of activated protein C (APC) based on the diagnosis of urosepsis. During the administration of rhAPC, the critical care nurse monitors the patient for signs of bleeding based on the knowledge that rhAPC increases

A. Thrombin activity
B. Coagulation
C. Platelet function
D. Fibrinolysis

2-63. The nurse is assigned an 82-year-old frail woman who is being transferred from the ICU to telemetry. She was admitted to the ICU for syncope and was later found to have taken her home medications incorrectly. The patient tells the nurse, "I just can't read the label like I used to; the printing is so faint." She lives alone and does not have children or relatives nearby. What intervention should the nurse consider?

    A. Contact her pharmacy to ask about provisions for vision-impaired patients
    B. Re-evaluate her medications for possible drug-drug interactions
    C. Contact the case manager for assistance in long-term placement
    D. Develop a plan of care that includes side effects of medications

2-64. Administration of thrombolytic therapy would be indicated for which of the following patients?

    A. Chest pain duration of 6 hours with ST elevation in leads II, III, aVF, and elevated troponin
    B. Chest pain duration 1 hour with new onset of LBBB and elevated troponin
    C. Chest pain less than 30 minutes with ST segment depression in leads II, III, aVF, and troponin level 0.1 ng/mL
    D. Chest pain with heart rate 150 beats/min, ST elevation in leads V_1-V_6, and troponin level 1.3 ng/mL

2-65. Patients with chronic pulmonary disease such as COPD may eventually develop cardiac dysfunction in the form of chronic cor pulmonale, which further limits their activity tolerance. Clinical manifestations of cor pulmonale that the nurse should look for to recognize this disorder include

    A. Fatigue and decreased CVP
    B. Distant heart sounds and jugular venous distention
    C. Exertional dyspnea and pedal edema
    D. Productive cough and hepatomegaly

2-66. Which of the following best describes how the nurse needs to administer sodium nitroprusside and esmolol in the preoperative care of a patient with aortic dissection?

    A. Titrate both nitroprusside and esmolol to maintain MAP of 70 mm Hg and HR of 70/min
    B. Titrate nitroprusside to keep SBP <140 mm Hg and infuse esmolol to maintain HR less than 100/min
    C. If more than 10 mcg/kg/min of nitroprusside is required to reduce SBP, add esmolol and titrate to reduce the MAP to 60 mm Hg
    D. Titrate esmolol to reduce SBP to 120-140 mm Hg. If heart rate decreases to 60 beats/min, stop esmolol and replace with nitroprusside infusion to achieve target BP

2-67. A newly admitted patient with traumatic brain injury (TBI) is experiencing increased intracranial pressure (ICP). At this point in the patient's care, the nurse should maintain the patient's arterial pCO_2 at a level

    A. Below 20 mm Hg
    B. Between 25 and 30 mm Hg
    C. Between 30 and 35 mm Hg
    D. Above 40 mm Hg

2-68. The permanent pacemaker rhythm strip below represents which of the following?

    A. Normal permanent pacemaker function
    B. Failure to sense
    C. Failure to pace
    D. Over-sensing

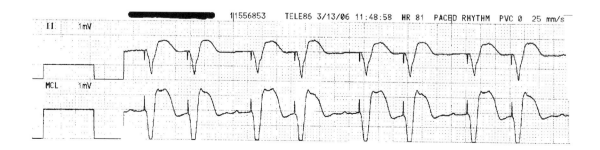

2-69. A 28-year-old woman with a history of mitral valve prolapse is admitted for dehydration following 48 hours of nausea and vomiting that began 5 hours after her employer's annual company picnic where she ate something that did not agree with her. Until 2 hours ago, the retching raised only bile, but the most recent episode evidenced bright red blood. While the physician is performing an endoscopy to determine the origin of the bleeding, it is especially important that the nurse

A. Monitor for cardiac ischemia
B. Administer IV fluids
C. Monitor blood gases and electrolytes
D. Institute warming procedures

2-70. After a motor vehicle collision, a teenager is admitted with chest pain and an ineffective cough with hemoptysis. The admission chest x-ray reveals consolidation and pulmonary infiltration, likely evidence of a severe pulmonary contusion. The patient's respiratory rate is 23/min, and his arterial blood gases on room air are pH 7.42, $PaCO_2$ 30 mm Hg, PaO_2 54 mm Hg, HCO_3 24 mEq/L. Which of the following pairs of interventions is most appropriate for this patient?

A. Administer an analgesic, apply 100% O_2 by face mask
B. Auscultate lung sounds, prepare for insertion of a chest tube
C. Prepare for immediate intubation and mechanical ventilation
D. Prepare for immediate thoracentesis and administer oxygen

2-71. A patient who was in a motor vehicle crash in which the airbag was deployed complains of sternal soreness. The 12-lead ECG indicates sinus tachycardia at a rate of 110 and development of right bundle branch block with occasional premature ventricular contractions. A bedside echocardiogram is performed that shows mild wall motion abnormalities. These findings are consistent with which of the following conditions?

A. Myocardial contusion
B. Pulmonary contusion
C. Cardiac chamber rupture
D. Cardiac tamponade

2-72. A patient with hemorrhagic stroke has been on a ventilator for approximately 1 week and remains unresponsive. While he is being cared for, approximately 10 visitors from his church arrive and ask the nurse if they can have a prayer service in his room. The nurse agrees to give them time to be alone with the patient. After about 30 minutes, the nurse enters the room and finds that the patient's bed has been pulled away from the wall, and the 10 visitors have formed a circle around the bed and ventilator and are praying, chanting, and humming while the patient is resting quietly. The nurse's best response would be to

A. Interrupt the prayer session to continue providing supportive patient care
B. Quietly close the door and allow the group to finish their prayer
C. Move into the circle and join the prayer group
D. Stand against the wall and observe the group to ensure patient safety

2-73. Which of the following electrolyte values would place the patient at risk for development of ventricular dysrhythmias?

A. Serum potassium 3.2 mEq/L
B. Serum sodium 124 mEq/L
C. Serum magnesium 2.0 mg/dL
D. Serum calcium 8.0 mg/dL

2-74. A patient is admitted to the ICU following ingestion of an unknown substance. The patient's arterial blood gas values are as follows: pH 7.50; pCO_2 22 mm Hg; pO_2 120 mmHg; HCO_3 15 mEq/L; anion gap >20. Based on these findings, the patient most likely ingested

A. Acetaminophen (Tylenol®)
B. Salicylates (aspirin)
C. Nonsteroidal anti-inflammatory medication (NSAID) (Advil®)
D. Benzodiazepine (Valium®)

2-75. A patient with epilepsy is admitted to the ICU after resection of a seizure focus for medically refractory seizures. For this patient, which of the following admission orders warrants an immediate hold until the nurse confers with the intensivist or neurosurgeon?

A. Neurological examination hourly
B. Lorazepam 1 mg IV prn for seizures lasting longer than 10 minutes
C. Phenobarbital 10-20 mg/kg IV for refractory seizures
D. Postoperative brain MRI upon admission

2-76. Which of the following vasopressors should the nurse anticipate using *first* for a patient with clinical evidence of pulmonary edema, signs and symptoms of shock, and systolic blood pressure less than 70 mm Hg?

A. Dopamine 20 mcg/kg/min
B. Dobutamine 25 mcg/kg/min
C. Nitroglycerin 9.9 mcg/min
D. Norepinephrine (Levophed) 10 mcg/min

2-77. A patient is 1 day post open heart surgery. The patient's spouse inquires about use of complementary therapies such as music to decrease pain. Which of the following is the nurse's best response?

A. "Use of music may reduce pain and tension."
B. "We will give your spouse as much pain medication as needed. Music therapy will not be necessary."
C. "While use of music does not pose a safety concern, there are no studies to suggest that it will help manage postoperative pain."
D. "We can try it, but the portable radio or CD player will require approval by the biomedical department before it can be used, and headphones will be needed."

2-78. A soldier is injured in a roadside blast, incurring blunt trauma to the upper chest. Which of the following clinical findings related to this type of injury does the nurse need to anticipate finding?

A. Chest wall asymmetry, diminished breath sounds, tachycardia
B. Hyporesonnance, dullness over lower thorax, peripheral vascular constriction
C. Unequal breath sounds, subcutaneous emphysema, peripheral vascular dilation
D. Tracheal deviation, reduction in oxygen saturation, bradycardia

2-79. A patient who develops cardiogenic shock after myocardial infarction with papillary muscle rupture would benefit most from which of the following immediate therapies?

A. Coronary artery bypass with mitral valve replacement
B. PTCA of occluded arteries and mitral valve replacement after the patient has stabilized
C. Thrombolytic therapy to reperfuse occluded coronary arteries and mitral valve repair after the patient has stabilized
D. Vasopressor support and intra-aortic balloon pump counterpulsation

2-80. A young adult patient was found unconscious at home after missing an important family celebration. The patient had complained of nausea earlier in the day and had a dry, hacking cough for the previous 5 days. The following were found upon assessment and receipt of laboratory values: temperature 101.1° F, pulse 110/min, respirations 26/min, BP 92/64 mm Hg, capillary glucose 304 mg/dL, pH 7.32, PO_2 98 mm Hg, PCO_2 32 mm Hg, and bicarbonate 18 mEq/L, with a urinary output of 20 mL in the previous hour. Which of the following should the nurse expect to administer at this time?

A. 50 mL bicarbonate intravenous push
B. 100 units glargine insulin subcutaneously
C. 1000 mL normal saline via intravenous bolus
D. 10 mEq KCL in 100 mL normal saline over 1 hour

2-81. Weaning a COPD patient from mechanical ventilation is often a difficult process. The nurse knows that decisions to extubate should be based on a patient's clinical status and his or her

A. Normal ABG values and chest x-ray findings
B. Ability to wean pressure support to less than +10 cm H_2O
C. Return to their own baseline pulmonary function and ABG values

D. Rapid Shallow Breathing Index (RSBI) score

2-82. An 80-year-old patient with heart failure and severe osteoarthritis complains of arthritic pain that prevents participation in a progressive exercise program. The most appropriate analgesic medication for this patient would be

A. A non-steroidal anti-inflammatory medication administered ½ to 1 hour prior to planned exercise
B. Daily administration of corticosteroids to reduce inflammation
C. Morphine sulfate 5 mg intravenously 10 minutes before planned exercise
D. Acetaminophen 650 mg orally ½ to 1 hour prior to planned exercise

2-83. A 75-year-old patient was struck by a motor vehicle, sustaining a head injury. The patient is sedated, intubated, and on mechanical ventilation. Vital signs are mean arterial pressure 60 mm Hg, HR 84/min, RR 18/min, ICP 14 mm Hg. Which of the following is indicated at this time?

A. Consult with the neurosurgeon regarding draining some fluid to decrease ICP
B. Speak with the attending physician regarding administering a fluid bolus to increase MAP
C. Call respiratory therapy to initiate hyperventilation to a pCO_2 of 30 mm Hg
D. No action is needed; these are acceptable values

2-84. An oncology patient is admitted to the critical care unit with a diagnosis of sepsis. The patient has a fever of 103° F with no other overt signs of infection. Multiple laboratory and diagnostic tests have been performed. On the complete blood count, the nurse notes a white blood count of 4000/mm³, segs 10%, bands 15%. To determine if the patient is severely immunosuppressed, requiring neutropenic precautions, the nurse must calculate an absolute neutrophil count (ANC). Based on the laboratory findings, this patient's ANC is

A. 0.6 or 600/mm³
B. 4.0 or 4000/mm³

C. 1.0 or 1000/mm³
D. 0.8 or 800/mm³

2-85. A patient in hypertensive crisis has a history of coronary artery disease and is complaining of angina. The most appropriate pharmacologic agent to lower blood pressure in this patient is

A. Sodium nitroprusside (Nipride)
B. Diazoxide (Proglycen)
C. Labetolol (Normodine, Trandate)
D. Nicardipine (Cardene)

2-86. A patient with esophageal cancer is admitted for vomiting bright red blood and is being resuscitated with IV fluids and blood products. His most recent laboratory results are as follows: hemoglobin 8 g/dL, hematocrit is 26 %, INR 1.7, PTT 22 sec, Na 135 mEq/L, K 3.2 mEq/L, creatinine 1.7 mg/dL, BUN 30 mg/dL, lactate 65 mg/dL. The nurse interprets these results as indicating

A. A potentially life-threatening condition requiring immediate correction
B. Findings expected at this stage of treatment for upper GI bleeding
C. Clear laboratory evidence of acute renal failure
D. Development of early stage DIC

2-87. A patient in the ICU is receiving high-dose diuretic therapy for fluid overload secondary to heart failure. The patient's ECG demonstrates prolonged PR and QT intervals, broad flat T waves, and multifocal PVCs. The initial management of this patient needs to include administration of

A. Magnesium
B. Hypertonic saline
C. Potassium
D. Acetazolamide

2-88. A patient is admitted with a COPD exacerbation and worsening dyspnea. His admission vital signs are temperature 38.1° C, HR 120/min, BP 180/80 mm Hg, SpO_2 90% on 2 L via nasal cannula (NC), RR 35/min and slightly labored. Initial ABGs are pH 7.33, $PaCO_2$ 57 mm Hg, PaO_2 61 mm Hg, SaO_2 87%, HCO_3 35 mEq/L. Which intervention should the nurse anticipate based on this assessment data?

A. Intubation related to the hypercarbia

B. Aggressive diuresis

C. Placing the patient on room air

D. Increasing O_2 to 4 L via NC

2-89. A 56-year-old man from Mexico is admitted to the ICU with hemodynamic instability related to urosepsis. Which of the following family members would be most appropriate for the nurse to include in teaching this patient about strategies to prevent future genitourinary tract problems?

A. 54-year-old wife

B. 59-year-old brother

C. 78-year-old mother

D. 82-year-old father

2-90. Two hours after femoral-popliteal bypass graft surgery, a patient complains of pain unrelieved by ordered narcotics. Neurovascular examination of the affected extremity reveals skin staples that are dry and intact. Skin is warm, pale, and dry. Capillary refill time is 2 seconds, and the popliteal and dorsalis pedis pulses are 2+. Motor strength is slightly decreased from the previous hourly assessment. The gastrocnemius muscle appears slightly swollen and is "doughy" to palpation. These findings indicate which of the following?

A. Compartment syndrome

B. Graft occlusion

C. Development of false aneurysm

D. Heparin-induced thrombocytopenia

2-91. A patient with chronic asthma was admitted 3 hours ago in marked respiratory distress owing to an acute exacerbation. The patient's most recent ABGs while on 40% facemask are pH 7.28, PCO_2 62 mm Hg, PO_2 58 mm Hg, HCO_3 23 mEq/L. Treatment has thus far included multiple doses of theophylline, albuterol, and ipratropium, and new medical orders are now pending. A medical order for which of the following should the nurse question as inappropriate for this patient?

A. Administration of a helium/oxygen mixture

B. Inhaled magnesium sulfate

C. Administration of broad-spectrum antibiotics

D. Inhaled general anesthetics

2-92. A 92-year-old female patient has a daughter who has been at her bedside since her admission for pulmonary edema. While the physician is making rounds, he suggests that the patient be discharged home on a dobutamine drip. The patient and daughter inform the physician that they do not want anything more done to prolong her life. Both the physician and the patient and her daughter continue to reiterate their opposing positions on this issue as the patient's nurse stands by observing this exchange. What is the nurse's best response upon entering this conversation?

A. " I have cared for her for the past week and I know she would want everything done."

B. "It is only right and fair that everything be done for this wonderful lady."

C. "It seems that the physician's wishes are in conflict due to his own need to do good."

D. "It would probably be best for you and your daughter to listen to the physician."

2-93. A patient admitted to the ICU with a diagnosis of unstable angina is receiving the following medications: low-molecular-weight heparin, aspirin, captopril, and continuous infusions of eptifibatide and nitroglycerin. Immediately after cardiac catheterization and percutaneous intervention, the patient is at high risk for which of the following?

A. Bleeding at groin access site

B. Coronary artery spasm

C. Restenosis

D. Heparin-induced thrombocytopenia

2-94. Carbon monoxide poisoning results in decreased oxygen-carrying capacity of blood and hypoxia. One of the primary reasons why tissue hypoxia occurs with this disorder is

A. Decreased affinity of Hb for carbon

monoxide molecules

B. Shift to the right in the oxyhemoglobin dissociation curve

C. Shift to the left in the oxyhemoglobin dissociation curve

D. Increased affinity of Hb for oxygen molecules

2-95. In caring for patients after coronary artery bypass surgery, the nurse knows the patient is most at risk for which of the following dysrhythmias within 1-3 days after surgery?

A. Atrial fibrillation

B. Supraventricular tachycardia

C. Atrial flutter

D. AV nodal re-entrant tachycardia

2-96. An 80-year-old immigrant from Taiwan who does not speak English was visiting her granddaughter and great-grandchildren 4 days prior to hospital admission and surgery for stomach cancer. For the past 4 days in the ICU, the patient has been alert and, when her granddaughter has been present to assist with translation, has appeared to be neurologically intact. The nightshift nurse now describes greater difficulty communicating with the patient, who remains awake and has become increasingly agitated throughout the night, repeating some phrases that staff cannot understand. When the granddaughter arrives, the day shift nurse verifies patient deficits in attention, cognition, and orientation, although her vital signs are stable and SaO_2 is 97% on room air. Which of the following should the nurse do to more fully appraise this patient's confusion?

A. Contact the hospital's Taiwanese interpreter

B. Ask the family to provide ongoing interpretation assistance

C. Educate the staff about Chinese values and communication patterns

D. Review the literature for a screening tool to detect confusion

2-97. A patient is admitted to the ICU following multiple stab wounds to the chest. His treatment has included placement of two chest tubes to the left anterior side and one chest tube to the right posterior. All are draining moderate amounts of serosanguinous fluid. The patient's hematocrit is 33%, and INR is 1.2. After several hours, the patient is intubated and on pressure support of +10, breathing comfortably with a respiratory rate of 20/min. He has received several doses of morphine and currently denies pain. After turning him onto his right side, the nurse notes that drainage from his right chest tube has suddenly stopped, his respiratory rate has increased to 35/min, and his oxygen saturation has decreased to 85%. What should be the first nursing actions for this patient?

A. Increase the FiO_2 and call respiratory therapy to change ventilator mode/settings

B. Draw an ABG and send specimens for hematocrit and coagulation studies

C. Turn the patient supine and assess patency of the right chest tube

D. Prepare for additional chest tube insertion to the right and notify the physician

2-98. After transfusion of 10 units of packed red blood cells for acute hemorrhagic shock, which of the following therapies is anticipated?

A. Fresh frozen plasma and platelets

B. Acetaminophen and diphenhydramine (Benadryl)

C. Furosemide (Lasix) and calcium chloride

D. Normal saline at 200 mL/hr and 50 mL of salt poor albumin

2-99. A patient has experienced a dominant hemisphere stroke following a motor vehicle collision that caused carotid artery dissection. The patient's GCS is 3, and she evidences no spontaneous movement. Other significant findings support a diagnosis of brain death. The patient's husband was informed of these findings earlier this evening, whereupon he abruptly departed the ICU. He has now returned to the ICU, where his behavior with staff is agitated, argumentative, and confrontational. In working with this patient's husband, which of the following actions should the nurse *avoid?*

A. Calling social services for assistance
B. Confronting the patient's husband about his aggressive and unacceptable behaviors
C. Speaking in a calm, gentle manner
D. Contacting the patient's sister to arrange a family conference

2-100. For a patient with a diagnosis of unstable angina, which of the following indicates that the patient is at risk for the development of acute myocardial infarction?

A. BNP 300 pg/mL
B. C-reactive protein 5.0 mg/dL
C. Total cholesterol 180 mg/dL
D. HDL 60 mg/dL

2-101. A patient in ICU is undergoing rotational therapy for respiratory failure. One very important clinical implication related to this therapy that the nurse needs to keep in mind is that while the patient is on rotational therapy

A. Hemodynamic monitoring with a pulmonary artery catheter will be unreliable in both lateral and prone positions
B. Enteral feedings should not be administered owing to a heightened risk of aspiration
C. A decrease in SpO_2 during lateral rotation will indicate the patient needs to be returned to the supine position
D. Hypotension and tachycardia that fail to return to baseline within 10 minutes of rotation will indicate the patient needs to be returned to the supine position

2-102. A 43-year-old patient with a BMI of 52 underwent bariatric surgery 2 months ago. He has not been taking his vitamin and mineral supplements. His vital signs are BP 133/87 mm Hg, pulse 78 beats/min, respirations 14 breaths/min. Which of the following clinical findings would the nurse expect to see as manifestations of this patient's vitamin and mineral deficiencies?

A. Vomiting, headache, diplopia, short-term memory loss
B. Thirst, increased urination, diploplia, fatigue
C. Jaundice, dark urine, gnawing epigastric pain relieved by bending forward
D. Irritability, disorientation, asterixis, slowed mentation

2-103. A 72-year-old man is admitted to the CCU with shortness of breath, chest pain, diaphoresis, and tachycardia. His history includes myocardial infarction 5 years ago with two stents, anorexia, hypertension, fatigue, hypercholesterolemia, and arthritis. He is currently on amiodarone, metoprolol, captopril, lovastatin, aspirin, multivitamin, an herbal remedy called cat's claw, and nitroglycerin. For the past 4 days, all cardiac labs, 12-lead ECG, and cardiac catheterization have been normal, whereas FT_4 has been elevated and TSH low. The patient's tachycardia persisted until hospital day 4, when he developed a junctional rhythm. Now that numerous differential diagnoses have been ruled out, how could the health care team determine whether one of his medications is causing these symptoms?

A. Hold one medication each day to see if symptoms resolve
B. Review the literature for drug-induced thyroid dysfunction
C. Obtain a thyroxine-binding globulin level
D. Assess for a Wolff-Chaikoff effect

2-104. After mitral valve replacement surgery, a patient has a right atrial pressure of 18 mm Hg and a pulmonary artery diastolic pressure (PAD) of 4 mm Hg. Initial treatment for this patient would include administration of which of the following?

A. Normal saline bolus 500 mL
B. Furosemide 40 mg
C. Norepineprine continuous infusion
D. Vasopressin 40 mg

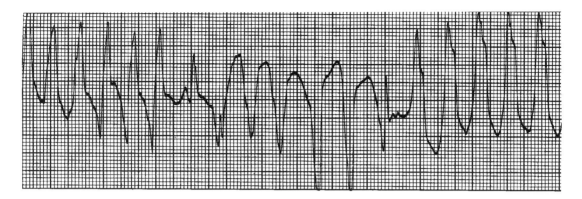

2-105. A patient with type 2 diabetes was found unresponsive, sitting at his desk at work. An admitting diagnosis of hyperglycemic, hyperosmolar, nonketotic coma was made in the emergency department. The nurse assigned to this patient anticipates his highest priority needs by preparing

A. Large amounts of intravenous normal saline for infusion
B. An insulin drip made with glargine insulin for infusion
C. Oxygen at 40% via mask
D. Padded side rails and a bite block

2-106. Pharmacologic therapy for the above rhythm would include

A. Procainamide
B. Lidocaine
C. Adenosine
D. Magnesium sulfate

2-107. The nurse admits a 50-year-old woman who complains of worsening dyspnea, a non-productive cough, and a recent weight loss of approximately 15 pounds. Her breath sounds reveal scattered inspiratory rales, and she quickly desaturates to 85% off her non-rebreather. Initial labs reveal a normal WBC with elevated sedimentation rate and C-reactive protein levels. Her chest x-ray shows diffuse, bilateral opacities. What interventions should the critical care nurse anticipate?

A. Pan-culturing the patient and initiating broad spectrum antibiotics as soon as possible
B. Pan culturing the patient and initiating corticosteroid therapy
C. Initiating aggressive diuretic therapy and antibiotic therapy
D. Obtaining an echocardiogram and initiating inotropic therapy

2-108. A patient newly diagnosed with leukemia suddenly develops a low platelet count. Patients with a low platelet count need to be instructed to avoid

A. Green, leafy vegetables
B. Aspirin
C. Fresh fruits
D. Prednisone

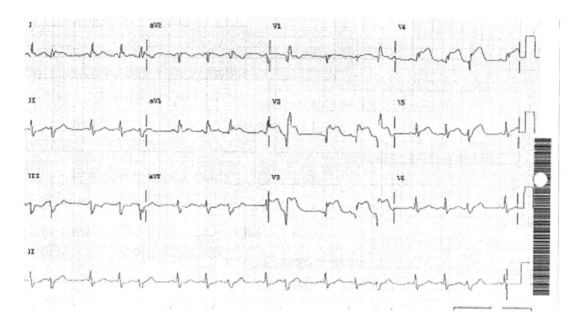

2-109. A patient complains of chest pain and palpitations, and the above 12-lead ECG is obtained. The most appropriate initial intervention the nurse should perform includes administration of oxygen 6 liters by nasal cannula and

    A. Obtain serum potassium level
    B. Administer nitroglycerin
    C. Obtain a coagulation panel
    D. Administer amiodarone

2-110. A patient is admitted to the ICU for hypovolemia secondary to lower GI bleed. On day 3, the patient's serum sodium is 115 mEq/L, and serum osmolality is 244 mOsm/Kg. Which of the following IV fluids is most likely responsible for these abnormalities?

    A. Half-strength saline solution (0.45% NaCl)
    B. Dextrose in water (D_5W)
    C. Normal saline solution (0.9% NaCl)
    D. Lactated ringer's solution (LR)

2-111. The nurse is assessing a postoperative patient who suffered a pulmonary embolism 3 days ago. Low-molecular-weight heparin was discontinued yesterday, and the patient is currently on warfarin. Recent arterial blood gas results are pH 7.44, PCO_s 35 mm Hg, PO_2 89 mm Hg. The physician orders pneumatic compression stockings, daily PT/INR, advancement of diet, and a reduction in her oxygen from 30% via facemask to 3 L/min by humidified nasal cannula. Which of these orders would the nurse put on hold until the physician is contacted?

    A. Daily PT/INR
    B. Pneumatic compression stockings
    C. Advancement of diet
    D. Reduction in oxygen

2-112. For an intubated patient with acute pulmonary edema who does *not* have a pulmonary artery catheter, adequate cardiac output is best indicated by which of the following findings?

    A. Ejection fraction greater than 50% on echocardiogram
    B. Respiratory rate 20/min with SpO_2 94%
    C. Absence of peripheral edema
    D. The patient is alert with a serum creatinine 1.0 mg/dL

2-113. A patient in the ICU was just admitted status post cardiac arrest. Management of this patient should include

    A. Rapidly cooling the patient to 33-35°C
    B. Monitoring for signs and symptoms of hyperkalemia
    C. Titrating insulin infusion to maintain serum glucose level 120-150 mg/dL
    D. Assessing for elevations in white blood cell and platelet counts

2-114. A patient with an implanted cardiovertor defibrillator has an episode of ventricular fibrillation that does not respond to implanted defibrillator shocks. Which of the following actions are most appropriate?

A. Allow the ICD to attempt to terminate the rhythm for at least three cycles
B. Place a magnet over the device prior to attempting manual defibrillation with 360 joules monophasic
C. Place defibrillator pads in the anterior-posterior position at least 2 inches away from the ICD generator and defibrillate with 360 joules monophasic
D. Place defibrillator pads to the left of the nipple at the 5th left interspace and just under the clavicle to the right of the sternum and defibrillate with 50 joules biphasic

2-115. After experiencing multiple admissions with increasing frequency related to complications of his underlying condition, a 30-year-old patient experiencing extreme shortness of breath related to a sickle cell anemia crisis states that he no longer wishes to be intubated and that he is tired of so many resources being used to keep him alive when these funds could be used to benefit others. Which of the following is the best response from the nurse?

A. "I am sure you won't feel that way after this exacerbation subsides."
B. "Look at all that you contribute to your community. What will they do without you?"
C. "Have you discussed this issue with your physician, friends, and family?"
D. "When you get well, you can draft an Advanced Directive."

2-116. The nurse administers glucagon to a hypoglycemic patient. Which of the following is the next most important nursing intervention?

A. Recheck the capillary glucose level in 30 minutes
B. Assess the patient's neurological status
C. Position the patient to avoid aspiration
D. Prepare nourishments to administer over the next hour

2-117. The intensivist wants to order new multichannel intravenous infusion pumps for the ICUs. A committee is to be assembled. The most appropriate initial action of the committee is to

A. Send for all literature on the available multichannel pumps
B. Include members of other units who may be using the new pump
C. Call other hospitals to determine their pros and cons for their pumps in use
D. Check for data on nationwide sentinel events involving all of the multichannel pumps

2-118. The health care team is making rounds on a patient with status asthmaticus who was intubated and placed on mechanical ventilation earlier that shift. The patient's most recent ABG findings reveal persistent hypoxemia, and the team is now considering whether to use neuromuscular blocking agents (NMBs) to help this patient. When an orientee asks his preceptor to clarify use of NMBs in this situation, the preceptor's best explanation would be that in patients with status asthmaticus who are experiencing hypoxia despite mechanical ventilation, neuromuscular blocking agents should

A. Never be administered while the patient is receiving steroids
B. Be used routinely for paralysis to control airway pressures
C. Be administered to augment smooth muscle relaxation
D. Be used with caution if other options are ineffective

2-119. The most likely reason a surgeon would use a left atrial line in a patient with pulmonary arterial hypertension undergoing mitral valve replacement and maze procedure would be to

A. Ensure accuracy of postoperative hemodynamic data
B. Enable evacuation of a left atrial air embolus
C. Provide a means of monitoring for cardiac tamponade more reliable than a PA line
D. Ensure continuous monitoring of chamber pressures during valve replacement

2-120. A patient in septic shock evidences the following hemodynamic parameters: HR 120/min; BP 80/40 mm Hg; PAP 25/10 mm Hg; CVP 4 mm Hg; CO 4.0 L/min; CI 2.1 L/min/m²; SVR 700 dynes/sec/cm⁻⁵; SVO_2 60%. Based on these hemodynamic values, which of the following interventions would *most* likely result in improving the patient's hemodynamic status?

   A. Norepinephrine 10 mcg/kg/min
   B. Metoprolol 2.5 mg IVP slowly
   C. 500 mL bolus of 0.9% normal saline
   D. Dobutamine 5 mcg/kg/min

2-121. A 70 kg patient with acute respiratory distress syndrome (ARDS) is intubated and mechanically ventilated. The patient is currently on a continuous vecuronium infusion titrated to maintain "0" twitch. Peak inspiratory pressure is 55 cm H_2O. The patient currently has a PaO_2 of 60 mm Hg, and the physician orders the following ventilator settings: SIMV; TV 700 mL; rate 12/min; FiO_2 100%; PEEP 15 cm H_2O. The nurse knows that

   A. SIMV is an inappropriate ventilator mode for a patient receiving vecuronium
   B. A tidal volume of 700 mL is inappropriate for this patient
   C. The PEEP should be increased to 20 cm H_2O to improve oxygenation
   D. The ordered ventilator settings are appropriate for this patient

2-122. When admitting a patient with hypertensive crisis, the nurse's immediate concern is to prevent which of the following complications?

   A. Stroke
   B. End organ failure
   C. Seizures
   D. Left ventricular hypertrophy

2-123. The physician is at the bedside of a patient who needs to go to the operating room for a perforated bowel. The physician explains the procedure to the family, indicates it will last about 2 hours, and relates that the patient will then return to the ICU. The physician then presents the informed consent form to the patient and says there should be no problem with the surgery as she has performed this procedure many times. The patient asks if there are any risks to this surgery. The physician states that there are minimal risks and then prepares to leave the room. What is the nurse's best next response?

   A. Allow the physician to leave, documenting the physician's visit in the nurse's notes
   B. Ask the physician to discuss risks of infection with the patient
   C. Call clergy to request consultation for a high-risk surgery
   D. Obtain a patient education brochure on the procedure for the family

2-124. A pregnant 26-year-old woman presents with a history of progressively increasing abdominal pain over her right upper abdomen and left lower abdomen for the past 5 days and vomiting of a primarily bile-colored fluid. Her current temperature is 100.8° F, and her only prior hospitalization was for an appendectomy when she was an adolescent. Obstetrical examination reveals gestation of 26 weeks and no problems with the active, alive fetus. As soon as the nurse inserts a nasogastric tube and initiates IV fluids, the nurse will tailor interventions for a patient with suspected

   A. Ectopic pregnancy
   B. Abruptio placenta
   C. Peptic ulcer disease
   D. Intestinal obstruction

2-125. Two days after abdominal aortic surgical repair, a patient develops hypotension, tachycardia, abdominal distension, diarrhea, and an elevated white blood cell count. The most likely cause of these findings is which of the following?

   A. Postoperative graft infection
   B. Ischemic colitis
   C. Aorto-enteric fistula
   D. Abdominal compartment syndrome

2-126. A patient involved in a motor vehicle crash who sustained a pelvic fracture, splenic laceration, and a compound fracture of the femur is admitted to the ICU following internal fixation of his femur. What should the nurse anticipate as the optimal method of deep vein thrombosis (DVT) prophylaxis for this patient?

A. Subcutaneous heparin administration
B. Elastic stockings
C. Mechanical compression devices
D. Early initiation of physical therapy

2-127. A patient with acute pulmonary edema is receiving furosemide (Lasix) 40 mg BID, captopril (Capoten) 50 mg TID, and morphine sulfate 2 mg every 2 hours and oxygen 70% by BiPAP mask. Current assessment data include HR 116/min, sinus rhythm with occasional APC, BP 100/70 mm Hg, and RR 25 with SpO$_2$ 97%. Which of the following findings should alert the nurse to a need to change the current treatment plan?

A. Serum creatinine 3.2 mg/dL
B. Serum potassium 3.8 mg/dL
C. SpO$_2$ 95%
D. HR 110/min with increasing atrial premature contractions

2-128. A 29-year-old woman is admitted to the ICU with exacerbation of systemic lupus erythematosa (SLE). Patient education regarding which of the following topics will help this patient avoid future rehospitalizations due to the major cause of morbidity associated with SLE?

A. Ulceration around the mouth
B. Anemia
C. Significant weight loss
D. Infection

2-129. The patient delivered a 5-pound infant via caesarean section after experiencing both pregnancy-induced hypertension and postpartum hemorrhage. Which of the following laboratory values would support the nurse's suspicion that this patient is exhibiting clinical evidence of HELLP syndrome?

A. Elevated liver enzymes and a decreased platelet count
B. Decreased hemoglobin and hematocrit

C. Elevated serum magnesium and albuminuria
D. Decreased blood urea nitrogen and increased serum creatinine

2-130. A patient with pulmonary edema has received 80 mg furosemide (Lasix). Arterial blood gas values include pH 7.60, PaO$_2$ 78 mm Hg, pCO$_2$ 42 mm Hg. The nurse anticipates which of the following interventions?

A. Administration of acetazolamide (Diamox)
B. Administration of additional furosemide (Lasix) 40 mg
C. Endotracheal intubation
D. Administration of hydrochlorthiazide

2-131. For patients with diabetes insipidus, which of the following statements regarding fluid management is accurate?

A. Electrolyte levels must be monitored to determine the correct IV fluids to administer
B. If the diabetes insipidus is nephrogenic, vasopressin will need to be adminsitered
C. If the diabetes insipidus is neurogenic, only fluids will need replacement
D. The patient's output must exceed his intake in order to prevent complications

2-132. A 58-year-old continuous ambulatory peritoneal dialysis (CAPD) patient is admitted to the ICU following a small bowel resection. The patient is hemodynamically stable and has a 3 L excess fluid balance. For these reasons, the critical care nurse anticipates the patient's end stage renal disease (ESRD) will be managed using

A. Peritoneal dialysis (PD)
B. Slow continuous ultrafiltration (SCUF)
C. Hemodialysis (HD)
D. Continuous venovenous hemofiltration (CVVH)

2-133. Following chest trauma associated with a recent motor vehicle collision, an ICU patient on mechanical ventilation has both right and left chest tubes in place with persistent bubbling throughout inspiration and expiration in the left chest tube. His breath sounds are clear and equal and the drainage system is working properly. The goal of ventilator management for this patient is to

A. Maximize PEEP
B. Minimize airway pressures
C. Minimize FiO_2
D. Maximize tidal volumes

2-134. Microbial translocation of normal gut flora into the systemic circulation can initiate and sustain inflammatory responses in critically ill patients that lead to sepsis in vulnerable patients. In an effort to minimize a patient's risk of developing the negative consequences associated with microbial translocation, which of the following interventions might *not* be implemented?

A. Mechanical ventilation
B. Inotropic therapy
C. Enteral nutrition
D. Histamine blockers

2-135. The nurse caring for a Hmong patient in the ICU is attempting to provide an environment conducive to healing. The Hmong people believe that illness can occur through the loss of souls and that souls may be lost through a variety of methods. The best intervention this patient's ICU nurse can implement to prevent the loss of a soul would be to

A. Provide a quiet environment
B. Offer the patient hot tea at regular intervals
C. Allow visitation by the shaman
D. Ensure that foods are cold or room temperature

2-136. A 60-year-old patient is transferred to the ICU with a new onset of fever, leukocytosis, and a cough productive of large amounts of rust-colored sputum. His vital signs are as follows: temperature 39.5° C, heart rate 120/min, respiratory rate 35/min, SO_2 90% on room air, BP 90/40 mm Hg. The critical care nurse knows that the highest priority interventions for this patient are to

A. Obtain sputum and blood cultures and start broad-spectrum antibiotics
B. Facilitate obtaining both a chest x-ray and a sputum culture
C. Administer acetaminophen and obtain a full set of cultures
D. Initiate administration of oxygen and IV fluids

2-137. A 28-year-old woman is in the ICU with a gunshot wound to the head. Surgery was performed to remove the bullet and to stop bleeding. The patient has been in the ICU for 2 weeks and remains unresponsive. An EEG is flat, and the physician has declared the patient brain dead. The nurse is present with the physician when the diagnosis is shared with the patient's mother. One of the first issues that the nurse needs to anticipate at this point is

A. That the family may request a second opinion
B. The need to document this physician-family discussion
C. The need to initiate discussion related to organ donation
D. That the hospital ethics committee should be contacted

2-138. Which of the following represents the only circumstances in which pericardiocentesis would be performed prior to emergency corrective surgery for a patient with suspected aortic dissection?

A. The patient has an elevated right atrial pressure
B. The patient demonstrates signs of cardiac tamponade with a stable blood pressure
C. The patient develops pulseless electrical activity (PEA)
D. Chest x-ray demonstrates indisputable evidence of mediastinal widening

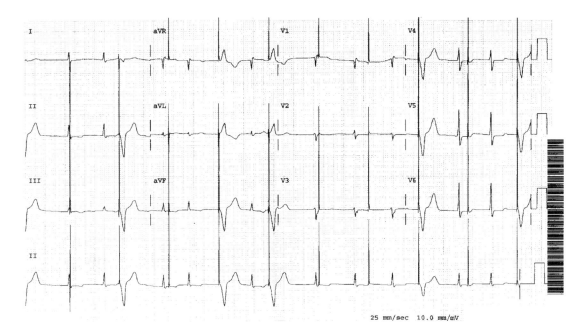

25 mm/sec   10.0 mm/mV

2-139. The 12-lead ECG above clearly demonstrates a ventricular pacemaker rate at 60 per minute with

    A. Complete capture
    B. Failure to capture
    C. Failure to sense
    D. Failure to output

2-140. A patient admitted to the ICU with a diagnosis of sepsis has the following urinary laboratory results: specific gravity 1.028, osmolality 362 mOsm/kg, sodium 15 mEq/L, and FENa 0.8%. Based on these findings, the critical care nurse anticipates which of the following actions?

    A. Administration of normal saline fluid bolus
    B. Fluid restriction of 1 L/24 hr
    C. Administration of furosemide (Lasix) 40 mg IVP
    D. Discontinued administration of cefazolin (Ancef)

2-141. A patient presents with new-onset seizures. Diagnostic imaging reveals a 4 cm right posterior frontal arteriovenous malformation. In planning this patient's nursing care needs, which of the following conditions should the nurse anticipate?

    A. Left-sided weakness
    B. Receptive aphasia

    C. Left homonymous hemianopsia
    D. Sensory deficits on the right face and arm

2-142. A patient was admitted with a history of blunt trauma to the head, chest, and abdomen related to a 30-foot fall. On admission, his vital signs were BP 148/82 mm Hg, pulse 120 beats/min, respirations 16 breaths/min. Over the past 45 minutes, the patient has become more agitated, pulse has risen to 135 beats/min, BP is now 100/60 mm Hg, and his skin is cool and clammy. The nurse's next interventions will be based on a high index of suspicion that the patient has sustained an acute

    A. Increase in intracranial pressure
    B. Myocardial infarction
    C. Intra-abdominal hemorrhage
    D. Pulmonary embolism

2-143. A patient is admitted to the ICU following extensive surgical repair of a perforated colon. He received a 15 L resuscitation with fluids and blood products perioperatively and still requires intermittent fluid boluses. He is intubated, and his chest x-ray shows diffuse bilateral infiltrates suggestive of ARDS. Ventilator settings are SIMV mode with a set rate of 18, tidal volume of 6 ml/kg, PEEP +10 and FiO_2 0.70. He is overbreathing to a rate of 30/min, and his latest ABG is pH 7.28, PaCO$_2$ 45 mm Hg, and PaO$_2$ 55 mm Hg. Pulmonary wheezes and crackles are audible bilaterally. He is grimacing and restless on the bed. In addition to having ventilator settings optimized, in what order does the nurse need to prioritize pharmacologic interventions?

A. IV steroids, sedation/analgesia, diuretic
B. Diuretic, bronchodilator, IV steroids
C. Bronchodilator, sedation, fluid bolus
D. Sedation/analgesia, bronchodilator, antibiotics

2-144. After implantation of a biventricular pacemaker for end-stage heart failure, ECG signs that the pacemaker is not functioning properly would include

A. A-V interval less than 0.20 sec
B. Widening of the QRS
C. T-wave inversion
D. More than one P wave for each QRS

2-145. The preceptor for a new ICU nurse notices that the orientee is taking a noninvasive blood pressure measurement using the patient's forearm rather than her upper arm. When questioned about this cuff placement, the orientee states that he had heard that the cuff could be placed on the forearm. The preceptor has never heard of using the forearm for this purpose and has no information on this change from standard practice BP technique. What should the preceptor do?

A. Instruct the new nurse on the standard BP protocol of using the upper arm
B. Take the blood pressure in both the upper and lower arms and then compare readings
C. Design a research study to compare the relationship between upper and lower arm BP measurements
D. Review the current literature to identify evidence and recommendations related to this change in practice

2-146. During the administration of packed red blood cells (PRBCs), the patient develops chills and a temperature of 102° F. The initial nursing intervention for this patient would be to

A. Obtain a urine specimen
B. Administer antipyretics
C. Call the physician
D. Stop the transfusion

2-147. A patient has undergone emergency coronary bypass within 2 hours after percutaneous coronary intervention with administration of GpIIb-IIIa inhibitors. Treatment of this patient's mediastinal oozing and chest tube output of 100 mL/hr should include administration of

A. Platelets
B. Protamine sulfate
C. Vitamin K
D. Agatroban

2-148. A patient is admitted to the ICU after respiratory arrest. The patient has a history of chronic obstructive bronchitis and was manually ventilated with 100% oxygen during transport to the ICU. The patient is placed on mechanical ventilation with the following settings: pressure regulated volume control (PRVC), FiO$_2$ 40%, rate 10/min. Arterial blood gases obtained 15 minutes later are pH 7.54, PaO$_2$ 76 mm Hg, PaCO$_2$ 45 mm Hg, saturation 90%. After reviewing these clinical findings and ventilatory settings, the nurse should conclude that the

A. Pressure ventilation is inappropriate for this COPD patient because it shortens expiratory time
B. Respiratory rate should be decreased to correct the pH
C. FiO$_2$ should be increased until the PaO$_2$ is at least 80%
D. Ordered ventilator settings are appropriate for this patient

2-149. A patient is newly admitted to the ICU with diabetic ketoacidosis. Aggressive fluid resuscitation is in progress. The family asks the nurse why the fluids are being administered so quickly. Which of the following is *not* part of the nurse's response? "In patients with very high blood glucose levels, rapid administration of fluids . . .

A. . . . helps to lower blood sugar."
B. . . . increases the volume of blood circulating to the body tissues."

C.   . . . decreases ketone levels from the breakdown of fats."

D.   . . . helps to return blood pressure to normal."

2-150. Which of the following patients is most at risk of developing heparin-induced thrombocytopenia after percutaneous coronary intervention?

A.   A patient with unstable angina who received unfractionated heparin several days prior to elective PCI

B.   A patient with diabetes, mild renal insufficiency, and multivessel coronary artery disease

C.   A patient who has steroid dependent asthma and RCA occlusion

D.   An obese patient with hypertension and left ventricular hypertrophy

2-1. **(A)** In patients with ARDS, pneumothorax is frequently related to the use of high PEEP and tidal volumes intended to promote oxygenation and is easily treated by insertion of a chest tube. Immediate treatment of pneumothorax is warranted to prevent further patient compromise. Although decreased urine output is of concern, improvement in oxygenation by relieving pneumothorax takes precedence. Although pneumonia may have contributed to sepsis, causing ARDS, sputum cultures would not be indicated for a patient with pneumothorax (indicated by the radiolucence in the right middle lobe). Administration of norepinephrine to increase blood pressure is not the immediate concern for this patient. Blood pressure may be improved via treatment of the pneumothorax.

> **Reference:** Hemmila, M. R., Napolitano, L. M. Severe respiratory failure: advanced treatment options. *Crit Care Med,* 34, S278-S290, 2006.

2-2. **(D)** Signs of brain death include the following: fixed pupils, no motor response to deep central pain, absent corneal reflexes, absent oculocephalic (doll's eyes) reflex, absent oculovestibular reflex (cold water calorics), positive apnea test (no spontaneous breaths with $PaCO_2$ >60 mm Hg and despite 100% FiO_2 ventilation 15 minutes prior). Loss of vascular tone (Option A) is not part of the diagnostic criteria for brain death, but hemodynamic instability can occur prior to or following diagnosis. Barbiturate infusion (Option B) is provided for refractory intracranial hypertension as a salvage measure. Lack of response to this treatment is not pathopneumonic for brain death, but many patients have a poor outcome. Barbiturates are metabolized slowly, so it can take days before they are cleared to subtherapeutic values, a prerequisite prior to testing for brain death. All diagnoses should be made in the absence of hypothermia, metabolic, or drug cause, shock or anoxia, or immediately post resuscitation. Responses of the spinal reflex arc (Option C)—elicited with infliction of peripheral noxious stimuli such as nail bed pressure—are commonly present after brain death.

> **References:** Bader, M. K., Littlejohns, L. R. (eds.). *AANN Core Curriculum for Neuroscience Nursing,* 4th ed. St. Louis, Elsevier, 2004.
>
> Wijdicks, E. F. M. *The Clinical Practice of Critical Care Neurology.* New York, Oxford University Press, 2003.

2-3. **(C)** Hyponatremia and hypokalemia result from prolonged vomiting. Changes in serum sodium concentration usually reflect changes in water balance. The signs and symptoms of hyponatremia are often nonspecific, and most are related to the changes in serum osmolality and consequent fluid shifts in the central nervous system. These can include headache, lethargy, disorientation, seizures, muscle cramps, or weakness. Hypokalemia can develop as a result of intracellular shifts of potassium or as a result of increased loss of or decreased ingestion or administration of potassium. Clinical signs of hypokalemia include weakness, paralysis, respiratory compromise, rhabdomyolysis, ECG changes, cardiac disrhythmias, and sudden death. Hyperglycemia may occur with extreme stress. Signs and symptoms of hyperkalemia (peaked T waves, diarrhea) are not associated with vomiting. These symptoms usually occur with ketoacidosis, tissue destruction, and renal failure and with certain medications such as beta-blockers. Hypoglycemia may occur with dehydration and protracted vomiting. However, symptoms of hyponatremia (headache, tremors, disorientation) occur with overuse of diuretics, certain psychoactive medications, inadequate dietary intake of sodium, water intoxication, or impaired adrenal or kidney function. Jaundice owing to hyperbilirubinemia, water retention and swelling, and muscle cramps owing to hypoalbuminemia, occur in patients with conditions such as cirrhosis.

Reference: Kraft, M. D., Btiache, I. F., Sacks, G. S., et. al. Treatment of electrolyte disorders in adult patients in the intensive care unit. *Am J Health-Syst Pharm,* 62, 1663-1682, 2005.

2-4. **(C)** Flail chest, caused by blunt trauma to the thoracic cavity, occurs when two or more adjacent ribs are fractured in two or more places. This flail segment moves independently from the rest of the thoracic cage and results in paradoxical chest wall movement during the respiratory cycle. Paradoxical motion refers to the movement of the flail segment in the direction *opposite* that of the intact chest wall. Instead of expanding outward with the rest of the thoracic wall during inspiration, the flail segment is drawn inward by the negative inspiratory pressure. Conversely, as this negative pressure falls during exhalation, the flail segment is pushed outward.

References: Newberry, L., Criddle, L. M., (eds.). *Sheehy's Manual of Emergency Care,* 6th ed. St. Louis, Elsevier, 2005, p 655.

Urden, L. D., Stacy, K. M., Lough, M. E. *Thelan's Critical Care Nursing, Diagnosis and Management,* 5th ed. St. Louis, Elsevier, 2006, pp 991-992.

2-5. **(A)** ST segment depression and T wave inversion indicate myocardial ischemia. Acute transmural infarction would be evidenced on 12-lead ECG as ST segment elevation (STEMI) or Q waves in indicative leads. Lateral wall ischemia or infarct is observed in leads I and aV_L or leads V_5 and V_6 on the 12-lead ECG. Anterior wall changes indicative of ischemia or infarct would be seen in leads V_3 and V_4.

Reference: Achar, S. A., Kundu, S., Norcross, W. A. Diagnosis of acute coronary syndrome. *Am Fam Phys,* 72, 119-1126, 2005.

2-6. **(D)** Late complications of renal injury include: hypertension, hydronephrosis, chronic pyelonephritis, calculus formation, and intrarenal calcification. Early complications include ileus, sepsis, shock, impairment or loss of renal function, perinephric or renal abscess, and fistula formation.

References: Adams, K., Johnson, K. Trauma. In Urden, L. D., Stacy, K. M., Lough, M. E. (eds.). *Thelan's Critical Care Nursing: Diagnosis and Management,* 5th ed. St. Louis, Elsevier, 2006, pp 969-1008.

Stark, J. L. The renal system. In J. G. Alspach (ed.). *Core Curriculum for Critical Care Nursing,* 6th ed. St. Louis, Elsevier, 2006, pp 525-607.

2-7. **(C)** Gastric irritation is a frequent adverse effect of immunosuppressive agents, so taking this medication with commercial chocolate milk (that contains algae derivatives for thickening) or food will help to prevent development of gastric ulcers. It is not safe to double the dose of immunosuppressive medications if a dose is missed because of the possibility of untoward effects. Resuming the normal dose as soon as possible will limit incidence of graft vs. host disease. Levels of immunosuppressive medications are not monitored using laboratory values, although antibody levels may be used to evaluate the effectiveness of immunosuppressive therapy. Elevated blood pressure represents a serious untoward effect of immunosuppressive agents and, if not monitored or reported to the primary health care provider, may lead to permanent neurological deficits.

References: Deglin, J. H., Vallerand, A. H. *Davis's Drug Guide For Nurses,* 10th ed. Philadelphia, F. A. Davis, 2007, pp 58-59, 336-339, 1100-1101.

Morton, P. G., Fontaine, D. K., Hudak, C. M., Gallo, B. M. *Critical Care Nursing: A Holistic Approach,* 8th ed. Philadelphia, Lippincott Williams & Wilkins, 2005, pp 1122-1128.

2-8. **(A)** Option A is correct because encouraging patients to recall past successes or reflect on the past may support adaptation to life changes. Option B is incorrect because a patient's views on these issues would not explain their current diagnosis. Option C might be an informative and reflective experience but would not necessarily have health implicatons for the future. Option D is not appropriate because the scenario described does not suggest this patient needs to focus on their mortality at this time.

References: Hardin, S. R. Caring practices. In S. R. Hardin, R. Kaplow (eds.). *Synergy for Clinical Excellence.* Sudbury, Jones & Bartlett, 2005, pp 69-74.

Rustoen, T., Howie, J., Eidsmo, I., Moum, T. Hope in patients hospitalized with heart failure. *Am J Crit Care,* 14(5), 417-425, 2005.

2-9. **(B)** In cases of acute hypoglycemia, treatment should be administered, then its effectiveness assessed through the use of capillary glucose measurement 15 minutes after administration of the glucose source. This timeframe should be adhered to regardless of whether or when circulation is restored or the patient is transferred between units.

References: Newberry, L., Criddle, L. *Sheehy's Manual of Emergency Care,* 6th ed. Philadelphia, Elsevier, 2006, pp 428-432.

Urden, L. D., Stacy, K. M., Lough, M. *Thelan's Critical Care Nursing: Diagnosis and Management,* 5th ed. St. Louis, Elsevier, 2006, p 926.

2-10. **(A)** The inferior wall is supplied by the right coronary artery, which also supplies the right ventricle. A right side ECG would demonstrate if RVMI has occurred. Treatment for RVMI requires fluid administration and perfusion and may be compromised by administration of vasodilators such as nitroglycerin. A second ECG in 30 minutes is not warranted and would delay treatment for this patient with acute inferior wall STEMI (ST segment elevation in leads II, III, and aVF). Although the heart rate is less than 50/min., transcutaneous pacing or administration of atropine would increase myocardial demand and potentially worsen

ischemia, so it should be withheld unless signs of decreased perfusion are present.

Reference: Woods, S. L., Froelicher, E. S., Motzer, S. U., Bridges, E. J. *Cardiac Nursing,* 5th ed. Philadelphia, Lippincott Williams & Wilkins, 2005.

2-11. **(A)** Chlorhexidine gluconate solutions used for vascular catheter site care reduce catheter-related bloodstream infections and catheter colonization more effectively than povidone iodine solutions. Data suggest that IV tubing containing crystalloids can be replaced every 72 to 96 hours, so Option B is not correct. Option C is not accurate because the transducer, tubing, flush device, and flush solution need to be replaced only every 96 hours. If aseptic technique during insertion cannot be ensured, the catheter should be replaced soon as possible, but within 48 hours, not within 72 hours as Option D suggests.

Reference: AACN Practice Alert. Preventing Catheter Related Bloodstream Infections. Available at www.aacn.org//AACN/practiceAlert.nsf/Files/Practice%20AlertCatherter%20Related%20BSI/$file/Practice%20AlertCatherter%20Related%20Blood%20Stream%20Infections.pdf. Retrieved on July 1, 2006.

2-12. **(D)** Pulse oximetry measures the percent of hemoglobin molecules that are saturated, but does not distinguish whether that saturation is with oxyhemoglobin or carboxyhemoglobin. During the initial management of patients with CO poisoning, arterial blood gas studies need to be used to evaluate a patient's oxygenation status. Poor tissue perfusion owing to hemodynamic instability leads to loss of pulsatile flow, signal failure, and unreliable readings. The cherry-red skin color is due to the binding of hemoglobin and CO in the blood. SaO_2 readings in the presence of carboxyhemoglobin are falsely elevated. The amount of oxygen a patient receives has no bearing on the accuracy of pulse oximetry.

Reference: Newberry, L., Criddle, L. M. (eds.). *Sheehy's Manual of Emergency Care,* 6th ed. Philadelphia, Elsevier, 2005, pp 470-471.

Urden, L. D., Stacy, K. M., Lough, M. E. *Thelan's Critical Care Nursing, Diagnosis and Management,* 5th ed. St. Louis, Elsevier, 2006, pp 616, 1057.

2-13. **(C)** Administration of agents that dilate the pulmonary arteries such as epoprostenol or calcium channel blocker agents will, in some cases, reduce right ventricular work and improve pulmonary blood flow and oxygenation. Phlebotomy may be considered in polycythemic patients with pulmonary hypertension when the hematocrit is greater than 60%. Fluid bolus may reduce blood viscosity but would not reduce symptoms owing to tricuspid valve incompetence. Increased cardiac contractility would not improve cardiac output in patients with tricuspid regurgitation.

Reference: Holcomb, S. S. Understanding pulmonary arterial hypertension. *Nurs Manage,* 3, 56A-56G, 2005.

2-14. **(A)** The body habitus of morbidly obese patients predisposes them to hypoventilation, particularly when in the supine position. Their body habitus does not lead to elevated intra-abdominal pressure (Option B), and their obesity does not alter immune responses (Option D). Option C is untrue.

Reference: Hurst, S., Blanco, K., Boyle, D., et al. Bariatric implications of critical care nursing. *Dimensions Crit Care Nurse,* 23, 76-83, 2004.

2-15. **(B)** The majority of postoperative complications in emergency hemicolectomy relate to infection, including sepsis, intra-abdominal abscess and wound infections. These complications are associated with increased morbidity and mortality. Using the sepsis bundle for early resuscitation, the intravascular volume needs to be re-established and the tissue beds need to be perfused to reduce tissue hypoxia. Lactate levels need to be kept less than 4 mmol/L. Normal central venous pressure is 5-8 mm Hg. A central venous pressure less than this indicates continued reduction in preload, which would not be an optimal response to the initiation of rapid fluid resuscitations. Urine output of 25 mL/hr is still below the norm of 30 mL/hr. This would not be an optimal response to rapid fluid administration. Cool, dry skin could indicate that the patient is experiencing peripheral vasoconstriction, suggesting continued hypovolemia and the need for further fluid resuscitation.

References: Dellinger, R. P., Vincent, J. L. The Surviving Sepsis Campaign sepsis change bundles and clinical practice. *Crit Care,* 9(6), 653-654, 2005.

Wyrzykowski, A. D., Feliciano, D. V., George, T. A., et al. Emergent right hemicolectomy. *Am Surg,* 71(8), 653-657, 2005.

2-16. **(A)** Dilated cardiomyopathy may be idiopathic or caused by toxic agents such as chemotherapy, alcohol, or cocaine. In dilated cardiomyopathy, death is usually related to the development of ventricular dysrhythmias, bradycardia, or thrombus formation in the dilated ventricle. Warfarin prevents clot formation and prevents death related to thrombus. Calcium channel blockers prevent supraventricular dysrhythmias, which are not common in dilated cardiomyopathy. Nitrates will improve coronary artery perfusion, but the primary defect in dilated cardiomyopathy is a structural defect in the ventricle that is not improved with administration of vasodilators. Digoxin improves contractility in cardiomyopathy but has no effect on the development of ventricular dysrhythmias, which may cause sudden death in this population. In addition, digoxin may contribute to the development of bradycardia, which could be detrimental.

Reference: Woods, S. L., Froelicher, E. S., Motzer, S. U., Bridges, E. J. *Cardiac Nursing,* 5th ed. Philadelphia, Lippincott Williams & Wilkins, 2005.

2-17. **(A)** Treprostinil sodium (Remodulin) is administered on a continuous subcutaneous basis, using a programmable pump. As a result, patients and caregivers must receive training in how to operate the pump. Treprostinil does not result in potential for pelvic bleeding. The drug is administered subcutaneously and does not interfere with digestion or cause indigestion. The pump does not use wireless technology.

Reference: Eells, P. L. Advances in prostacyclin therapy for pulmonary arterial hypertension. *Crit Care Nurse,* 24(2), 42-54, 2004.

2-18. **(C)** Transfusion of two units of packed red blood cells should increase the hemoglobin by 2 g/dL and the hematocrit by 4-6% in this patient with anemia. Patients with end-stage renal disease (ESRD) experience anemia secondary to a decrease in production of erythropoietin; as a result, there is diminished stimulation of the bone marrow to produce red blood cells. Transfusion of one unit of packed red blood cells will not sufficiently increase the patient's hemoglobin and hematocrit. Administration of Epoetin Alfa takes weeks to increase the hemoglobin and hematocrit and is contraindicated in patients with uncontrolled hypertension. Decreasing the dose of Epoetin Alpha will not address the problems of low hemoglobin and hematocrit.

References: Dressler, D. K. Hematology and immunology systems. In M. Chulay, S. M. Burns (eds.). *AACN Essentials of Critical Care Nursing.* New York, McGraw-Hill, 2006, pp 305-316.

Mayer, B. Hematologic disorders and oncologic emergencies. In L. D. Urden, K. M. Stacy, M. E. Lough (eds.). *Thelan's Critical Care Nursing: Diagnosis and Management,* 5ᵗʰ ed. St. Louis, Elsevier, 2006, pp 1128-1144.

Stark, J. L. The renal system. In J. G. Alspach (ed.). *Core Curriculum for Critical Care Nursing,* 6ᵗʰ ed. St. Louis, Elsevier, 2006, pp 525-607.

2-19. **(D)** An invasive strategy is preferred if the onset of symptoms and signs of acute MI have persisted for more than 3 hours from the time of presentation. Since the availability of open heart surgery as an intervention would cause further delay in treatment, percutaneous coronary intervention is the preferred therapy for this patient. Administration of thrombolytic therapy is contraindicated in a patient who has exhibited symptoms for longer than 3 hours. The patient has evidence of STEMI. Heparin and G IIb/IIIa inhibitors are indicated for patients with acute coronary syndrome.

Reference: Field, J. M., Hazinski, M. F., Gilmore, D. (eds.). *Handbook of Emergency Cardiovascular Care for Healthcare Providers.* Dallas, American Heart Association, 2006.

2-20. **(C)** Maintaining glucose levels <150 mg/dL has been shown to reduce morbidity in critically ill medical patients with sepsis. In a large double-blind study, human recombinant activated protein C decreased mortality by 6% in patients with severe sepsis and decreased mortality by 13% for patients at high risk for death (i.e., patients having an APACHE II score of 25 or greater), but there is no indication that this patient had severe sepsis, so Option A is not correct. When a patient is hypotensive, fluid replacement should be optimized before vasopressors

are started. Option B is incorrect because aggressive volume resuscitation is an essential early intervention for sepsis so that the hemodynamics altered by the inflammatory response are corrected prior to use of vasopressors. Option D is incorrect as two meta-analyses have concluded that high-dose corticosteroids are of no benefit or may be detrimental to patients with septic shock.

Reference: AACN Practice Alert. Severe Sepsis. Available at www.aacn.org/AACN/practiceAlert.nsf/Files/ss/$file/Severe%20Sepsis.pdf Retrieved July 1, 2006.

2-21. **(D)** Linear fracture of the temporal bone leading to laceration of the middle meningeal artery is the most common cause of epidural hematoma. Classically, these patients present with a history of a brief loss of consciousness immediately after the injury with a subsequent period of lucidity. Subsequently, these patients often deteriorate owing to the expanding arterial bleed. Epidural hematoma is a neurosurgical emergency. Urgent non-contrast head CT scan may be considered, but this patient's history would most likely result in immediate operative intervention for this surgical emergency. Option A, cerebral angiography and coil embolization, would be indicated for a cerebral aneurysm, not a traumatic brain injury (TBI). This patient was noted to have a linear left temporal skull fracture. Once the likely underlying epidural hematoma is evacuated, the patient should significantly improve and is unlikely to need (Option B) ventriculostomy and CSF drainage. If there were additional intracranial findings, these actions may be indicated. Option C, osmotic diuretic, may be given to patients with known head injury and focal neurologic deficits. However, corticosteroids are not indicated in traumatic brain injury.

References: Alspach, J. G. (ed.). *Core Curriculum for Critical Care Nursing,* 6ᵗʰ ed. St. Louis, Elsevier, 2006, p 475.

Bader, M. K., Littlejohns, L. R. (eds.). *AANN Core Curriculum for Neuroscience Nursing,* 4ᵗʰ ed. St. Louis, Elsevier, 2004.

Greenberg, M. S. (ed.). *Handbook of Neurosurgery,* 6ᵗʰ ed. New York, Thieme Medical Publishers, 2006.

2-22. **(D)** Sore throats, aching joints, and painful urination all signal activity of opportunistic bacteria and fungal growth associated with taking immunosuppressive medications to protect donor organs. Rapid recognition and intervention will help to avoid damage and potentially lethal infections. Neither restricted physical activity nor dietary restrictions will help avoid future infections. Drinking plenty of liquids will help avoid dehydration and infection, but this is not the best reply for avoiding delays in treatment.

References: Newberry, L., Criddle, L. *Sheehy's Manual of Emergency Care,* 6th ed. Philadelphia, Elsevier, 2006, pp 681-682.

Urden, L. D., Stacy, K. M., Lough, M. E. *Thelan's Critical Care Nursing: Diagnosis and Management,* 5th ed. St. Louis, Elsevier, 2006, pp 1105.

2-23. **(C)** The chest-x-ray demonstrates atelectasis, which may be due to obesity hypoventilation syndrome. Another common finding related to this syndrome is loss of hypoxic drive. Addition of CPAP will assist in opening the alveoli and decreasing atelectasis. Decreasing the FiO_2 may help to increase this patient's respiratory drive and reduce ventilator dependence. It should be anticipated that the patient may have sleep apnea after extubation and would benefit from Bi-PAP, but due to the difficulty in intubating the patient, immediate extubation prior to correcting atelectasis should occur. T-piece would not be an effective weaning strategy for this patient because inspiratory volumes would not be predictable owing to the restrictive effects of obesity, and positioning of bariatric patients may present challenges to effective ventilation owing to abdominal size and pressure on the diaphragm. Pressure support may not be an effective weaning mode for morbidly obese patients because of the increase in weight on the thorax preventing delivery of adequate tidal volumes.

Reference: Blouw, E. L., Rudolph, A. D., Narr, B. J., Sarr, M. G. The frequency of respiratory failure in patients with morbid obesity undergoing gastric bypass. *AANA J,* 71, 45-50, 2003.

2-24. **(D)** Data suggest that both low dose unfractionated heparin (UFH) and low molecular weight heparin (LMWH) are effective in preventing DVT in moderate-risk critical care patients. For patients at higher risk, such as those who have experienced major trauma or orthopedic surgery, LMWH has been shown to provide better protection than low dose UFH (Option B). Direct thrombin inhibitors may be used in place of LMWH or UFH for patients with documented or suspected heparin induced thrombocytopenia. In general, mechanical prophylaxis (Options A and C) is less effective when compared with anticoagulation-based therapy. Data suggest that there is a high risk of noncompliance with pneumatic compression devices. In one study involving below-the-knee graded stockings (Option C), 98% of commercially available stockings failed to produce an ideal pressure gradient, and 54% were found to produce a dangerous reverse pressure gradient.

Reference: AACN Practice Alert. Deep Vein Thrombosis Prevention. Available at www.aacn.org/AACN/practiceAlert.nsf/Files/dvt/$file/DVT.pdf Retrieved on July 1, 2006.

2-25. **(D)** Enterocutaneous fistulas can result in major fluid losses. The low serum albumin contributes to the development of edema and further increases intravascular fluid loss. Replacement of albumin is the most appropriate method to increase intravascular volume and blood pressure. The hematocrit is 30%, and blood replacement is not indicated until the hematocrit is decreased to 28% or less. The patient is on hyperalimentation, which contains glucose, and the serum glucose is low normal, so D50% is not indicated. Since the serum sodium is already elevated, fluid replacement with normal saline would be controversial. ½ normal saline may be preferred for fluid replacement in the hypernatremic patient.

Reference: Baird, M. S., Keen, J. H., Swearingen, P. L. *Manual of Critical Care Nursing.* St. Louis, Elsevier, 2005.

2-26. **(C)** The patient is exhibiting findings characteristic of an arthropod-borne encephalitis. CSF cultures would be most beneficial in identifying the causative organism. While (Option A) serologic tests may be of help, the nurse would not obtain a specimen while the patient is experiencing a grand mal seizure. Nor would the nurse (Option B) wait to intervene until the seizure is completed, as prolonged seizure activity is life-threatening. If a standing order for a benzo-diazepine is available for the patient, then the nurse would be able to quickly provide treatment to stop the seizure activity. If no order is available, the nurse should notify the physician to inform of the situation and obtain further orders. While it is important to protect the patient from injury, restraints (Option D) are not appropriate in this circumstance. Padded side rails would be most appropriate.

References: Alspach, J. G. (ed.). *Core Curriculum for Critical Care Nursing,* 6th ed. St. Louis, Elsevier, 2006.

Bader, M. K., Littlejohns, L. R. (eds.). *AANN Core Curriculum for Neuroscience Nursing,* 4th ed. St. Louis, Elsevier, 2004.

2-27. **(C)** Compared with Caucasians, all ethnic groups are more sensitive to the effects of central nervous system drugs and require lower doses. Asians metabolize CNS drugs more slowly than other groups and therefore require lower doses of antidepressants. Chinese in particular require lower doses of haloperidol. There are no data in the case to suggest the patient's symptoms are related to hypovolemia, as described in Option A. Option A also will not protect the patient from potentially getting too high a dose of medication. Option B is incorrect because it suggests the patient will receive a larger loading dose of this medication, which may cause harm. Option D is not the best choice because this test is not readily available in hospital laboratories and will not address the underlying issue of the patient requiring a lower dose of medication; in addition, this deficiency is not associated with metabolism of haloperidol.

Reference: Burroughs, V., Maxey, R., Crawley, L., et al. Cultural and Genetic Diversity in America: The Need for Individualized Pharmaceutical Treatment. Available at www.npcnow.org. Retrieved on July 1, 2006.

2-28. **(D)** Morphine sulfate is the most appropriate medication to relieve chest pain due to myocarditis. In myocarditis, pain is due to inflammation of the myocardium and is often related to autoimmune infiltration. Nitroglycerin is not effective in relieving the pain of myocarditis because the pain is not related to coronary blood flow. Diuret-ics may be effective to relieve symptoms of heart failure associated with myocarditis, but they would not relieve pain. Non-steroidal anti-inflammatory medications are contraindicated in chest pain associated with myocarditis because they may induce complications such as bleeding and tamponade.

References: Deason, J., Hope, B. A 23 year old man with chest pressure, pallor, tachypnea and tonsillitis. *J Emerg Nurs,* 31, 199-202, 2005.

Magnani, J. W., William, D. Myocarditis current trends in diagnosis and treatment. *Circulation,* 113, 876-890, 2006.

2-29. **(D)** In patients with liver dysfunction, an altered level of consciousness occurs due to the development of hepatic encephalopathy, which occurs when the detoxification functions of the liver are lost, resulting in impairment of the central nervous system. Hepatic encephalopathy is a neuropsychiatric disorder associated with portal hypertension. In the patient with acute liver failure, the development of encephalopathy follows the development of jaundice. An additional concern is that when patients develops encephalopathy, their ability to maintain a patent airway may become compromised. Hypotension is not a clinical feature of patients with hepatic dysfunction; hyperdynamic circulation is more likely with liver disorders. While esophageal bleeding is a potential complication with liver failure, this patient evidences no indications of that problem. Although the patient has elevated liver enzymes, there are no findings that specifically reflect the presence of systemic infection.

References: Hays, P. C., Simpson K. J. Approach to the patient with fulminant (acute) liver failure. In T. Yamada (ed.).*Textbook of Gastroenterology,* 4th ed. Philadelphia, Lippincott Williams & Wilkins, 2003.

Stewart, C. A., Cerhan, J. Hepatic encephalopathy: a dynamic or static condition. *Metab Brain Dis,* 20, 193-204, 2005.

2-30. **(C)** On the 12-lead ECG, posterior wall MI presents as tall, broad R waves and ST depression in leads V_1 and V_2. When reversed and rotated 180 degrees, these findings appear as deep Q waves and ST segment elevation. Unstable angina presents on the 12-lead ECG as transient ST depression and T wave inversion. Anterior septal MI presents with ST segment elevation in leads V_1-V_3. Pericarditis would present on the 12-lead ECG as ST segment elevation in the anterior leads V_1-V_6.

Reference: Sole, M. L., Klein, D. G., Moseley, M. J. *Introduction to Critical Care Nursing*, 4th ed. St. Louis, Elsevier, 2005.

2-31. **(A)** Social support can be emotional or instrumental in facilitating a need. Emotional support consists of receiving comforting gestures and knowing that someone is available. The patient does not appear to be experiencing anxiety (Option B). Patient needs related to Options C and D can be met through other activities, such as watching TV or reading.

References: Finfgeld-Connett, D. Clarification of social support. *J Nurs Scholarship*, 37(1), 4-9, 2005.

Hardin, S. R. Caring practices. In Hardin, S. R., Kaplow, R. (eds.). *Synergy for Clinical Excellence*. Sudbury, Jones & Bartlett, 2005, pp 69-74.

2-32. **(B)** Cautious use of antihypertensives (such as labetolol and hydralazine) and diuretics (such as furosemide) to decrease blood pressure without causing hypotension will help to maintain blood flow to the fetus and represent the goals of therapy in peripartum cardiomyopathy. Immediate C-section is not indicated unless the fetus demonstrates distress such as deceleration of fetal heart rate. ACE inhibitors are contraindicated in the antepartum period because they may cause birth defects, spontaneous abortions, stillbirth, and low birth weight due to fetal hypotension. Chronic use of beta blockers in pregnancy is associated with low birth weight, but beta blockers such as labetolol are frequently used to treat hypertensive emergencies in pregnancy.

Reference: Tidswell, M. Peripartum cardiomyopathy. *Crit Care Clin*, 20, 777-786, 2004.

2-33. **(B)** Patients with longstanding COPD have difficulty maintaining adequate nutritional intake owing to the caloric demands inflicted by increased work of breathing and by the great effort required to breathe and eat simultaneously. Cor pulmonale demonstrates as right heart failure and causes edema with weight gain. The weight loss may be associated with weaker thoracic excur-

sion and diminished ventilation and is not usually related to dehydration.

Reference: Nici, L., Donner, C., Wouters, E., et al. American Thoracic Society/European Respiratory Society statement on pulmonary rehabilitation. *Am J Respir Crit Care Med*, 173, 1390-1413, 2006.

2-34. **(D)** Data support that pulmonary embolus, anastomotic leaks, and respiratory failure account for 80% of all deaths within 30 days after bariatric surgery. These data need to be incorporated in the assessment and plan of care of these patients. Appropriate prophylaxis for venous thrombotic events usually includes low-molecular-weight heparin. Option A reflects some of the common short-term complications of bariatric surgery, which include wound infection, stomal stenosis, marginal ulceration, and constipation. Options B and C relate to some long-term complications of this surgery, including symptomatic cholelithiasis, dumping syndrome, persistent vomiting, and nutritional deficiencies.

Reference: Virji, A., Murr, M. M. Caring for patients after bariatric surgery. *Am Fam Physician*, 73(8), 1403-1408, 2006.

2-35. **(B)** Vasovagal reaction may occur during sheath removal and resolve rapidly after administration of atropine. If decreased blood pressure occurs without bradycardia, a normal saline bolus may be administered. Nausea occurs due to decreased blood pressure. Prochlorperazine (Compazine) is associated with vasodilation and would cause a further decrease in blood pressure. Retroperitoneal bleeding generally becomes evident after sheath removal when the puncture site is no longer protected by the sheath.

Reference: Baird, M. S., Keen, J. H., Swearingen, D. L. *Manual of Critical Care Nursing: Nursing Interventions and Collaborative Management*. St. Louis, Elsevier, 2005.

2-36. **(B)** Use of garlic may increase bleeding time. This can pose problems in patients undergoing invasive procedures. Not respecting a patient's desire to use complementary therapies, if not contraindicated, demonstrates a low level of caring practices. Option A is incorrect because the patient should not be taking garlic on the day of the procedure. Option C does not respect the patient's choice to use complementary therapies. Option D is not correct because patients are usually instructed to take their cardiac medications on the day of the procedure, and beta blocker therapy should continue unless contraindicated.

References: Agency for Healthcare Research and Quality: Garlic: Effects on cardiovascular risks and disease, protective effects against cancer, and clinical adverse effects. Evidence Report/Technology Assessment: Number 20. Rockville, MD, Author. Available at http://www.ahrq.gov/clinic/epcsums/garlicsum.htm. Retrieved on July 1, 2006.

Eschiti, V. S. A closing word: critically ill patients' use of complementary and alternative modalities. *Dimens Crit Care Nurs,* 25(1): 52-53, 2006.

2-37. **(B)** In right ventricular myocardial infarction, the right ventricle is unable to maintain forward flow to the lungs without adequate preload. Intravenous fluid administration increases right ventricular volume and promotes forward flow to the lungs. Diuretics would diminish circulating volume and preload, and so would aggravate the problem. Nitroglycerin and morphine cause vasodilation which decreases preload and would diminish right ventricular filling and output, thus worsening myocardial ischemia.

Reference: Woods, S. L., Froelicher, E. S., Motzer, S. U., Bridges, E. J. *Cardiac Nursing,* 5th ed. Philadelphia, Lippincott Williams & Wilkins, 2005.

2-38. **(A)** *Anterior cord syndrome* is commonly caused by flexion injuries as seen in head-on collisions or by acute herniation of an intervertebral disk. It is associated with injury to the anterior gray horn (motor) cells, the spinothalamic tracts (pain), the anterior spinothalamic tract (light touch), and the corticospinal tracts (temperature). This type of injury results in a loss of motor function and the ability to sense pain and temperature with intact position sense and sensation to pressure and vibration below the level of the injury. *Central cord syndrome* produces a motor and sensory deficit more pronounced in the upper extremities than in the lower extremities. *Brown-Sequard syndrome* presents as loss of voluntary motor movement on the same side as the injury with loss of pain, temperature, and sensation on the opposite side. *Posterior cord syndrome* results

in loss of position sense, pressure, and vibration below the level of injury with intact motor function and sensation of pain and temperature.

Reference: Urden, L. D., Stacy, K. M., Lough, M. E. *Thelan's Critical Care Nursing, Diagnosis and Management,* 5th ed. St. Louis, Elsevier, 2006, pp 981-984.

2-39. **(C)** Delivery of a succession of shocks by the AICD is termed *implantable cardioverter defibrillator storm.* After interrogation, if no mechanical error is found, the patient should be assessed for electrolyte imbalance, medication compliance and activities that may have induced the dysrhythmia. Since the device functioned appropriately, lead fracture is not suspected. EP testing would be indicated prior to device implant if the dysrhythmia required ablation.

Reference: O'Brien, M. C., Langberg, J., Valderrama, A. L., et al. Implantable cardioverter defibrillator storm: nursing care issues for patients and families. *Crit Care Nurs Clin North Am,* 17, 9-16, 2005.

2-40. **(C)** The earliest indication that aspiration may have occurred would be the development of tachypnea and tachycardia. The PaCO$_2$ may decrease with tachypnea associated with aspiration, and the tachypnea associated with aspiration is generally the reason an arterial blood gas is obtained. Chest x-ray findings are later signs and may be seen in the right middle lobe owing to the angle of the right mainstem bronchus, although infiltrates associated with aspiration may be located in any dependent lung field. This patient's cough reflex may be suppressed, and positive sputum cultures associated with bacterial infections may take up to 3 days to develop.

Reference: Myrianthefs, P. M., Kalafati, M., Samara, I., Baltopoulos, G. J. Nosocomial pneumonia. *Crit Care Nurs Q,* 27, 241-257, 2004.

2-41. **(C)** The patient failed to respond to the initial insulin infusion dose, which should have caused the serum glucose to drop by 50 mg/dL after each hour of therapy. Doubling the hourly infusion rate and continuing to monitor is the appropriate intervention under such a circumstance. Simply documenting and monitoring the patient will not achieve desirable results, as the patient will continue to produce ketone bodies. Increasing by 2 units/hr is inadequate because the client is failing to respond to a rate of 4 units/hr, and doubling the dose is the acceptable intervention. In this acute phase, it is too early to move to subcutaneous insulin, which has a slower rate of absorption than the intravenous route.

References: Newberry, L., Criddle, L. *Sheehy's Manual of Emergency Care,* 6th ed. Philadelphia, Elsevier, 2006, pp 426-431.

Urden, L. D., Stacy, K. M., Lough, M. E. *Thelan's Critical Care Nursing: Diagnosis and Management,* 5th ed. St. Louis, Elsevier, 2006, pp 934-937.

2-42. **(C)** The 12-lead ECG does not demonstrate evidence of ischemia or infarction, and the troponin level is within normal limits. This patient would benefit from serial ECGs and serum markers to determine if evolving myocardial ischemia is present. Immediate PCI or thrombolytic therapy is indicated if the patient has evidence of myocardial ischemia. Administration of aspirin should occur as soon as possible after the onset of chest pain. Administration of heparin and ACE inhibitors is indicated for patients at high or intermediate risk of cardiac ischemia.

Reference: Field, J. M., Hazinski, M. F., Gilmore, D. (eds.). *Handbook of Emergency Cardiovascular Care for Healthcare Providers.* Dallas, American Heart Association, 2006.

2-43. **(B)** The most appropriate action is Option B, because the most reliable source of information would be a chart audit to objectively quantify the number of cases and the specific outcome indicators for each. This option could also be accomplished quickly. Option A will delay securing data to determine the nature and extent of any problem for 6 months; if a problem were identified, its solution would be even further delayed, possibly compromising patient outcomes. Options C and D afford purely subjective discussions rather than the facts needed for future decision making at the organizational level.

Reference: Molter, N. Professional caring and ethical practice. In J. G. Alspach (ed.). *Core Curriculum for Critical Care Nursing,* 6th ed. St. Louis, Elsevier, 2006, pp 1-44.

2-44. **(C)** The primary goals of emergency management of intracerebral hemorrhage (ICH) are to prevent subsequent damage from rebleeding, edema, or hypoxia and to identify the cause, site and extent of the hemorrhage. If coagulopathies are present, these must be corrected in order to prevent further bleeding. In patients with ICH, BP reduction (Option A) should be gradual and controlled because acute BP normalization may reduce local cerebral perfusion pressure and cerebral blood flow to ischemic levels; in chronically hypertensive patients, it may shift the autoregulatory curve to higher pressures. BP treatment must be tailored to the needs of the individual patient. As a guide, for patients with a history of significant hypertension, the MAP should initially be maintained in the range of 120 mm Hg. In formerly nonhypertensive patients, lowering SBP to less than 160 mm Hg in the first hours after ICH may prevent additional bleeding. CT scan of the head is the primary imaging modality used for these patients, whereas cerebral angiography (Option B) is not commonly performed in this patient population. Size and location of an ICH are used to judge the usefulness of surgical interventions (Option D). While surgical intervention may be beneficial for noncomatose patients with large or enlarging superficial clots, traditional craniotomy with evacuation of spontaneous supratentorial hematomas has been shown to be ineffective in reducing mortality or disability in this patient population as a whole. Infratentorial hematomas, which often present with signs of brain stem compression, are often treated with surgical evacuation and have significantly decreased mortality in this subgroup.

References: Adams, H., Adams, R., Del Zoppo, G., Goldstein L. B. Guidelines for the early management of patients with ischemic stroke: 2005 guidelines update. A scientific statement from the Stroke Council of the American Heart Association/American Stroke Association. *Stroke,* 36: 916-923, 2005.

Grotta, J. C. Management of primary hypertensive hemorrhage of the brain. *Curr Treat Options Neurol,* 6(6), 435-442, 2004.

2-45. **(A)** There should be bubbling in the water seal chamber when the patient exhales to indicate that air is escaping from the pleural space. A large amount of bubbling that does not coincide with the patient's phase of ventilation suggests a large air leak in the system. Bubbling in the water seal chamber will disappear slowly as the lung re-expands to fill the pleural space and air stops leaking. There should not be any dependent loops in the chest drainage tubing system, as these may inhibit drainage. If suction is ordered, it will be a negative pressure. Positive pressure is not applied to a closed drainage system. A chest tube is not to be clamped unless specifically ordered by the physician or unless unit procedure calls for clamping as part of replacing or changing the system.

References: Ellstrom, K. Pulmonary system. In J. G. Alspach (ed.). *Core Curriculum for Critical Care Nursing,* 6th ed. St. Louis, Elsevier, 2006, p 151.
Roman, M., Mercado, D. Review of chest tube use. *Med-Surg Nurs,* 15(1), 41-43, 2006.

2-46. **(C)** Norepinephrine would be the vasopressor of choice in this particular patient. Norepinephrine is a positive inotrope and increases mean arterial pressure due to its vasoconstrictive effects, with little change in heart rate and less increase in stroke volume compared with dopamine. Because the patient is experiencing tachycardia with a heart rate of 110, dopamine would not be the initial choice. Epinephrine also has strong positive chronotropic effects, so would not be the preferred agent. Vasopressin is a direct vasoconstrictor and a negative inotrope. Use of vasopressin can lead to coronary artery and splanchnic ischemia, resulting in further compromise of a critically ill patient.

Reference: Dellinger, R. P., Carlet, J. M., Masur, H., et al. Surviving Sepsis Campaign guidelines for management of severe sepsis and septic shock. *Crit Care Med* 32(3), 858-873, 2004.

2-47. **(A)** Patients receiving a large volume of fluids and blood components are at high risk for dilutional coagulopathy, which is accentuated with hypothermia (temperature less than 36.5° C or 97.7° F); therefore, warming blood components and fluids will help control factors altering coagulopathy. Monitoring laboratory values alone will not prevent the development of complications. Antihistamine and anti-inflammatory medication will help to decrease immune

responses to blood transfusions, including febrile incidents and pruritis, but these are not life-threatening complications. In times of trauma and shock, intramuscular injections are poorly absorbed.

References: Newberry, L., Criddle, L. *Sheehy's Manual of Emergency Care,* 6th ed. Philadelphia, Elsevier, 2006, pp 117-122.
Schell, H., Puntillo, K. A. *Critical Care Nursing Secrets,* 2nd ed. St. Louis, Elsevier, 2006, p 433.

2-48. **(A)** Mediastinal bleeding is very common in the early postoperative period after VAD implantation. The extracorporeal circuits and anticoagulation for the procedure increase coagulopathy. VADs may be pulsatile or continuous flow. Flow rates are generally maintained high enough to prevent thrombus formation, so anticoagulants may not be necessary, but blood contact with the circuits increases the risk of thrombus formation. Ventricular assist devices are now portable so patients are not restricted from contact with others (except those with infections). Neutropenia does not occur with VAD implantation unless the patient receives immunosuppression in the immediate pretransplant period. Although the patient may become immunologically sensitized, this does not prevent future transplant.

Reference: Bojar, R. M. *Manual of Perioperative Care in Adult Cardiac Surgery*, 4th ed. Berlin, VT, Blackwell, 2005.

2-49. **(D)** Blood pressure reductions that occur after bariatric surgery and substantial weight loss depend on the blood pressure status of patients before surgery: normotensive patients and hypertensive patients taking antihypertensive medications show small postsurgical pressure reductions, while patients with elevated blood pressure before surgery show notable postsurgical pressure drops. Option A does not answer the patient's question directly even though it illustrates the nurse's ability to collaborate with other members of the multidisciplinary team. Option B describes gastric banding, which is not the procedure the patient had. Gastric leakage does not necessarily cause a change in a patient's blood pressure.

Reference: Fernstrom, J. D., Courcoulas, A. P., Houck, P. R., Fernstrom, M. H. Long-term changes in blood pressure in extremely obese patients who have undergone bariatric surgery. *Arch Surg,* 141(3), 276-283, 2006.

2-50. **(D)** After turning a postoperative coronary artery bypass patient, it is common to have an increase in chest tube drainage, from blood which has pooled. The nurse should continue to monitor drainage, and if drainage continues at 200 mL/hr after the patient is turned, the physician should be notified. Autotransfusion is generally performed when there is greater than 400 mL of blood in the autotransfusion apparatus. Stripping of chest tubes is controversial. Aggressive stripping may damage the myocardial or pleural tissue. Coagulation studies are not indicated unless the patient exhibits continued bleeding.

Reference: Bojar, R. M. *Manual of Perioperative Care in Adult Cardiac Surgery*, 4th ed. Berlin, VT, Blackwell, 2005.

2-51. **(C)** The resuscitation of a patient in severe sepsis or sepsis-induced tissue hypoperfusion (hypotension or lactic acidosis) should begin as soon as the syndrome is recognized. An elevated serum lactate concentration identifies tissue hypoperfusion in patients at risk who are not hypotensive. Early goal-directed therapy has been shown to improve survival for patients presenting with septic shock. Resuscitation directed toward the following four goals for the initial 6-hour period of the resuscitation reduced 28-day mortality: (1) CVP 8-12 mm Hg (in ventilated patients: 12-15 mm Hg); (2) mean arterial pressure ≥65 mm Hg; (3) urine output ≥ 0.5 mL/kg/hr; (4) continuous central venous oxygen saturation ($ScVO_2$) ≥70% (normal 70% to 80%).

References: Alspach, J. G. (ed.). *Core Curriculum for Critical Care Nursing,* 6th ed. St. Louis, Elsevier, 2006, p 768.

Dellinger, R. P., Carlet, J. M., Masur, H., et al. Surviving Sepsis Campaign guidelines for management of severe sepsis and septic shock. *Crit Care Med* 32(3), 858-873, 2004.

2-52. **(A)** Nesiritide (Natrecor) is a potent vasodilator used in the treatment of heart failure that may cause profound hypotension. It should be withheld if the patient's blood pressure is below 90 mm Hg. Although placing the patient flat in bed would improve blood pressure, it would likely increase respiratory distress and lower the SpO_2. A fluid bolus is inappropriate in this instance as it would likely worsen the patient's heart failure. The diuresis resulting from furosemide (Lasix) administration may further decrease blood pressure.

Reference: Smith, A. L., Brown, C. S. New advances and novel treatments in heart failure. *Crit Care Nurs,* 23, S11-S20, 2003.

2-53. **(B)** Alleviation of postoperative pain will allow the patient to perform breathing exercises focused on prevention of atelectasis. Although the patient may require increased oxygen, the breathing exercises will likely restore his oxygen saturation to acceptable levels. There is no clinical evidence of hemothorax; breath sounds are diminished owing to lobe removal on the right and atelectasis on the left. Anxiety management alone would be insufficient to improve this patient's pulmonary status.

References: Alspach, J. G. (ed.). *Core Curriculum for Critical Care Nursing,* 6th ed. St. Louis, Elsevier, 2006.

Brunner, Suddarth (eds.). *Textbook of Medical-Surgical Nursing,* 10th ed. Philadelphia, Lippincott Williams & Wilkins, 2004.

2-54. **(C)** Pleural effusion and pain are complications of pancreatitis that can negatively affect management of ARDS. Pancreatic enzymes released into the circulation damage pulmonary vasculature and stimulate inflammation, leading to intrapulmonary shunt and hypoxemia. Exudates may then cross the diaphragm and enter the pleural space via lymphatic channels, causing pleural effusions. Pleural effusions can reduce pulmonary compliance and limit lung expansion. The hypovolemia experienced by patients with acute peritonitis is typically a relative form owing to third-spacing of fluids within the abdomen and can be managed with fluids to optimize preload and circulating volume. Autodigestion of body tissues by pancreatic enzymes can lead to fistula formation and impaired skin integrity, but these problems do not significantly affect pulmonary function. The pain associated with acute pancreatitis is often characterized as "the worst ever" and could compromise pulmonary function via limited lung expansion and guarding. Effective, aggressive, and continual pain management should enable avoidance of additional pulmonary compromise owing to pain.

Reference: Pastor, C. M., Matthay, M. A., Frossard, J. L. Pancreatitis associated acute lung injury: new insights. *Chest,* 124, 2341-2351, 2003.

2-55. **(C)** Pericardial tamponade from lead perforation would result in symptoms of JVD and hypotension with narrowed pulse pressure. Hemothorax or pneumothorax may cause diminished breath sounds on the affected side. Pacemaker syndrome results from loss of atrial kick during pacing and may cause altered mental status and hypotension, but not narrowed pulse pressure or JVD.

Reference: Howell, C., Bergin, J. D. A case report of pacemaker lead perforation causing late pericardial effusion and subacute cardiac tamponade. *J Cardiovasc Nurs,* 20, 271-275, 2005.

2-56. **(D)** The preceptor needs to use evidence-based interventions such as testing via pH paper to assess nasogastric tube placement and prevent potential harm. Option A is refuted by case reports in which bubbling did not occur despite malpositioning of the tube within the airways. Option B is incorrect because the literature contains numerous reports of the ineffectiveness of air insufflation and auscultation for verification of tube location. Option C is also not optimal. Although observing for respiratory distress may be useful, there have been reports of failures of this method such that 16 Fr to 18 Fr NG tubes malpositioned in the respiratory tract did not induce immediate respiratory distress in patients with neurologic debilitation or advanced respiratory disease.

Reference: AACN Practice Alert. Verification of Feeding Tube Placement. Available at www.aacn.org/AACN/practiceAlert.nsf/Files/FTP/$file/Verification%20of%20Feeding%20Tube%20Placement.pdf Retrieved on July 1, 2006

2-57. **(C)** The diet plan for patients with acute renal failure is restricted in intake of fluid, protein, phosphorus, and potassium, making an adequate intake of calories, vitamins, and minerals difficult. Protein is restricted on a renal diet to prevent increasing the patient's BUN. This restriction is necessary despite the renal patient's increased requirements for protein secondary to metabolic acidosis, catabolic conditions, and losses from dialysis, wounds, or corticosteroid drugs. The protein deficit weakens muscles and increases the patient's susceptibility to infection. Carbohydrates are encouraged in the renal diet to provide energy for metabolism and healing. Fluid overload may be the precursor of other conditions, such as heart failure and respiratory failure, which may lead to risk for infection. Fluid restriction is a requirement of the renal diet and does not place the patient at risk for infection.

Reference: Mitchell, J. G. Renal disorders and therapeutic management. In L. D. Urden, K. M. Stacy, M. E. Lough (eds.). *Priorities in Critical Care Nursing,* 4th ed. St. Louis, Elsevier, 2004, pp 333-356.
Moore, M. C. Nutritional alterations. In L. D. Urden, K. M. Stacy, M E. Lough (eds.). *Priorities in Critical Care Nursing,* 4th ed. St. Louis, Elsevier, 2004, pp 51-64.

2-58. **(C)** In patients on diuretic therapy, the vascular system may be depleted and need fluid augmentation despite the presence of rales and heart failure. This patient has an elevated HCT suggesting hypovolemia, a low serum albumin that would contribute to loss of fluid into the interstitial spaces, and a BUN/creatinine ratio greater than 20:1, indicating hypovolemia. Dobutamine infusion would increase the force of ventricular contraction but would not raise BP if the stroke volume remained low owing to intravascular volume depletion. Norepinephrine (Levophed) could temporarily increase BP via vasoconstriction, but vasopressors should be used only after volume deficits are corrected. Furosemide (Lasix) would further decrease intravascular volume.

Reference: Baird, M. S., Keen, J. H., Swearingen, P. L. *Manual of Critical Care Nursing.* St. Louis, Elsevier, 2005.

2-59. **(D)** Insofar as it is possible, allowing patients to continue their customary routines and practices while in the hospital is the best approach because it offers COPD patients the greatest amount of control, which can lessen anxiety and maintain a more positive outlook. A mental health consult may be advisable for some COPD patients but is not warranted for others. The health care team should consider continuing antidepressants and other medications during the exacerbation, but benzodiazepines are not indicated for all COPD patients.

References: Hynninen, K. M., Bretieve, M. H., Wiborg, A. B., et al. Clinical characteristics of patients with chronic obstructive pulmonary disease: a review. *J Psychosomatic Res,* 59, 429-443, 2005.

Nici, L., Donner, C., Wouters E., et al. American Thoracic Society/European Respiratory Society statement on pulmonary rehabilitation. *Am J Respir Crit Care Med,* 173, 1390-1413, 2006.

2-60. **(C)** Spirituality has potential importance for acute and critically ill patients and families. Spirituality may influence understanding of suffering and illness and how a patient or family copes with the situation. By addressing spiritual issues, critical care nurses can create more holistic and compassionate systems of care. Option A is incorrect since spirituality may promote a patient's clinical stability. Option B is incorrect because spirituality issues can be addressed during all phases of health and illness. Option D is incorrect and demonstrates lack of respect for a patient's beliefs.

Reference: Puchalski, C. Spirituality in health: the role of spirituality in critical care. *Crit Care Clin,* 20(3), 487-504, 2004.

2-61. **(B)** Intra-aortic balloon counterpulsation increases myocardial oxygen supply by increasing coronary artery perfusion when balloon inflation occurs during diastole. Just prior to ventricular systole, the balloon is deflated, allowing the left ventricle to eject against a low volume in the aorta. This reduction of afterload effectively decreases the left ventricular workload. Balloon augmentation improves contractility by supporting more efficient left ventricular emptying, thus increasing cardiac output. Neither myocardial oxygen supply nor left ventricular filling volume is directly affected. Although the balloon-augmented systolic pressure is higher than the aortic systolic pressure, left ventricular systolic pressure is not increased.

Reference: Woods, S. L., Froelicher, E. S., Motzer, S. U., Bridges, E. J. *Cardiac Nursing,* 5th ed. Philadelphia, Lippincott Williams & Wilkins, 2005.

2-62. **(D)** In sepsis, activated protein C is used to *increase* fibrinolysis, *decrease* coagula-

tion, and *decrease* inflammation. Protein C is a natural component of the *anticoagulant* system. In sepsis, decreased levels of circulating APC result in increased formation of clots and decreased fibrinolysis. Thrombin plays a role in activating the inactive form of protein C by binding with thrombomodulin. Owing to the decreased levels of protein C during sepsis, increased thrombin activity will not increase the risk of bleeding in this patient. Increased platelet activity and coagulation will propagate the formation of clots.

References: Dellinger, R. P., Carlet, J. M., Masur, H., et al. Surviving Sepsis Campaign guidelines for management of severe sepsis and septic shock. *Crit Care Med* 32(3), 858-873, 2004.

Tazhir, J. Sepsis and the role of activated protein C. *Crit Care Nurse* 24(6), 40-45, 2004.

2-63. **(A)** Option A shows the nurse taking the initiative to find a solution to the patient's problem with compliance in medication administration. Neither Option B nor Option D helps the patient with her vision problem. Option C might be considered as collaboration; however, this patient does not warrant long-term placement until all possible solutions to keep her independent have been exhausted.

References: Molter, N. Professional caring and ethical practice. In J. G. Alspach (ed.). *Core Curriculum for Critical Care Nursing,* 6th ed. St. Louis, Elsevier, 2006, pp 1-44.

2-64. **(B)** Thrombolytic therapy is indicated in patients with chest pain onset of less than 3 hours associated with ST segment elevation in indicative leads or new onset of LBBB and positive serum markers. The normal value for troponin I is less than 0.1 ng/mL. Troponin levels do not rise after myocardial injury until 4 hours after onset of symptoms. ST segment elevation in leads V_1-V_6 indicates pericarditis. Thrombolytic therapy is contraindicated in pericarditis as it may cause bleeding and cardiac tamponade.

Reference: Field, J. M., Hazinski, M. F., Gilmore, D. (eds.). *Handbook of Emergency Cardiovascular Care for Healthcare Providers.* Dallas, American Heart Association, 2006.

2-65. **(C)** The most common symptom of pulmonary hypertension associated with cor pulmonale is exertional dyspnea. Other clinical manifestations include those characteristic of right heart failure (i.e., fatigue, increased central venous pressures, jugular venous distention, hepatomegaly, splenomegaly, and peripheral edema, especially in dependent areas). Distant heart sounds are heard in pericardial tamponade or effusion. Although patients with COPD may experience cough, that finding reflects their pulmonary rather than cardiac disorder.

References: Calverley, P. Chronic obstructive pulmonary diseases. In M. P. Fink, E. Abraham, J. L. Vincent, P. M. Kochanek (eds.). *Textbook of Critical Care,* 5th ed. Philadelphia, Elsevier, 2005.

Ellstrom, K. The pulmonary system. In J. G. Alspach (ed.). *Core Curriculum for Critical Care Nursing,* 6th ed. St. Louis, Elsevier, 2006.

2-66. **(A)** Sodium nitroprusside and esmolol are used in combination to achieve blood pressure reduction, heart rate control, and decreased contractility. Titration of infusions is typically ordered to achieve a MAP of 70 mm Hg and heart rate of 70/min.

Reference: Stone, C. K., Humphries, R. L. *Current Emergency Diagnosis and Treatment,* 5th ed. New York, McGraw-Hill, 2004.

2-67. **(C)** Normal arterial pCO_2 is 35 to 45 mm Hg. Generally, hyperventilation is avoided in the early hours after head injury in order to prevent ischemia and worsening of related secondary injury. Chronic prophylactic hyperventilation therapy should be avoided during the first 5 days after severe TBI, particularly during the first 24 hours. Mild hyperventilation (arterial pCO_2 30 to 35 mm Hg) is considered for management of intracranial hypertension when measures such as osmotic therapy (mannitol), cerebrospinal fluid drainage (in patients with an external ventricular drain), sedation, and chemical paralysis are ineffective. More severe hyperventilation resulting in severe hypocapnia (Options A and B) is generally avoided to prevent ischemia. Higher levels of hyperventilation (Option D) can cause vasodilation, increasing cerebral blood volume and raising ICP.

References: Bullock, R., Chesnut, R. M., Clifton, G., et al. Guidelines for the management and prognosis of severe traumatic brain injury. *J Neurotrauma,* 17, 451–553, 2000.

Robertson, C. Critical care management of traumatic brain injury. In H. R. Winn (ed.). *Youmans Neurological Surgery,* 5th ed. Philadelphia, Elsevier, 2004.

2-68. **(A)** Permanent pacemakers have a pre-set delay after a sensed P wave called the AV delay, in which there is a longer interval allowed after an intrinsic P wave for the P wave to conduct to the ventricle. If no P wave is sensed, the pacemaker will pace the ventricle in a shorter time period. This rhythm strip demonstrates the occurrence of paced ventricular impulses occurring at a later time period when no intrinsic SA node activity is present. Failure to sense would result in inappropriate pacemaker discharge. Failure to pace would be demonstrated by the presence of a pacemaker artifact without a corresponding paced P or QRS. Over-sensing would be demonstrated by an interval where a pacemaker artifact would be anticipated but is absent.

Reference: Woods, S. L., Froelicher, E. S., Motzer, S. U., Bridges, E. J. *Cardiac Nursing,* 5th ed. Philadelphia, Lippincott Williams & Wilkins, 2005.

2-69. **(A)** The endoscopy procedure may evoke patient responses that include tachycardia, dysrhymias, and hypoxia. As a result, it is important to monitor for cardiac ischemia during the examination. In patients such as this with known heart disease, there is an increased risk of these cardiovascular effects. IV fluids should be administered as indicated by the patient's hemodynamic status; however, during endoscopy, risk of a cardiopulmonary event is a greater concern than fluid monitoring. The need to monitor this patient's ABGs and electrolytes is part of overall patient assessment and is not heightened by the endoscopy procedure. Maintenance of normothermia is not a particular concern for this patient.

Reference: Krumberger, J., Parrish, C. R., Krenitsky, J. Gastrointestinal system. In M. Chulay, S. Burns (eds.). *AACN Essentials of Critical Care Nursing.* New York, McGraw-Hill, 2006, p 321.

2-70. **(A)** Pulmonary contusion causes impairment of gas exchange at the gas tissue interface. The most common etiology of pulmonary contusion is trauma related to a motor vehicle crash. The greater the degree of pulmonary contusion, the greater the degree of ventilatory impairment. Administration of pain medication will improve ventilation and decrease splinting, and the administration of oxygen will improve oxygenation and gas exchange. Auscultation of lung sounds is appropriate; however, pulmonary contusions do not require insertion of chest tubes as there is no hemothorax or pneumothorax. Patients can be managed without mechanical ventilation if their PaO_2 is greater than 60 mm Hg on 50% FiO_2, their respiratory rate is less than 24 breaths/min, spontaneous tidal volume is more than 5 mL/kg, and vital capacity exceeds 10 mL/kg. There is no evidence of a pleural effusion. A subsequent intervention would be to obtain a chest x-ray. If a chest x-ray revealed a pleural effusion, then a thoracentesis would be done if the effusion was significantly impairing the patient's ventilatory status.

References: Ellstrom, K. Pulmonary system. In J. G. Alspach (ed.). *Core Curriculum for Critical Care Nursing,* 6th ed. St. Louis, Elsevier, 2006, p 149.

Yamamoto, L., Schroeder, C., Morely, D., Beiveau, C. Thoracic trauma: The deadly dozen. *Crit Care Nurse Q,* 28(1), 22-40, 2005.

2-71. **(A)** Myocardial contusion may result from blunt cardiac trauma. Hypotension and cardiac dysrhythmias place the patient at high risk of complications. Diagnostic findings of myocardial contusion include chest pain, ECG changes including tachycardia, bundle branch block, and dysrhythmias. Echocardiogram findings are generally nonspecific in myocardial contusion and include wall motion abnormalities. Pulmonary contusion may lead to ARDS, and symptoms include respiratory failure and hypoxia. Cardiac chamber rupture would result in the development of a murmur and signs of cardiogenic shock. Cardiac tamponade would cause decreased QRS amplitude on the 12-lead ECG, muffled heart tones, JVD and hypotension.

Reference: American College of Surgeons Committee on Trauma. *Advanced Trauma Life Support for Doctors,* 7th ed. Chicago, American College of Surgeons, 2004.

2-72. **(B)** Allowing the group to complete their prayer session supports the patient's cultural and perhaps religious beliefs and displays cultural sensitivity. Interrupting the prayer (Option B) is inappropriate, unwarranted, and insensitive to the patient's belief system. Option C would not be appropriate as movement into the group could disrupt the prayer session. Observing the session (Option D) appears unwarranted as there is no indication that patient safety has been jeopardized in any way.

References: Hardin, S. R. Response to diversity. In S. R. Hardin, R. Kaplow, R. (eds.). *Synergy for Clinical Excellence.* Sudbury, Jones & Bartlett, 2005, pp 91-96.

Molter, N. Professional caring and ethical practice. In J. G. Alspach (ed.). *Core Curriculum for Critical Care Nursing,* 6th ed. St. Louis, Elsevier, 2006, pp 1-44.

2-73. **(A)** Hypokalemia predisposes the patient to development of ventricular dysrhythmias. The normal values for serum potassium are 3.5-5.0 mEq/L. The normal serum sodium is 135-145 mEq/L, and abnormal sodium levels generally have effects on blood pressure, muscle strength, and sensorium but do not predispose to ventricular dysrhythmias. Magnesium is used in the treatment of ventricular tachyarrythmias and may be beneficial even when serum magnesium levels are normal. Low serum calcium may have a negative inotropic effect on the myocardium but does not affect the ventricular rate unless the dysrhythmia is caused by calcium channel blocker toxicity and resulted in heart block.

Reference: Sole, M. L., Klein, D. G., Moseley, M. J. *Introduction to Critical Care Nursing,* 4th ed. St. Louis, Elsevier, 2005.

2-74. **(B)** The combination of respiratory alkalosis and metabolic acidosis, as evidenced by an elevated anion gap, is the hallmark of salicylate toxicity. Salicylates such as aspirin (acetylsalicylic acid) stimulate the respiratory center, causing hyperventilation that results in respiratory alkalosis along with a compensatory renal loss of bicarbonate. Salicylates also cause the uncoupling of oxidative phosphorylation, which leads to deceased ATP production, increased oxygen consumption, increased CO_2 production, and increased heat production. Derangements in the Krebs cycle and in carbohydrate metabolism leads to an accumulation of organic acids, including pyruvate, lactate, and acetoacetate, resulting in a metabolic acidosis. Acetaminophen toxicity leads to hepatic necrosis and massive liver damage. Patients will present with GI irritation, lethargy, and diaphoresis/pallor and, in rare cases of massive poisoning, will develop metabolic acidosis (low pH and low HCO_3) within the first 24 hours. Signs and symptoms of NSAID toxicity include metabolic acidosis (low pH and low HCO_3), lethargy, hypotension, bradycardia, apnea, renal failure and hepatotoxicity. Benzodiazepine overdose manifests as behavior associated with excessive alcohol ingestion, respiratory depression, dilated pupils, and weak and rapid pulse. ABG results would show a respiratory acidosis (low pH and elevated pCO_2) secondary to respiratory depression.

Reference: Newberry, L., Criddle, L. M. (eds.). *Sheehy's Manual of Emergency Care,* 6th ed. Philadelphia, Elsevier, 2005, pp 464-465.

2-75. **(B)** Seizures are defined as a discrete event characterized by an excessive and disorderly discharge of cerebral neurons with associated sensory, motor, and/or behavioral changes. Seizures warrant treatment when they last longer than 3 minutes in order to avoid the possibility of permanent neurological injury. Frequent neurological examinations (Option A) are appropriate in the early postoperative period. High-dose phenobarbital (Option C) may be given if seizures are refractory to other medications. A postoperative imaging study (Option D) may be obtained to evaluate structural changes after surgery and to identify any complications, such as a blood clot.

References: Bader, M. K., Littlejohns, L. R. (eds.). *AANN Core Curriculum for Neuroscience Nursing,* 4th ed. St. Louis, Elsevier, 2004.
Greenberg, M. S. (ed.). *Handbook of Neurosurgery,* 6th ed. New York, Thieme Medical Publishers, 2006.

2-76. **(D)** Norepinephrine (Levophed) is a potent vasoconstricting agent that rapidly increases blood pressure. Dopamine is indicated in pulmonary edema when blood pressure is at least 70 mm Hg. Dobutamine is a positive inotropic agent that is indicated in pulmonary edema when the blood pressure is 70 to 100 mm Hg and signs of shock are *not* present. Nitroglycerin may be indicated in pulmonary edema to reduce systemic vascular resistance and cardiac work when the systolic blood pressure is greater than 90-100 mm Hg.

Reference: Field, J. M., Hazinski, M. F., Gilmore, D. (eds.). *Handbook of Emergency Cardiovascular Care for Healthcare Providers.* Dallas, American Heart Association, 2006.

2-77. **(A)** Complementary therapy (such as music or touch) has not been shown to be associated with safety concerns and appears to reduce pain and tension during early recovery from open heart surgery. Option B is incorrect because it negates the family's interest in providing a therapy that may assist the patient. The first portion of Option C and Option D are untrue (there are no biomedical or electrical safety concerns) for battery-operated music players, but the latter portion of Option C is not true, as there are data to suggest that pain may be reduced in the immediate postoperative period with use of complementary therapies.

Reference: Kshettry, V. R., Carole, L. F., Henly, S. J., et al. Complementary alternative medical therapies for heart surgery patients: feasibility, safety, and impact. *Ann Thor Surg,* 81(1), 201-205, 2006.

2-78. **(D)** Blunt traumatic injuries include lung contusion, spontaneous pneumothorax, myocardial contusion, and rupture of trachea, as well as soft tissue injuries such as abrasions, lacerations, burns, and hematomas. Frequent evaluation of breath sounds, thoracic symmetry, and tracheal position is important for the early identification of secondary injury development such a spontaneous or tension pneumothorax. Reduction in oxygen saturation can indicate the development of pulmonary barotrauma, the most common fatal primary blast injury, evidenced clinically with chest wall motion changes, unequal breath sounds, decreased pulmonary compliance, subcutaneous emphysema, decreased oxygenation, pulmonary embolism, or pneumothorax. Thoracic blast injury produces a unique cardiovascular response that may cause death in the absence of any demonstrable physical injury. The immediate cardiovascular response to pulmonary blast injury is a decrease in heart rate, stroke volume, and cardiac index. The normal reflex increase in systemic vascular resistance does not occur, so blood pressure falls. This effect occurs within seconds and, if it is not fatal, recovery usually occurs within 15 minutes to 3 hours.

References: Ellstrom, K. Pulmonary system. In J. G. Alspach (ed.). *Core Curriculum for Critical Care Nursing*, 6th ed. St. Louis, Elsevier, 2006, p 140.

Lavonis, E., Pennardt, A. Blast Injuries. Accessed October 17, 2006 at ttp://www.emedicine.com/emerg/topic63.htm

Yamamoto, L., Schroeder, C., Morely, D., Beiveau, C. Thoracic trauma: the deadly dozen. *Crit Care Nurse Q,* 28(1), 2005, 22-40.

2-79. **(A)** Acute MI with papillary muscle rupture requires both revascularization and valve repair or replacement. Immediate treatment may be accomplished with open heart surgery. If immediate cardiac surgery is not available, PTCA and IABP may stabilize the patient until transfer to a facility that performs cardiac valve repair can occur. IABP therapy decreases afterload and reduces mitral valve regurgitation. Thrombolytics should not be administered to the patient with papillary muscle rupture because that would delay valve replacement surgery and allow cardiogenic shock to continue without definitive treatment until the half-life of the thrombolytics has transpired. IABP and vasopressor support may be used to stabilize the patient until surgery but will not reperfuse the occluded coronary artery.

Reference: Woods, S. L., Froelicher, E. S., Motzer, S. U., Bridges, E. J. *Cardiac Nursing,* 5th ed. Philadelphia, Lippincott Williams & Wilkins, 2005.

2-80. **(C)** Administration of normal saline will help replace fluids, providing volume to improve the blood pressure and urinary output, while helping to dilute glucose levels and blood viscosity. Administration of bicarbonate would fail to benefit the patient in that it would result in alkalemia, too rapid a shift of potassium back into the cells, and potentially cause cerebral edema, central acidosis, and death. Glargine insulin is a long acting, basal analog preparation that provides a more physiologic control of glucose; however, it would not provide the rapid correction required for this patient. Correction of serum potassium will be needed as glucose is corrected; however, it would be inappropriate to administer it while the patient is oliguric.

References: Newberry, L., Criddle, L. *Sheehy's Manual of Emergency Care,* 6th ed. Philadelphia, Elsevier, 2006, pp 426-431.

Urden, L. D., Stacy, K. M., and Lough, M. E. *Thelan's Critical Care Nursing: Diagnosis and Management,* 5th ed. St. Louis, Elsevier, 2006, pp 934-937.

2-81. **(C)** Patients with COPD have some degree of nonreversible damage to their lungs, so, rather than regaining textbook "normal" function or laboratory or diagnostic study values (Option A), COPD patients—in the best of situations—will regain their former baseline function and laboratory values. Pressure support and spontaneous breathing trials are both used for weaning COPD patients from mechanical ventilation.

Reference: Calverley, P. Chronic obstructive pulmonary diseases. In M. P. Fink, E. Abraham, J. L. Vincent, P. M. Kochanek (eds.). *Textbook of Critical Care,* 5th ed. Philadelphia, Elsevier, 2005.

2-82. **(D)** Acetaminophen is the most appropriate medication to administer to this elderly patient to reduce pain and permit participation with planned exercise. It will not cloud sensorium and does not affect blood pressure or sodium reabsorption. Nonsteroidal anti-inflammatory medications are contraindicated in heart failure because they may cause sodium and water retention, which would exacerbate symptoms of failure. Corticosteroids also cause sodium and water retention. Morphine sulfate 5 mg is a large dose for an 80-year-old patient and may cause hypotension and drowsiness, which would impede participation in the exercise program.

Reference: Wheeler, M., Wingate, S. Managing non-cardiac pain in heart failure patients. *J Cardiovasc Nurs,* 19, S75-S83, 2004.

2-83. **(D)** No action is needed for this patient as all of the parameters are within acceptable range. Normal cerebral perfusion pressure decreases from 80 mL/min/100 g at age 30 years to 40 mL/min/100 g at age 70 years. Normal intracranial pressure is up to 15 mm Hg. Option D is incorrect because even if ICP were elevated, hyperventilation down to a p_aCO_2 of 30 mm Hg is no longer recommended based on research findings.

Reference: Kane R. L., Ouslander, J. G., Abrass, I. B. *Essentials of Clinical Geriatrics,* 5th ed. New York, McGraw-Hill, 2003.

2-84. **(C)** The absolute neutrophil count (ANC) is calculated by multiplying the total WBC by the percentage of neutrophils in the differential WBC count. The percentage of neutrophils consists of the segmented (fully mature) + the bands (almost mature neutrophils). The normal range for the ANC = 1.5 to 8.0 (1,500 to 8,000/mm³). Below 1.5 indicates that the patient is severely immunosuppressed and will require neutropenic precautions to prevent the development of overwhelming infection. In this patient, $4000 \times 25\%$ (10% + 15%) = 1000/mm³ or an ANC of 1.0.

Reference: Marr, J. A. Care of patients with neutropenia. *Clin J Oncol Nurs* 10(2), 164-166, 2006.

2-85. **(C)** Labetolol (Normodine, Trandate), an alpha- and beta-blocking agent, would be the most appropriate medication to lower blood pressure in a patient with hypertensive crisis, tachycardia, and chest pain. Nitroprusside (Nipride) could increase tachycardia owing to decreased preload, thus increasing myocardial ischemia. Although diazoxide (Proglycen) can lower BP via arteriolar dilation, it is contraindicated here because it may also precipitate a reflex sympathetic response that can provoke angina, ischemia, and cardiac failure in patients with ischemic heart disease. Nicardipine (Cardene) is a calcium channel blocker; its side effects include tachycardia, which could worsen angina.

Reference: Chulay, M., Burns, S. M. *AACN Essentials of Critical Care Nursing.* New York, McGraw-Hill, 2006.

2-86. **(B)** These laboratory results reflect a patient with active hemorrhage and hypovolemia resulting in dropping hemoglobin/hematocrit, elevation of creatinine, and increase in lactate levels owing to tissue hypoxia. In patients with active hemorrhage, the laboratory results may lag behind the patient's current condition prior to or after resuscitation. With resolution of the hemorrhage and stabilization of the patient, a majority of the laboratory results should return to normal ranges. The patient is still being resuscitated; if the still-abnormal values are corrected at this time, overcorrection and introduction of new problems may occur. It is normal for serum creatinine to become transiently elevated in hypovolemic shock, so the patient does not likely have acute renal failure. Diagnosis of DIC requires evaluation of fibrinogen and fibrin split products, not elevation of INR.

Reference: Krumberger, J., Parrish, C. R., Krenitsky, J. Gastrointestinal system. In M. Chulay, S. Burns (eds.). *AACN Essentials of Critical Care Nursing.* New York, McGraw Hill, 2006, p 320.

2-87. **(A)** Magnesium needs to be administered because this patient is exhibiting ECG evidence that suggests hypomagnesemia. Although the patient may be hypokalemic and/or hypocalcemic owing to diuretic therapy, the patient's ECG changes are consistent with hypomagnesemia. Hypertonic saline would be administered for hypoosmolar disorders such as syndrome of inappropriate ADH (SIADH). Potassium would be administered for hypokalemia, and acetazolamide is used to treat hyperphosphatemia.

References: Hinkle, C. Renal system. In M. Chulay, S. Burns (eds.). *AACN Essentials of Critical Care Nursing.* New York, McGraw-Hill, 2006, pp 341-355.
Lough, M. E. Renal disorders and therapeutic management. In L. D. Urden, K. M. Stacy, M. E. Lough (eds.). *Thelan's Critical Care Nursing: Diagnosis and Management,* 5th ed. St. Louis, Elsevier, 2006, pp 813-846.
Stark, J. L. The renal system. In J. G. Alspach (ed.). *Core Curriculum for Critical Care Nursing,* 6th ed. St. Louis, Elsevier, 2006, pp 525-607.

2-88. **(D)** This patient's ABG shows hypoxemia that may respond to judicious increases in FiO_2. The elevated $PaCO_2$ is not accompanied by a commensurately acidotic pH, so the patient likely retains high levels of CO_2 on a chronic basis, negating any need for intubation. Since the patient is tachypneic, the CO_2 level does not reflect a diminished respiratory drive. There are no data provided that suggest a need for diuresis.

Reference: Calverley, P. Chronic obstructive pulmonary diseases. In M. P. Fink, E. Abraham E, J. L. Vincent, P. M. Kochanek (eds.). *Textbook of Critical Care,* 5th ed. Philadelphia, Elsevier, 2005.

2-89. **(B)** In general, Mexican families do not discuss sexual or genitourinary issues across genders or age groups. Based on this, the best person with whom to discuss the patient's condition would be his brother who is close to the patient's age.

Reference: Chang, M., Harden, J. Meeting the challenge of the new millennium: caring for culturally diverse patients. *Urol Nurs,* 22(6), 372-377, 2002.

2-90. **(A)** The hallmark symptom of compartment syndrome is pain not controlled by narcotic administration. Other symptoms in compartment syndrome are subtle and include a doughy muscle mass. Pulse pressure decrease and loss of motor function are usually late signs. Graft occlusion would cause loss or decrease of distal pulses and signs of poor perfusion in the extremity, such as increased capillary refill time, pallor, paresthesia, and weakness. False aneurysm would cause a pulsatile mass at the suture site, hematoma, and a tense thigh or calf. Signs of heparin-induced thrombocytopenia include oozing at the sutures sites, petechiae, and decreased platelet count.

Reference: Fahey, V. A. *Vascular Nursing,* 4th ed. St. Louis, Elsevier, 2004.

2-91. **(C)** Although the usefulness of antibiotics for treatment of acute exacerbations of asthma continues to be debated, there is no consensus advocating their use, and treatment aims primarily toward relieving the bronchoconstriction experienced by patients with status asthmaticus (Option C). All of the other interventions (Heliox, magnesium, and general anesthetics) can be used effectively to relax the airways (Options A, B, D).

References: Corbridge, T., Corbridge, S. J. Severe asthma exacerbation. In M. P. Fink, E. Abraham, J. L. Vincent, P. M. Kochanek (eds.). *Textbook of Critical Care,* 5th ed. Philadelphia, Elsevier, 2005.

Ellstrom, K. The pulmonary system. In J. G. Alspach (ed.). *Core Curriculum for Critical Care Nursing,* 6th ed. St. Louis, Elsevier, 2006.

Little, F. Treating acute asthma with antibiotics—Not quite yet. *N Engl J Med,* 354, 1632-1634, 2006.

2-92. **(C)** A major source of common ethical conflict occurs when the physician and patient or patient surrogate disagree. With beneficence, the person is trying to do good for the other person as the physician is attempting to do in this situation. Option A is incorrect

because the nurse is acting as a surrogate. Option B is incorrect because the nurse is displaying justice in her comments but is not advocating according to the family's expressed wishes. Option D is incorrect in that the nurse is advocating for the physician rather than the patient.

Reference: Molter, N. Professional caring and ethical practice. In J. G. Alspach (ed.). *Core Curriculum for Critical Care Nursing,* 6th ed. St. Louis, Elsevier, 2006, pp 1-44.

2-93. **(A)** The combination of heparin, eptifibatide, and aspirin increases the risk of bleeding. Cardiac catheterization and PCI use the groin for access, and the groin site may exhibit signs of bleeding such as oozing and hematoma formation. Risk of coronary artery spasm is reduced with infusion of nitroglycerin. Abrupt closure may be seen in the immediate post-PCI period. Restenosis may occur days to years after PCI. Heparin-induced thrombocytopenia may occur in a patient who has received prior heparin therapy, or after receiving heparin therapy for greater than 24 hours.

Reference: Woods, S. L., Froelicher, E. S., Motzer, S. U., Bridges, E. J. *Cardiac Nursing,* 5th ed. Philadelphia, Lippincott Williams & Wilkins, 2005.

2-94. **(C)** CO-Hb binding causes a shift to the left in the oxyhemoglobin dissociation curve, resulting in hemoglobin not releasing oxygen and impeding oxygen delivery to the tissues. The affinity of hemoglobin molecules for carbon monoxide is approximately 200 times greater than that for oxygen. Inhalation of carbon monoxide (CO) results in its bonding to available hemoglobin, producing carboxyhemoglobin (HbCO), which effectively decreases oxygen saturation of hemoglobin. Carboxyhemoglobin binds poorly with oxygen, reducing oxygen-carrying capacity of blood and leading to hypoxia.

Reference: Urden, L. D., Stacy, K. M., Lough, M. E. *Thelan's Critical Care Nursing: Diagnosis and Management,* 5th ed. St. Louis, Elsevier, 2006, p 1057.

2-95. **(A)** Atrial fibrillation commonly occurs within 3 days after open heart surgery. Multiple trials have compared the effects of various pharmacologic agents to treat or prevent the occurrence of atrial fibrillation, including digoxin, beta blockers, amiodarone, and magnesium, but none has been shown to be clearly superior. Supraventricular dysrhythmias such as AVNRT and SVT may occur after coronary artery bypass surgery, but more commonly occur with surgery involving the cardiac septum. Atrial flutter may occur with digoxin toxicity.

> **Reference:** Hilleman, D. E., Hunter, C. B., Mohiuddin, S. M., Maciejewski, S. Pharmacological management of atrial fibrillation following cardiac surgery. *Am J Cardiovasc Drugs,* 6, 361-369, 2005.

2-96. **(D)** Option D is the best response because early detection of acute confusion is best evaluated with a screening tool. The nurse should seek to apply research findings and to evaluate current literature and research on complex issues such as acute confusion in diverse patient populations. Screening tools can be useful to identify and more thoroughly assess specific clinical problems. For example, the Hartford Institute for Geriatric Nursing recommends the Confusion Assessment Method (CAM) as a screening tool. Interpreters can offer only limited help in more fully understanding the patient's status for this problem. The clinical problem is not directly related to cultural values or communication patterns.

> **References** Molter, N. Professional caring and ethical practice. In J. G. Alspach (ed.). *Core Curriculum for Critical Care Nursing,* 6th ed. St. Louis, Elsevier, 2006, pp 1-44.
>
> Wang, J., Mentes, C. Detection of acute confusion in Taiwanese elderly individuals. *J Gerontol Nurs,* 32(6), 7-12, 2006.
>
> Waszynski, C. M. Confusion Assessment Method (CAM). Try This: Best Practices in Nursing Care to Older Adults, Issue 13, November 2001. Hartford Institute for Geriatric Nursing. Access at www.hartfordign.org/publications/trythis/issue13.pdf

2-97. **(A)** Administration of additional oxygen is the first priority in this situation. The patient may be found to need placement of a new right chest tube (Option D) or adjustment of the existing chest tube (Option C), but meanwhile requires more oxygen and either an increase in pressure support or placement on mechanically controlled ventilation. Drawing laboratory studies will likely provide useful data but is secondary in impor-

tance to supporting this patient's oxygenation.

> **Reference:** Alspach, J. G. (ed.). *Core Curriculum for Critical Care Nursing,* 6th ed. St. Louis, Elsevier, 2006.

2-98. **(A)** Packed red blood cells do not contain clotting factors, so replacement of clotting factors with transfusion of fresh frozen plasma and platelets should occur after administration of each five units of packed red blood cells. Acetaminophen and diphenhydramine (Benadryl) are generally administered prior to transfusion to prevent transfusion reaction. Furosemide (Lasix) is indicated if pulmonary congestion is apparent after transfusion. Normal saline is administered concurrently with transfusion to prevent hemolysis and increased blood viscosity. Salt poor albumin is indicated to increase blood volume in hypovolemic patients with excess interstitial fluid volume and is not indicated if blood replacement has been adequate. Calcium chloride is sometimes administered to patients who receive large volumes of banked blood containing citrate as a preservative.

> **Reference:** Woods, S. L., Froelicher, E. S., Motzer, S. U., Bridges, E. J. *Cardiac Nursing,* 5th ed. Philadelphia, Lippincott Williams & Wilkins, 2005.

2-99. **(B)** The nurse could appropriately implement any of these activities, except pointing out to the husband that his current behavior is inappropriate and unacceptable. Under the circumstances, the husband may be lashing out from anger at his wife's status and his own difficulty coping with that situation. Confrontation without accompanying empathy may just escalate the behavior. Indeed, his anger may represent a step in the grieving process. Certainly, social services (Option A) could provide supportive resources and assistance to both the staff and the patient's spouse in such a difficult situation. The nurse should speak calmly and directly to the patient's husband regarding the situation (Option C), acknowledging the impact of the situation and what he may be experiencing. Arranging for a family conference (Option D) may be an appropriate way to provide information to the family, share the husband's burden of repeated retelling about the situation from him alone to the family, and provide the husband some support during this difficult time.

Reference: Henneman, E. A. Psychosocial aspects of critical care. In J. G. Alspach (ed.). *Core Curriculum for Critical Care Nursing,* 6ᵗʰ ed. St. Louis, Elsevier, 2006.

2-100. **(B)** The normal C-reactive protein level is 0.03 to 1.1 mg/dL. C-reactive protein elevation indicates the presence of inflammation in the coronary arteries due to plaque, which may be ready to embolize. The normal brain natriuretic peptide (BNP) is less than100 pg/mL. BNP elevation indicates LV dysfunction owing to strain on the ventricle from volume or pressure overload and indicates risk of heart failure. The desired cholesterol level to reduce risk of CAD is less than 200 mg/dL. The desired value of HDL to reduce risk of coronary artery disease is greater than 40 mg/dL. Total cholesterol value of 180 mg/dL and HDL of 60 mg/dL indicate low risk of coronary artery disease.

Reference: Baird, M. S., Keen, J. H., Swearingen, D. L. *Manual of Critical Care Nursing: Nursing Interventions and Collaborative Management.* St. Louis, Elsevier, 2005.

2-101. **(D)** Hemodynamic instability, as demonstrated by tachycardia and hypotension, indicates that the patient is not tolerating rotational therapy and should be returned to a supine position. Hemodynamic values obtained while the patient is in the lateral or prone position are reliable as long as the zero level is maintained at the phlebostatic axis. Neither side lying nor prone positioning increase the risk of aspiration. SpO_2 is not a good indicator of positioning tolerance and for this reason, arterial blood gases are used to gauge the effectiveness of rotational therapy.

Reference: Wiegand, D. J., Carlson, D. J. (ed.). *AACN Procedure Manual for Critical Care,* 5ᵗʰ ed. St. Louis, Elsevier, 2005.

2-102. **(A)** Patients who have undergone bariatric surgery may develop deficiencies in calcium, iron, vitamin B_{12}, and folate owing to the bypassing of the gastric fundus, body, and antrum, as well as the duodenum and variable lengths of the proximal jejunum. Bypassing these structures results in mal-

absorption. Option B identifies symptoms characteristic of hyperglycemia. Option C lists symptoms associated with pancreatic cancer. Option D includes findings associated with hepatic encephalopathy.

Reference: Elliot, K. Nutritional considerations after bariatric surgery. *Crit Care Nurse Q,* 26(2), 133-138, 2003.

2-103. **(B)** Since the patient has an elevated FT_4 and low TSH, the nurse needs to search the literature to identify drugs associated with thyroid dysfunction. Nurses should be vigilant in seeking information on drug-drug and drug-food interactions. Clinical inquiry seeks to validate whether available literature can answer the clinical question. Holding medications one at a time (Option A) could be both time-consuming and dangerous and suggests a lack of direction in searching for relevant evidence. Option C would not afford sufficient information to identify the problem. Option D is inappropriate because Wolf-Chaikoff is a protective mechanism against the development of hyperthyroidism.

References: Molter, N. Professional caring and ethical practice. In J. G. Alspach (ed.). *Core Curriculum for Critical Care Nursing,* 6ᵗʰ ed. St. Louis, Elsevier, 2006, pp 1-44.

Porsche, R., Brenner, Z. R. Amiodarone-induced thyroid dysfunction. *Crit Care Nurse,* 26(3), 34-42, 2006.

2-104. **(A)** Right ventricular failure may occur after mitral valve replacement in patients with pulmonary hypertension. When the right ventricle fails it requires larger volumes to ensure adequate output. This is easily accomplished with crystalloid fluid boluses to maintain the pulmonary artery diastolic or wedge pressure at 15-18 mm Hg. Nesiritide or nitroglycerin may be ordered with fluid bolus to reduce right ventricular afterload. Furosemide would decrease preload and worsen right ventricular failure. Norepinephrine or vasopressin would increase vasoconstriction and worsen right ventricular failure. .

Reference: Bojar, R. M. *Manual of Perioperative Care in Adult Cardiac Surgery,* 4ᵗʰ ed. Berlin, VT, Blackwell, 2005.

2-105. **(A)** Because complications from HHNK result from an increase in blood viscosity, IV normal saline will help to replace fluids lost to polyuria, diminish blood viscosity, and improve perfusion. Regular insulin, rather than glargine, would be used in insulin drips since regular insulin does not promote antigen development and is short acting. Unless the patient has other concurrent health problems, oxygen administration and seizure precautions are usually not needed for hyperosmolar patients.

References: Newberry, L., Criddle, L. *Sheehy's Manual of Emergency Care,* 6th ed. Philadelphia, Elsevier, 2006, pp 431-433.

Urden, L. D., Stacy, K. M., Lough, M. E. *Thelan's Critical Care Nursing: Diagnosis and Management,* 5th ed. St. Louis, Elsevier, 2006, p 934.

2-106. **(D)** Torsades de pointes is a polymorphic ventricular rhythm characterized by varying QRS morphology and is associated with prolonged QT intervals. Magnesium sulfate is the medication utilized to treat dysrhythmias associated with long QT syndromes. Medications such as procainamide and lidocaine prolong the QT interval and may potentiate the development of torsades de pointes in patients with pre-existing prolonged QT intervals. Adenosine is used to manage supraventricular tachycardias.

Reference: Stone, C. K., Humphries, R. L. *Current Emergency Diagnosis and Treatment*, 5th ed. New York, Lange Medical Books, 2004.

2-107. **(B)** The patient is presenting with the hallmarks of cryptogenic organizing pneumonia (COP), previously termed bronchiolitis obliterating organizing pneumonia (BOOP). Her laboratory results suggest an inflammatory rather than an infectious process (Option A), and there is no evidence suggesting cardiac failure (Options C and D). Since certain infections may be contributive factors to COP, Option B is the best answer.

Reference: Cordier, J. F. Cryptogenic organizing pneumonia. *Clin Chest Med,* 25, 727-737, 2004.

2-108. **(B)** This patient should avoid taking aspirin because both aspirin and a low platelet count predispose the patient to potential bleeding. Green, leafy vegetables need to be avoided when a patient is on warfarin, not aspirin. Individuals on reverse isolation for leukemia may have fruit restricted, but this patient's immediate concern is the low platelet count. Prednisone is not prohibited with a low platelet count.

Reference: Cheek, D. J., Hall, M. A. Hematologic and immunologic systems. In J. G. Alspach (ed.). *Core Curriculum for Critical Care Nursing,* 6th ed. St. Louis, Elsevier, 2006, pp 671-673.

2-109. **(B)** The ECG demonstrates premature ventricular contractions and ST segment elevation in leads V_1, V_2, V_3, and V_4, indicating acute anterior wall myocardial infarction. Administration of nitroglycerin may vasodilate the affected coronary artery and reperfuse the myocardium. Reperfusion may eliminate myocardial irritability, causing PVCs. Although low potassium may cause development of PVCs, initial laboratory studies for this patient should include cardiac biomarkers. A coagulation panel should be drawn if nitroglycerin is ineffective and thrombolytic therapy is ordered. Amiodarone is not indicated unless PVCs continue after interventions directed at reperfusion.

Reference: Sole, M. L., Klein, D. G., Moseley, M. J. *Introduction to Critical Care Nursing,* 4th ed. St. Louis, Elsevier, 2005.

2-110. **(B)** Dextrose in water (D_5W) is the IV solution most often associated with aggressive fluid resuscitation. This fluid can be used to replace mild volume loss and provide calories to the patient. Extremely common in critically ill patients, hypoosmolar disorders are the result of an excess of water and can be caused by replacement of fluid loss with pure water. Patients who have experienced volume loss, such as the patient with a GI bleed, require balanced fluid replacement. Half-strength saline solution is indicated for free water replacement, correction of mild hyponatremia, and free water/electrolyte replacement. Normal saline solution is used to maintain fluid volume, replace mild fluid loss, and correct mild hyponatremia. Lactated ringer's solution is indicated in fluid and electrolyte replacement but is contraindicated for patients with renal or liver disease or lactic acidosis.

Reference: Hinkle, C. Renal system. In M. Chulay, S. M. Burns (eds.). *AACN Essentials of Critical Care Nursing.* New York, McGraw-Hill, 2006, pp 341-355.

Stark, J. L. The renal system. In J. G. Alspach (ed.). *Core Curriculum for Critical Care Nursing,* 6th ed. St. Louis, Elsevier, 2006, pp 525-607.

2-111. **(B)** The physician should be contacted regarding the use of pneumatic compression stockings owing to the use of warfarin in this patient. The warfarin may contribute to bruising and increased risk of bleeding when using the pneumatic compression stockings. Monitoring the PT/INR daily is appropriate until a stable level is reached, which is usually 1.5 to 2 times the normal ratio. If the patient is able to protect his/her airway, there is no contraindication for advancement of diet. The reduction in oxygenation is appropriate based on the recent arterial blood gas results.

Reference: Ellstrom, K. Pulmonary system. In J. G. Alspach (ed.). *Core Curriculum for Critical Care Nursing,* 6th ed. St. Louis, Elsevier, 2006, p 148.

2-112. **(D)** Mental status and renal perfusion are the best indicators of cardiac output as the brain and kidneys receive one fourth of the cardiac output. Patients with pulmonary edema due to diastolic dysfunction may have normal ejection fractions. Peripheral edema may be absent in left ventricular failure if it is not accompanied by right ventricular failure. Although a respiratory rate of 20 or less and an SpO_2 of 94% may be therapeutic target goals for this patient, they do not indicate cardiac output adequacy in the mechanically ventilated patient.

Reference: Baird, M. S., Keen, J. H., Swearingen, D. L. *Manual of Critical Care Nursing: Nursing Interventions and Collaborative Management.* St. Louis, Elsevier, 2005.

2-113. **(A)** Recent data suggest that clinically chilled hypothermia to 33-35° C can improve neurologic outcomes and survival after hospital discharge. These patients are at risk for a decrease in white blood cell and platelet counts owing to immune response suppression from hypothermia. Blood sugar levels are ideally maintained at 80-110 mg/dL. Option B is incorrect as, based on the data provided, the patient is not at risk for development of hyperkalemia.

Reference: Holden, M., Makic, M. B. Clinically induced hypothermia. Why chill your patient? *AACN Adv Crit Care,* 17(2), 125-32, 2006.

2-114. **(C)** If the implanted cardioverter defibrillator fails to terminate the rhythm, the nurse should institute ACLS measures that include

prompt defibrillation with 360 joules monophasic or 120 to 200 joules biphasic. It is not necessary to turn the ICD off with a magnet prior to performing manual defibrillation. Placement of defibrillation paddles may be anterior–anterior or anterior–posterior, but the pads should be at least 2 inches away from the ICD generator, and 360 joules should be delivered.

References: Field, J. M., Hazinski, M. F., Gilmore, D. (eds.). *Handbook of Emergency Cardiovascular Care for Healthcare Providers.* Dallas, American Heart Association, 2006.

Wiegand, D. J., Carlson, K. K. *AACN Procedure Manual for Critical Care,* 5th ed. St. Louis, Elsevier, 2005.

2-115. **(C)** While the decision to draft an advanced directive should have been made prior to this admission, that is not the issue at this time. The patient has a need to confer with his family, physician, and significant others so that they understand his wishes. Attempting to placate the patient by saying he will probably change his mind later belittles the decision-making process that led to this conclusion. While he is experiencing an alteration in oxygenation, he may not be legally responsible to make such a decision; however, he may have been thinking about and discussing this issue over a period of time. Ascertaining the patient's true wishes and supporting that decision will enable the nurse to serve more effectively as an advocate for the needs of patients and their families.

References: Nettina, S. M. *The Lippincott Manual of Nursing Practice,* 7th ed. Philadelphia, Lippincott Williams & Wilkins, 2000, p 192.

Urden, L. D., Stacy, K. M., Lough, M. E. *Thelan's Critical Care Nursing: Diagnosis and Management,* 5th ed. St. Louis, Elsevier, 2006, p 163.

2-116. **(C)** It is common for persons treated with glucagon to vomit, so positioning the patient to avoid aspiration would be the next most important nursing measure. Each of the other choices can be appropriate measures at a later time. Ongoing assessment of neurological status would represent the next appropriate intervention, with a recheck of capillary glucose to evaluate the effectiveness of the glucagon dose in 30 minutes, and then preparation to feed the patient after he or she regains conciousness.

References: Newberry, L., Criddle, L. *Sheehy's Manual of Emergency Care,* 6th ed. Philadelphia, Elsevier, 2006, pp 428-432.

Urden, L. D., Stacy, K. M., Lough, M. E. *Thelan's Critical Care Nursing: Diagnosis and Management,* 5th ed. St. Louis, Elsevier, 2006, p 926.

2-117. **(B)** Each of the options will be part of the process, but it is important for all of the units who will be using the new equipment to be part of the evaluation process from the beginning. Central to any successful change process are communication and input. As multiple units may be involved in the change, it is essential that the decision be based on input from each of the involved areas.

Reference: Bacal, R. Managing change—step by step change implementation for change leaders. Available at www.work911.com/managing change/stepbystepchange.htm. Retrieved September 2, 2006.

2-118. **(D)** Neuromuscular blocking agents may cause prolonged myopathy in any patient, so their relative benefit must always be weighed against their potential for harm. As a result, NMBs should be used with caution and only after other options have proven ineffective. The myopathy associated with NMBs is particularly problematic for patients concomitantly receiving steroids (Option A), so NMB use would only be as a last resort. Because of the risks associated with NMBs, they are not used routinely (Option B). NMBs act on skeletal, rather than smooth, muscle (Option C).

References: Corbridge, T., Corbridge, S. J. Severe asthma exacerbation. In M. P. Fink, E. Abraham, J. L. Vincent, P. M. Kochanek (eds.). *Textbook of Critical Care,* 5th ed. Philadelphia, Elsevier, 2005.

Ellstrom, K. The pulmonary system. In J. G. Alspach (ed.). *Core Curriculum for Critical Care Nursing,* 6th ed. St. Louis, Elsevier, 2006.

2-119. **(A)** Pulmonary artery hypertension causes enlargement of the pulmonary artery, which makes obtaining PCWP pressures unreliable or unobtainable. Therefore, a left atrial line is used to obtain left ventricular end diastolic pressures to reflect preload status. Left atrial lines predispose the patient to development of air embolus but are not used to evacuate left atrial air emboli. A left atrial line is not superior to a pulmonary artery catheter in diagnosing pericardial tamponade. During cardiac surgery, there is no need for continuous monitoring of cardiac chambers since the patient is on cardiopulmonary bypass.

Reference: Bojar, R. M. *Manual of Perioperative Care in Adult Cardiac Surgery,* 4th ed. Berlin, VT, Blackwell, 2005.

2-120. **(C)** The hemodynamic values indicate that the patient is experiencing a decrease in cardiac output (in relation to the SVR) as a result of decreased preload (CVP: 4 mm Hg). Administering a fluid bolus of normal saline is the most appropriate intervention that would improve the patient's hemodynamic status. If the patient were anemic, then the fluid of choice would be PRBCs. Based on the Society of Critical Care Medicine guidelines for patient management for sepsis and septic shock, the preload (as measured by CVP) should be at least 8 to 12 mm Hg. Other hemodynamic values that reflect the patient's inadequate fluid resuscitation are HR, BP, and PAP. Norepinephrine would increase the patient's BP and SVR but would likely increase rather than reduce the patient's tachycardia. Administering fluid would lessen the need for vasopressor therapy. Metoprolol is a negative chronotropic and inotropic agent (β-blocker) that is not indicated for this patient. The patient is hypotensive and would not tolerate the administration of a β-blocker. Dobutamine results in a positive inotropic and chronotropic effect with afterload reduction. The patient is tachycardic and has a low SVR secondary to the septic shock. Administering dobutamine would result in an increased HR and lower SVR, which would further compromise the patient's clinical status.

References: Dellinger, R. P., Carlet, J. M., Masur, H., et al. Surviving Sepsis Campaign guidelines for management of severe sepsis and septic shock. *Crit Care Med,* 32(3), 858-873, 2004.

Urden, L. D., Stacy, K. M., Lough, M. E. *Thelan's Critical Care Nursing: Diagnosis and Management,* 5th ed. St. Louis, Elsevier, 2006, pp 1023-1030.

2-121. **(B)** The tidal volume settings for a patient with ARDS should be 5-8 mL/kg. An optimal tidal volume for this patient, then, is 350 to 560 mL. Excessive tidal volumes and high PEEP levels increase the risk of volutrauma and barotrauma, so the PEEP should not be increased until the tidal volume is adjusted and PaO_2 levels do not improve. SIMV is an acceptable mode for the patient because the rate of 12/min ensures that the patient will receive at least 12 breaths per minute. Pressure control ventilation may be used in ARDS to prevent volutrauma, but other modes of ventilation are also acceptable.

Reference: Chulay, M., Burns, S. M. *AACN Essentials of Critical Care Nursing*. New York, McGraw-Hill, 2006.

2-122. **(A)** Prevention of stroke is the primary concern when a patient presents with hypertensive crisis. Prevention centers around rapid lowering of systolic blood pressure. End organ failure is generally preventable when blood pressure and vasoconstriction are reduced in a timely manner. Renal failure from chronic hypertension may precipitate the hypertensive event. Seizures are not common with hypertensive crisis but may occur if there is intracerebral bleeding or encephalopathy. Left ventricular hypertrophy is common in patients with chronic hypertension and may result in heart failure.

Reference: Baird, M. S., Keen, J. H., Swearingen, D. L. *Manual of Critical Care Nursing: Nursing Interventions and Collaborative Management.* St: Louis, Elsevier, 2005.

2-123. **(B)** The nurse recognizes that explanation of significant risks should be discussed with the patient and family to ensure informed consent. Allowing the physician to leave without discussing the risks of the procedure does not advocate for the patient. Option C provides collaboration with another discipline but does not provide informed consent. Option D facilitates knowledge of the family but does not ensure that the risks of the procedure are reviewed by the physician prior to signing consent.

References: Molter, N. Professional caring and ethical practice. In J. G. Alspach (ed.). *Core Curriculum for Critical Care Nursing,* 6th ed. St. Louis, Elsevier, 2006, pp 1-44.
Stannard, D., Hardin S. R. Advocacy and moral agency. In S. R. Hardin, K. Kaplow (eds.). *Synergy for Clinical Excellence,* Sudbury, Jones & Bartlett, 2005, pp 63-68.

2-124. **(D)** Intestinal obstruction can occur in pregnant patients who have had prior operative procedures and may result from the enlarging uterus exerting pressure on preexisting adhesions. Obstruction of this nature is most common in the third trimester, and the symptoms are similar to those of a nonpregnant patient. Ectopic pregnancy would have evidenced and been detected before 26 weeks' gestation. If an ectopic pregnancy goes undetected for 6 to 8 weeks, there is severe lower abdominal pain and fainting. These symptoms indicate rupture of the fallopian tube and hemorrhage. Abruptio placenta would present with fetal cardiac distress and maternal shock. Peptic ulcer disease presents with intermittent colicky pain, which increases 2 to 3 hours after meals. It can also occur in the middle of the night. Eating usually decreases the symptoms. It is not associated with fever.

References: Charles, A., Domingo, S., Goldfadden, A., et al. Small bowel ischema after roux-en-y gastric bypass complicated by pregnancy: a case report. *Am Surg,* 71(3), 231-235, 2005.
Pakfetrat, M. A pregnant lady with abdominal pain. *Shiraz E-Medical J,* 6, 1-2, 2005.

2-125. **(B)** Ischemic colitis may occur after aortic surgery owing to embolization, occlusion, or ligation of mesenteric vessels, or hypoperfusion from long aortic cross-clamp times or hypovolemia. Initial symptoms of ischemic colitis may include edema, elevated white count, tachycardia, pain, acidosis, hypotension, and diarrhea. Graft infection is not usually evident within 2 days, but symptoms would include tachycardia, hypotension, and elevated white count without GI symptoms. Fistula formation is also a late-onset finding and may cause signs of peritonitis, GI bleeding, or visible fistula formation. Abdominal compartment syndrome may present as abdominal pain, rigidity, and myoglobinuria.

Reference: Fahey, V. A. *Vascular Nursing,* 4th ed. St. Louis, Elsevier, 2004.

2-126. **(C)** The use of mechanical compression devices should be initiated. The devices will not increase the risk of bleeding, yet will provide prophylaxis for deep vein thrombosis. The pelvic fracture, splenic laceration, and compound fracture of the femur would prevent the use of low-molecular-weight heparin in the early stages of this patient's treatment because the risk of increased bleeding is too great. Once it can be verified that there is no active bleeding, low-molecular-weight heparin may be administered. Elastic stockings could be used on the uninjured extremity; however, mechanical compression devices have been found to be more effective for this purpose. Physical therapy can be initiated but will be limited on the injured extremity and is only provided intermittently, so it is not likely to be as effective as continuous mechanical compression devices.

References: Ellstrom, K. Pulmonary system. In J. G. Alspach (ed.). *Core Curriculum for Critical Care Nursing,* 6th ed. St. Louis, Elsevier, 2006, p 146.

Yang, J. C. Prevention and treatment of deep vein thrombosis and pulmonary embolism in critically ill patients. *Crit Care Nurse Q,* 28(1), 72-79, 2005.

2-127. **(A)** ACE inhibitors should be discontinued if the serum creatinine level increases above 3.0 mg/dL because they prevent conversion of angiotensin I to angiotensin II, which decreases glomerular filtration and may potentiate renal insufficiency. Serum creatinine is an indicator of renal function. Serum potassium levels less than 3.5 mEq/L indicate a need for potassium replacement. An SpO_2 of 95% is still adequate to maintain oxygenation. An increased number of atrial premature contractions could herald the onset of atrial fibrillation and warrants continued monitoring, but a reduced heart rate indicates that therapy is appropriate.

Reference: Woods, S. L., Froelicher, E. S., Motzer, S. U., Bridges, E. J. *Cardiac Nursing,* 5th ed. Philadelphia, Lippincott Williams & Wilkins, 2005.

2-128. **(D)** Infection is the leading cause of morbidity associated with SLE. Ulcers around the mouth could become infected but are not, in themselves, a major cause of morbidity for SLE. Anemia and weight loss can be effectively treated on an outpatient basis.

Reference: Lash, A. A., Lusk, B. Systemic lupus erythematosus in the intensive care unit. *Crit Care Nurse,* 24(2), 56-65, 2004.

2-129. **(A)** HELLP syndrome derives its name from severe preeclampsia characterized by

hemolytic anemia, elevated liver enzymes, and a low platelet count. Decreased hemoglobin and hematocrit are related to blood loss and hemodilution owing to crystalloid and colloidal infusions to replace depleted circulating volume. Magnesium levels rise if a magnesium drip is used to slow electrical impulses and prevent seizure activity; however, this laboratory value increases secondary to magnesium administration, not from pathophysiology. Albuminuria and increased serum creatinine levels occur related to the renal response to hypertension. Generally, BUN is elevated rather than decreased with renal impairment.

References: Newberry, L., Criddle, L. *Sheehy's Manual of Emergency Care,* 6th ed. Philadelphia, Elsevier, 2006, p 804.

Urden, L. D., Stacy, K. M., Lough, M. E. *Thelan's Critical Care Nursing: Diagnosis and Management,* 5th ed. St. Louis, Elsevier, 2006, pp 214-215.

2-130. **(A)** The patient is alkalotic with a pH of 7.60. Acetazolamide (Diamox) is a diuretic used in alkalosis to decrease hydrogen ion loss that may occur with diuresis. Alkalosis hinders release of oxygen to tissues, and so should be avoided in patients with pulmonary edema, who may be hypoxemic. Additional furosemide (Lasix) will continue diuresis without correcting alkalosis. Endotracheal intubation will improve oxygenation but is not indicated when PaO_2 is 78 mm Hg and pCO_2 is normal. Hydrochlorthiazide is a thiazide diuretic that will induce diuresis but not preserve hydrogen ions and thus would increase alkalosis.

Reference: The Task Force on Acute Heart Failure of the European Society of Cardiology. Executive summary of the guidelines on the diagnosis and treatment of heart failure. *Eur Heart J,* 26, 384-416, 2005.

2-131. **(A)** Regardless of the cause or type of diabetes insipidus, the patient's electrolyte values will govern appropriate treatment for this disorder. In nephrogenic diabetes insipidus, the kidney has been damaged and no longer responds to vasopressin, so aggressive replacement of fluids is required to sustain life. Neurogenic diabetes insipidus is a problem caused when too little vasopressin is released by the pituitary gland, possibly due to increased intracranial pressure; therefore, supplemental vasopressin administration sustains life. Whether because of a lack of vasopressin or a lack of response, urinary output exceeds 500 mL/hr, resulting in dehydration and altered electrolytes. The goal of therapy is to reestablish and maintain a normal fluid and electrolyte balance.

References: Newberry, L., Criddle, L. *Sheehy's Manual of Emergency Care,* 6th ed. Philadelphia, Elsevier, 2006, pp 433-434.

Urden, L. D., Stacy, K. M., Lough, M. E. *Thelan's Critical Care Nursing: Diagnosis and Management,* 5th ed. St. Louis, Elsevier, 2006, pp 952-953.

2-132. **(C)** Hemodialysis is the "gold standard" for management of chronic renal failure because it is the most effective of all renal replacement therapies. Although the patient managed her renal failure using CAPD at home, peritoneal dialysis is not currently an option due to the patient's abdominal surgery. SCUF is used in patients with volume overload and some degree of renal function, but it has minimal impact on urea and creatinine levels. CVVH is used for patients who require fluid removal and are hemodynamically unstable.

Reference: ANNA. *Continuous Renal Replacement Therapy.* Pitman, NJ, American Nephrology Nurses Association, 2005, pp 1-12.

Hinkle, C. Renal system. In M. Chulay, S. M. Burns (eds). *AACN Essentials of Critical Care Nursing.* New York, McGraw-Hill, 2006, pp 341-355.

Mitchell, J. K. Renal disorders and therapeutic management. In L. D. Urden, K. M. Stacy, M. E. Lough (eds). *Priorities in Critical Care Nursing,* 4th ed. St. Louis, Elsevier, 2005, pp 333-356.

2-133. **(B)** The goal of ventilator management with persistent air leaks is to minimize airway pressures in order to prevent further injury to the affected area (Option B). Maximizing PEEP or using large tidal volumes may worsen the clinical situation by increasing the volume lost through the air leak (Options A and D). Using the minimal effective FiO_2 is always a good idea, but it will not aid management of an air leak (Option C).

Reference: Lois, M., Noppen, M. Bronchopleural fistulas: An overview of the problem with special attention to endoscopic management. *Chest,* 128, 3955-3965, 2005.

2-134. **(D)** The GI tract harbors organisms that may trigger an inflammatory focus if they are translocated from the gut into the portal circulation, where they may not be adequately cleared by the liver. Common enteric organisms with this potential include *Enterococcus, Escherichia coli, Clostridium perfringens,* and *Enterobactor cloacae.* Bacterial translocation has been associated with paralytic ileus and with drugs commonly used in critically ill patients such as antibiotics, antacids, and histamine blockers. Antibiotics alter the function of normal protective bacteria located in the gut. Antacids and histamine blockers increase the intragastric pH, allowing ingested bacteria to survive in the GI tract and potentially become pathologic. Conditions thought to increase gut permeability and microbial translocation include mucosal ischemia, mucosal hypoperfusion, immunoglobulin A deficit (associated with TPN), thermal injury, glucocorticoid administration, endotoxin release, glutamine, and fiber deficiencies. The use of mechanical ventilation prevents ischemia by increasing arterial oxygenation. Inotropic agents increase oxygen delivery and prevent hypoperfusion of the gut by increasing cardiac output. Enteral feeding prevents the development of microbial translocation by maintaining the gastrointestinal mucosal barrier, immune function, and blood flow to the GI tract.

References: Alspach, J. G. (ed.). *Core Curriculum for Critical Care Nursing,* 6th ed. St. Louis, Elsevier, 2006, p 762.

Urden, L. D., Stacy, K. M., Lough, M. E. *Thelan's Critical Care Nursing: Diagnosis and Management,* 5th ed. St. Louis, Elsevier, 2006, pp 1040-1041.

2-135. **(A)** The Hmong believe that a soul may be lost through sudden fright, such as from loud noises or a fall; fear or excessive grief; capture by an evil spirit; or one soul transferring to another. Providing a quiet environment is therefore important in caring for members of the Hmong culture. Hot tea, visit by a shaman, and food temperature are not associated with prevention of loss of souls in the Hmong culture.

Reference: Cheng, H., Culhane-Pera, K. Culturally responsive care for Hmong patients. *Postgrad Med,* 116(6), 39-45, 2004.

2-136. **(D)** Rapid culture and antibiotic administration (Option A) are important interventions in treating any pneumonia; however, preventing hypoxia and hypoperfusion are the priorities (Option D) for this patient. Completing confirmatory diagnostic tests such as a chest x-ray and treating the patient's fever are secondary priorities (Options B and C).

> **References:** American Thoracic Society. Guidelines for the management of adults with hospital-acquired, ventilator-associated and healthcare-associated pneumonia. *Am J Respir Crit Care Med*, 171, 388-416, 2005.
>
> Ellstrom, K. The pulmonary system. In J. G. Alspach (ed.). *Core Curriculum for Critical Care Nursing*, 6th ed. St. Louis, Elsevier, 2006.

2-137. **(A)** The nurse knows that sensitivity to family needs is required when brain death is declared. Family members have the option to obtain a second opinion about brain death. Documentation of the discussion (Option B) is an important aspect but is superceded by the need to advocate on behalf of the family during a time of crisis. Options C and D may come later in the course of this patient's care. Organ donation should not be discussed immediately after the family has just learned of a flat EEG. Option D is inappropriate because there is no apparent conflict in this situation that needs to be resolved.

> **Reference:** Molter, N. Professional caring and ethical practice. In J. G. Alspach (ed.). *Core Curriculum for Critical Care Nursing*, 6th ed. St. Louis, Elsevier, 2006, p 31.

2-138. **(C)** Ideally, corrective surgery for aortic dissection should not be delayed. One exception is when a patient with aortic dissection develops profound hypotension or pulseless electrical activity (PEA). In this instance, emergency pericardiocentesis may be performed prior to surgery. Pericardial tamponade is an anticipated complication of aortic dissection, so clinical evidence of this disorder as increased right atrial pressure or widened mediastinum on chest x-ray would not represent reasons for delay. Stable patients should proceed directly to surgery.

> **Reference:** Zipes, D. P., Libby, P., Bonow, R. O., Braunwald, E. (eds.). *Braunwald's Heart Disease: A Textbook of Cardiovascular Medicine*, 7th ed. Philadelphia, Elsevier, 2005.

2-139. **(C)** The presence of pacemaker artifacts following intrinsic QRS complexes demonstrates failure to sense. Several pacemaker artifacts fall within the refractory period following the intrinsic QRS when, as expected, they would not result in capture. If the pacemaker artifact occurred slightly later on the T wave, however, it might produce R on T phenomenon, precipitating ventricular tachycardia or fibrillation. Failure of the pacemaker to output would be evidenced on the ECG by the absence of pacemaker artifacts where a pacemaker output would be expected.

> **Reference:** Woods, S. L., Froelicher, E. S., Motzer, S. U., Bridges, E. J. *Cardiac Nursing*, 5th ed. Philadelphia, Lippincott Williams & Wilkins, 2005.

2-140. **(A)** Administration of normal saline fluid bolus is used to treat prerenal acute renal failure (ARF). The fluid bolus will increase the patient's blood pressure and renal perfusion. Urine in prerenal ARF is concentrated with low sodium. Restricting the patient's fluid or administering a diuretic such as furosemide will further exacerbate the patient's prerenal condition. Both fluid restriction and administration of diuretics are used for patients who are in ARF and are fluid overloaded. Discontinuing the administration of cefazolin, which is nephrotoxic, would be appropriate if the patient was in intrarenal ARF.

> **References:** Mitchell, J. G. Renal disorders and therapeutic management. In L. D. Urden, K. M. Stacy, M. E. Lough (eds.). *Priorities in Critical Care Nursing*, 4th ed. St. Louis, Elsevier, 2004, pp 333-356.
>
> Schera, M. Renal assessment and diagnostic procedures. In L. D. Urden, K. M. Stacy, M. E. Lough (eds.). *Priorities in Critical Care Nursing*, 4th ed. St. Louis, Elsevier, 2004, pp 323-332.
>
> Stark, J. L. The renal system. In J. G. Alspach (ed.). *Core Curriculum for Critical Care Nursing*, 6th ed. St. Louis, Elsevier, 2006, pp 525-607.

2-141. **(A)** The location of the AVM suggests which deficit the nurse needs to anticipate. A lesion in the right frontal area would be expected to affect voluntary motor control on the left side of the body. Comprehension of spoken language (Option B) is controlled in the dominant temporal lobe; in most patients, this would be in the left hemisphere. A visual field deficit such as a homonymous hemianopsia (Option C) would result from a temporal lobe or optic tract disorder. The sensory deficits described in Option D would most likely result from a lesion in the parietal lobe. AVMs are abnormal vascular networks connecting arteries directly to veins. The lack of a capillary network bridging the high-pressure arterial system to the low-pressure venous system creates a risk of bleeding at that junction, where aneurysms are found in these malformations. Small AVMs commonly present with intracranial hemorrhage, whereas large AVMs present most often with seizures.

References: McQuillan, K. A. Table 4-1: functional localization in the cerebral cortex. Alspach, J. G. (ed.). *Core Curriculum for Critical Care Nursing,* 6th ed. St. Louis, Elsevier, 2006, p 384.
Alspach, J. G. (ed.). *Core Curriculum for Critical Care Nursing,* 6th ed. St. Louis, Elsevier, 2006, pp 484-487.

2-142. **(C)** Acute intra-abdominal blood loss results in decreased venous return to the heart and reduces preload and thus cardiac output. This reduction in cardiac output results in the clinical signs of hypovolemia, hypotension, and diminished cerebral blood flow and triggers compensatory changes such as tachycardia and narrow pulse pressure. The compensatory vasoconstriction that increases blood flow to vital organs also reduces blood flow to peripheral tissues, causing cold, clammy, pale skin. Increased intracranial pressure is often associated with a widened pulse pressure and the development of bradycardia. In this scenario, the patient's pulse pressure narrows and the heart rate increases, reflective of a hypovolemic shock state. In acute MI, the patient typically exhibits chest pain, diaphoresis, nausea, vomiting, and shortness of breath. A patient suffering from pulmonary embolism will exhibit symptoms of tachypnea, anxiety, light-headedness, sharp chest pain, hemoptysis, and rales.

Reference: Krumberger, J., Parrish, C. R., Krenitsky, J. Gastrointestinal system. In M. Chulay, S. M. Burns. *AACN Essentials of Critical Care Nursing.* New York, McGraw-Hill, 2006, p 317.

2-143. **(D)** Administration of sedation/analgesia will treat operative pain and allow the patient to tolerate mechanical ventilation; a bronchodilator can help to open constricted airways to improve ventilation and oxygenation; and postoperative antibiotics are a standard treatment following contaminated bowel surgery. IV steroids (Option A) have not demonstrated definitive benefits in patients with ARDS and are not a priority intervention for this patient. Diuretics (Option B) are not indicated in a fresh postoperative patient who has no evidence of fluid overload. Volume status needs to be assessed before administration of additional fluids (Option C) to minimize volume overload in ARDS.

References: Alspach, J. G. (ed.). *Core Curriculum for Critical Care Nursing,* 6th ed. St. Louis, Elsevier, 2006.
Steinberg, K. P., et al. Efficacy and safety of corticosteroids for persistent acute respiratory distress syndrome. *N Engl J Med,* 354(16), 1671-1684, 2006.

2-144. **(B)** Increased QRS duration indicates loss of capture in one of the ventricles. In biventricular pacing, the programmed A-V interval is shorter than 0.20 owing to asynchronous conduction. The shorter A-V interval accommodates the ventricular conduction defect to ensure synchronous ventricular conduction. T-wave inversion is common in ventricular pacing. Since atrial fibrillation is common in heart failure, the presence of more P waves than QRS complexes is to be expected.

Reference: Carey, M. G., Pelter, M. M. Resynchronization therapy. *Am J Crit Care,* 15, 103-104, 2006.

2-145. **(D)** The nurse competency of clinical inquiry relates to the nurse applying a change in practice when evidence exists to support the change. Especially since the preceptor is not familiar with the practice change, the best course is for the nurse to conduct a literature review to identify studies that support or refute the use of the lower arm for noninvasive blood pressure monitoring. Option A is likely not necessary since there is no evidence that the orientee does not know how to perform standard BP measurement. Option B would be of limited value since it affords a single set of measurements, though current literature indicates that upper and lower arm readings are not interchangeable in either the supine position or with the head of bed elevated 45 degrees. Rather, a difference in measurements of up to 33 mm Hg can exist between the upper arm and lower arm locations. Designing a research study would be a time-consuming activity that may not be justified if literature addressing the issue is already available.

References: Molter, N. Professional caring and ethical practice. In J. G. Alspach (ed.). *Core Curriculum for Critical Care Nursing,* 6th ed. St. Louis, Elsevier, 2006, pp 1-44.

Schell, K., Lyons, D., Bradley, E., et al. Clinical comparison of autonomic, noninvasive measurements of blood pressure in the forearm and upper arm with the patient supine or with the head of the bead raised 45°: A follow-up study. *Am J Crit Care,* 15(2),196-205, 2006.

2-146. **(D)** Febrile nonhemolytic reactions occur in about 1% of transfusions and manifest with a temperature increase of more than 1° C (2° F) during or shortly following a transfusion. The reaction is thought to represent the action of antibodies against white cells or the actions of cytokines either present in the transfused component or generated by the recipient to the transfused component. The initial nursing intervention for this patient would be to immediately stop the transfusion to prevent additional exposure to the offending antigen or infectious agent. Following the termination of the transfusion, the physician would be contacted for additional orders to administer antipyretics and/or antihistamines. Individual institutions have policies and procedures regarding the disposition of the remaining unit contents and post reaction testing.

Reference: Lynn-McHale Wiegand, D. J., Carlson, K. K. (eds.). *AACN Procedure Manual for Critical Care,* 5th ed. St. Louis, Elsevier, 2005, pp 1024-1030.

2-147. **(A)** Aspirin and GpIIb-IIIa inhibitors have antiplatelet activities. There is no antidote, but transfusion of platelets may reverse bleeding caused by platelet dysfunction. Packed red blood cells do not contain clotting factors and are used to increase hematocrit and red cell volume. Protamine sulfate is an antidote for heparin and may be used after coronary artery bypass surgery to reverse heparin administered during bypass. Vitamin K is the reversal agent used when the patient has received warfarin/Coumadin. Agatroban is used for patients with heparin-induced thrombocytopenia.

Reference: Whitlock, R., Crowther, M. A., Heng, J. M. Bleeding in cardiac surgery: its prevention and treatment—an evidence based review. *Crit Care Clin,* 21, 589-610, 2005.

2-148. **(D)** Pressure regulated volume controlled ventilation is an appropriate choice for a patient with chronic obstructive bronchitis because it prevents hyperventilation and barotrauma by adjusting flow rates to provide consistent tidal volumes. A rate of 10/min permits the patient to have a physiologically regulated exhalation time. Patients with obstructive disoders may develop lung injury with volume cycle modes of ventilation. Chronic obstructive disease generally results in elevated $PaCO_2$,which is compensated by elevated bicarbonate. When the CO_2 is corrected, this results in a metabolic alkalosis, which is to be expected in this patient. Increasing the FiO_2 in this patient may decrease the patient's respiratory drive and prevent weaning. Short-term ventilation while the obstruction causing respiratory failure is relieved is the goal for the patient. Increasing FiO_2 would delay the patient's spontaneous respiratory drive and prolong mechanical ventilation.

Reference: Diepenbrock, N. H. *Quick Reference to Critical Care.* Philadelphia, Lippincott Williams & Wilkins, 2004.

2-149. **(C)** The family has expressed a need for information, and the nurse is responsible for providing answers to questions posed. Using knowledge of the disease process, the nurse explains that fluid repletion decreases blood sugar levels independently of insulin administration (Option A), prevents/treats intravascular collapse (Option D), and improves organ perfusion (Option B). Option C is the incorrect reply because fluid resuscitation does not affect fat breakdown.

Reference: Brenner, Z. R. Management of hyperglycemic emergencies. *AACN Clin Issues,* 17(1), 56–65, 2006.

2-150. **(A)** A patient who has received heparin in the past has an increased risk of developing heparin-induced thrombocytopenia because prior exposure causes development of antibodies that are already present when the patient is next exposed to heparin. Patients undergoing cardiac catheterization and PCI receive heparin during the procedure. Chronic conditions such as asthma, diabetes, hypertension, and renal failure do not influence the development of heparin-induced thrombocytopenia.

Reference: Baird, M. S., Keen, J. H., Swearingen, D .L. *Manual of Critical Care Nursing: Nursing Interventions and Collaborative Management.* St. Louis, Elsevier, 2005.

3 Core Review Test 3

3-1. Which of the following assessment findings would the nurse anticipate in patients with *both* right- and left-sided heart failure?

A. S_3 and S_4 heart sounds
B. Orthopnea
C. Basilar crackles
D. Elevated PA pressures

3-2. A patient is admitted to the ICU after attempted drug overdose. He develops generalized muscle rigidity followed by a rhythmic muscle jerking. The nurse observes this activity for 1 minute and pages the physician managing the patient's care. The activity continues for 10 minutes despite administration of lorazepam 4 mg IV. The next course of action the nurse should anticipate is

A. STAT EEG to confirm that the patient is having a seizure and to localize foci
B. STAT serum and urine labs including myoglobin
C. Infusion of lorazepam with phenytoin 15 mg/kg IV
D. Infusion of pentobarbital 20 mg/kg IV

3-3. A patient is admitted after exhibiting several neuropsychiatric symptoms including motor coordination difficulties, delayed reaction times, headache, and impaired cognitive skills. During the nurse's conversations with the family to secure a patient history, the patient's spouse mentioned that they are in the process of renovating a home that has been in the family for over 50 years. This information suggests that the most likely etiology for this patient's symptoms is

A. Cyanide poisoning
B. Carbon monoxide exposure
C. Exposure to pesticides
D. Lead poisoning

3-4. Occlusion of the left anterior descending coronary artery is associated with which of the following complications?

A. Papillary muscle dysfunction
B. Left ventricular aneurysm
C. Bradycardia
D. Pulmonary edema

3-5. A patient from the Mediterranean is admitted for unstable angina. The patient reports substernal chest pain 7/10, radiating down his left arm. Vital signs are 136/78 mm Hg, HR 106 beats/min, RR 24/min, temp 98.6° F (37° C). Which of the following medications should be administered with caution to this patient?

A. Aspirin
B. Metoprolol (Lopressor®)
C. Nitroglycerin
D. Morphine

3-6. Two hours after open surgical repair of an abdominal aortic aneurysm, a patient is hemodynamically stable and mechanically ventilated. Nursing care of the patient at this time should focus on

A. Preventing peripheral vascular damage with a bed cradle and toe padding
B. Ensuring return of bowel function by instituting a bowel protocol
C. Frequent suctioning to prevent pneumonia
D. Pain control

3-7. A patient with acute exacerbation of COPD is minimally responsive, tachypneic, and tachycardic. Arterial blood gas results include pH 7.20, PaO_2 55 mm Hg, and $PaCO_2$ 68 mm Hg. The nurse anticipates that the next intervention will be

A. Instituting BiPAP
B. Endotracheal intubation
C. Application of low flow oxygen by nasal cannula
D. Administration of 50 mg sodium bicarbonate to correct acidosis

3-8. A 35-year-old Asian man is admitted with jaundice, elevated liver enzyme levels, malaise, and lack of appetite. His total bilirubin is 34 mg/dL; aspartate aminotransferase (AST) 874 U/L; alanine aminotransferase (ALT) 789 IU/L; prothrombin time (PT) 23 sec; international ratio (INR) 3.2. His HAV IgM is negative; HAV IgG is positive; HCV Ab is negative; HBVsAg is positive; HBVs-Ab is negative. The probable cause of these findings is

A. Hepatitis A
B. Hepatitis B
C. Hepatitis C
D. Hepatitis D

3-9. Which of the following findings indicates that end organ dysfunction has occurred in a patient undergoing treatment for hypertensive crisis?

A. Blurred vision
B. BUN 20 mg/dL
C. Patient complaints of lethargy
D. Tall R waves in V_5 and V_6 higher than 30 mm

3-10. A patient is admitted from the operating room after aneurysmal subarachnoid hemorrhage and has been stable since her cra-

niotomy for left middle cerebral artery aneurysm clipping. On the nurse's most recent assessment, he notices that the patient has developed new right lower extremity weakness, perseveration, and a rather flat affect. Which of the following interpretations of these new findings will best aid the nurse in planning appropriate care?

A. Hyponatremia related to cerebral salt wasting
B. Rebleeding of the left middle cerebral artery aneurysm
C. New onset of hydrocephalus
D. Vasospasm of the left anterior cerebral artery

3-11. After a motor vehicle crash, a patient undergoes repair of an aortic rupture that extends from just distal to the subclavian artery to 8 cm above the renal artery. During the immediate postoperative period, this patient is at highest risk for development of which of the following?

A. Coagulopathy
B. Failure to wean from mechanical ventilation
C. Myocardial infarction
D. Stroke

3-12. Which of the following hemodynamic profiles would the nurse anticipate for a patient with a pulmonary history of COPD?

A. PAP 40/20 mm Hg, PAOP 20 mm Hg, CVP 18 mm Hg, CI 1.8 L/min/m²
B. PAP 20/7 mm Hg, PAOP 4 mm Hg, CVP 1 mm Hg, CI 1.8 L/min/m²
C. PAP 35/20 mm Hg, PAOP 7 mm Hg, CVP 4 mm Hg, CI 1.8 L/min/m²
D. PAP 30/15 mm Hg, PAOP 14 mm Hg, CVP 4 mm Hg, CI 1.8 L/min/m²

3-13. A patient diagnosed with acute myocardial infarction suddenly develops hypotension with a blood pressure of 76/58 mm Hg, shortness of breath, and JVD. A loud, high-pitched pansystolic murmur is auscultated. Immediate treatment for the patient would include

A. Transfer to the operating room for CABG surgery
B. Administration of IV nitroglycerin and insertion of intra-aortic balloon pump

C. Transfer to the cardiac catheterization suite for PCI

D. Administration of IV norepinephrine at a rate to maintain systolic BP greater than 90 mm Hg

3-14. A patient was in the ICU with newly diagnosed diabetes and diabetic ketoacidosis and is now ready for discharge. The patient lives alone and is unable to see the numbers on the syringes to self-administer insulin. Which of the following is indicated at this time to decrease the chance of hospital readmission?

A. Determine if the patient may be placed in a skilled nursing facility

B. Provide the patient with a video on insulin administration to reinforce the information.

C. Consult with the case manager for a visiting nurse to see this patient

D. Request that the patient's daughter live with the patient until she can self-administer her insulin

3-15. Three days ago, an older patient was admitted to the ICU following abdominal surgery for a perforated bowel. During the past 4 hours, the patient has developed progressive hypotension unresponsive to fluid boluses, has become oliguric, and demonstrates signs of MODS. The nurse's priority for care now centers on which of the following as the *most* important intervention in reducing mortality of patients with SIRS and/or MODS?

A. Pain management

B. Maintenance of tissue oxygenation

C. Nutritional and metabolic support

D. Identification and treatment of underlying source

3-16. A patient with an intra-aortic balloon pump, intubated on mechanical ventilation, is receiving inotropic support with norepinephrine for cardiogenic shock. The patient is hemodynamically stable. Physical assessment findings include bilateral rales, pale dry skin, right radial pulse 1+, left radial pulse absent, right and left dorsalis pedis pulses 1+. Bowel sounds are hypoactive, and urine output is 30 mL/hr. These findings indicate that the intra-aortic balloon is

A. Malpositioned caudally

B. Obstructing the renal artery

C. Timed incorrectly

D. Obstructing flow along the insertion extremity

3-17. A challenge in nursing care of patients undergoing bariatric surgery is adequately meeting the patient's psychosocial needs. In caring for this patient population, the nurse can anticipate needs related to

A. Low self-esteem

B. Dependence

C. Personal autonomy

D. Trusting others

3-18. The nurse is conducting discharge teaching for a patient newly diagnosed with COPD. Among the recommendations are smoking cessation, pulmonary rehabilitation therapy, and counseling. At the end of the session, the patient asks if giving up cigarettes will make the COPD "go away." What is the nurse's best response?

A. "Yes, if you stop smoking, your lungs will slowly but eventually return to normal."

B. "Most of the damage is permanent, so stopping smoking won't affect your COPD."

C. "If you stop smoking, the rate of damage slows, but your lungs will not be normal again."

D. "As long as you don't have alpha-1 antitrypsin deficiency, cessation of smoking can restore nearly normal lung tissues after about 2 years."

3-19. After abdominal aortic surgery, a patient develops paralytic ileus. Current vital signs include temperature 36.6° C, heart rate 122/min, sinus tachycardia, BP 82/64 mm Hg, respiratory rate 30/min and shallow owing to abdominal distention. SpO_2 is 94% on 4 L oxygen by nasal prongs. Lungs are clear with decreased sounds in the bases. Urine output is 30 mL and 26 mL for the last 2 hours. The patient is restless and complains of abdominal pain. The most likely cause of these findings is

A. Sepsis

B. Hypovolemia

C. GI hemorrhage

D. Acute respiratory failure

3-20. A 67-year-old with type 2 diabetes is scheduled for an intravenous pyelogram (IVP). To reduce the potentially toxic effects of contrast dye on the kidney, which of the following medical orders should *not* be implemented until the nurse has conferred with the intensivist?

A. Administer N-Acetylcysteine (Mucomyst) in AM

B. Hold furosemide (Lasix) in AM

C. Administer metformin (Glucophage) in AM

D. Discontinue renal-dose dopamine

3-21. An unresponsive patient in the ICU is at end of life. The family has requested that no heroic measures be initiated, that no unnecessary monitoring be used, and that withdrawal of support be initiated. One family member asks why the Bispectral Index Monitor (BIS monitor) is still in use. The nurse's best response is that

A. "It will tell us when your loved one is brain dead."

B. "It is used to ensure that the patient is not experiencing any pain."

C. "We used it to measure pressures inside the skull."

D. "It's used routinely on all comatose patients."

3-22. Which of the following clinical situations places the patient at high risk for the development of pericardial tamponade?

A. Acute renal failure with hemodialysis

B. STEMI with administration of thrombolytic therapy

C. Pericardial effusion with friction rub

D. Insertion of intra-aortic balloon pump

3-23. A patient admitted with necrotizing pancreatitis and has just returned from the operating room where aggressive debridement of peripancreatic tissue was performed. The patient's postoperative care includes antibiotics, IV fluids, and mechanical ventilation. In managing care for this patient over the next few days, which of the following findings should the nurse recognize as the most

reliable indicator of a poor prognosis for this patient?

A. Elevated serum amylase

B. Elevated APACHE-II score

C. Decreased PaO$_2$ level

D. Decreased serum C-reactive protein (CPR) level

3-24. A patient comes to ICU following left pneumonectomy for a hilar mass. The patient has stable vital signs and is awake, oriented, intubated, and ventilated on assist-control mode at a rate of 18, tidal volume 8 mL/kg, PEEP +5, and FiO$_2$ .40. The patient's heart rate and respiratory rate suddenly increase, and his oxygen saturation decreases. The nurse notes that a new central line was placed to the right subclavian site. While increasing the oxygen and preparing for chest tube insertion, the nurse formulates an ongoing plan of care. Which of the following interventions is *least likely* to be helpful in preventing further pulmonary complications in this patient?

A. Prompt ventilator weaning

B. Aggressive pulmonary toilet

C. Increase PEEP

D. Pain management

3-25. A combination of furosemide (Lasix) infusion at 8 mg/hr and bumetanide (Bumex) 10 mg fails to produce urine output greater than 25 mL/hr in a hypertensive patient with pulmonary edema. Which of the following interventions does the nurse now anticipate for this patient?

A. Increase furosemide (Lasix) infusion to 10 mg/hr

B. Discontinue furosemide (Lasix) and administer another 10 mg of bumetanide (Bumex) IV

C. Institute continuous arterial venous hemofiltration (CAVH)

D. Initiate dopamine infusion at 10 mg/kg/hr

3-26. Anemia and coagulation abnormalities are common hematologic findings in the patient with SIRS/MODS. Which of the following sets of laboratory findings suggests that a patient with SIRS/MODS has now developed one of these coagulation disorders?

A. ↑aPTT, ↑PT, ↓Platelets, ↑FDPs (fibrin degradation products)
B. ↓aPTT, ↓PT, ↑Platelets, ↓FDPs
C. ↑aPTT, ↑PT, ↑Platelets, ↑FDPs
D. ↓aPTT, ↓PT, ↓Platelets, ↓FDPs

3-27. The clinical pathway for a cardiac surgery patient states that today the epicardial pacing wires are to be removed by the nurse. Which of the following conditions would indicate that the nurse should obtain an order to leave the epicardial wires in place?

A. The patient's heart rate is 58 BPM and BP is 122/68 mm Hg
B. The patient received low-molecular-weight heparin, 30 mg, 14 hours prior to planned removal time
C. The INR is 1.1
D. The aPTT is 74 seconds

3-28. A patient with advanced heart failure is deciding whether or not to consent to placement of a ventricular assist device (VAD) and asks for information. Which of the following should the nurse include?

A. A VAD may not improve quality of life but will improve symptoms
B. The pump is placed in the upper chest, like a pacemaker
C. Most VADs are used temporarily until transplant
D. Once the VAD is in place, you will be hospitalized and bedridden

3-29. After ethanol ablation is performed for a patient with hypertrophic cardiomyopathy, which of the following should the nurse anticipate performing?

A. Administration of amiodarone to treat atrial fibrillation
B. Administration of calcium channel blockers to treat supraventricular dysrhythmias
C. Use of temporary cardiac pacing
D. Obtaining serial cardiac troponin and CPK studies

3-30. In the early stages of idiopathic thrombocytopenic purpura (ITP), nursing interventions primarily focus on

A. Maintaining a patent airway
B. Controlling the respiratory rate

C. Replenishing circulating blood volume
D. Coping with alterations in body image

3-31. Patients who are older or malnourished, as well as those with impaired host defense systems or severe illness, are all at increased risk of developing central venous catheter (CVC) infections. Prevention is the most effective means of avoiding infection from this source. Which of the following interventions accurately reflects current guidelines for prevention and management of CVC infections?

A. Routine change of catheter using guidewire exchange technique
B. Application of topical antibiotic ointment or cream at insertion site
C. Maximum sterile precautions during catheter insertion
D. Use of gauze and transparent dressing to maintain sterile environment

3-32. A patient is admitted to the ICU following surgery to remove a bullet from a gunshot wound to the chest. The patient remains intubated on mechanical ventilation and stabilizes with chest tube drainage averaging 75 mL/hr. Two hours later, the nurse notes that the patient's tidal volumes are decreasing, chest tube output has increased to 300 mL/hr, and BP has decreased from 123/78 to 70/50 mm Hg. After notification of the trauma surgeon, the nurse immediately prepares for

A. Insertion of a second chest tube
B. Returning the patient to the operating room
C. Hanging a dopamine drip
D. Assisting with a bronchoscopy

3-33. An ICU patient has become confused and lethargic 5 days after aneurysmal subarachnoid hemorrhage and aneurysm coil embolization. Which of the following approaches should the nurse anticipate discussing with the acute care nurse practitioner managing this patient's care?

A. Increase the nimodipine dose to 60 mg every two hours
B. Reduce the volume of IV fluids to prevent hyperemia and risk of rebleed

C. Perform angiography to evaluate evidence of vasospasm and treat with transluminal ballooning.

D. Prepare for lumbar puncture to evaluate for evidence of meningitis

3-34. An 83-year-old patient with a history of chronic heart failure, longstanding COPD, and osteoarthritis is admitted to the ICU with pneumonia. The patient has undergone tracheostomy and has since failed at three attempts to wean. Although the patient is alert and oriented, he seems too fatigued to assist with the weaning process. Nursing staff are feeling increasingly frustrated in their attempts to help this patient progress. Which of the following would likely help the ICU nursing staff improve outcomes for this patient?

A. Contact the social worker to help prepare the patient for discharge to a long-term acute care facility

B. Suggest that the intensivist request a consult from the multidisciplinary ventilator team

C. Speak with the family to determine feasibility of taking the patient home on a ventilator

D. Suggest a nutrition team consult to build the patient's strength for successful weaning

3-35. Following left heart cardiac catheterization, which of the following complications would the nurse be vigilant for?

A. Stroke
B. Pulmonary embolus
C. Flushing and nausea
D. Bradycardia and vagal responses

3-36. A patient with type 1 diabetes is frequently rehospitalized for diabetic ketoacidosis. The patient refuses to administer insulin, perform capillary glucose measurement, or follow the diabetic diet since initial diagnosis of the disease. This admission's initial laboratory results are as follows: glucose 200 mg/dL, pH 6.9, PCO_2 25.7 mm Hg, PaO_2 94 mm Hg, and bicarbonate 7.0 mEq/L. Which of the following orders should the nurse perform first?

A. Administer 8 units of NPH insulin subcutaneously using a sliding scale

B. Encourage oral clear liquids in order to maintain nutritional status

C. Obtain specimen for blood gas interpretation and chemistry in 1 hour

D. Administer 50 mmol bicarbonate in 200 mL intravenously over 1 hour

3-37. Which of the following conditions most predisposes the intubated patient to develop ventilator-associated pneumonia (VAP)?

A. Endotracheal tube cuff leak
B. Presence of enteral feedings
C. Glasgow coma scale score of 9
D. Presence of an NG tube

3-38. A 12-lead ECG is performed on a patient with wide complex tachycardia demonstrating QS complexes (negative concordance) in all precordial leads. This finding is consistent with which of the following?

A. Pericarditis
B. Right bundle branch block
C. Left bundle branch block
D. Ventricular tachycardia

3-39. Patients who experience cardiac arrest related to trauma prior to arriving at the hospital rarely survive despite rapid and effective emergency management. Among the interventions designed to improve survival for these patients, which of the following is *most* important?

A. Performing the primary and secondary survey

B. Determining the extent of injury by removing the patient's clothing

C. Providing aggressive IV fluid resuscitation

D. Transporting the patient to the ER or tertiary care facility

3-40. An elevated level of which of the following serum values represents the most specific finding in the diagnosis of perioperative myocardial infarction?

A. Troponin
B. Total CK
C. C-reactive protein
D. Myoglobin

3-41. A patient is in the ICU with septic shock from toxoplasmosis. The patient has a history of AIDS and is intubated and on mechanical ventilation. The patient communicates concern over having not taken antiretroviral treatment since being intubated. The nurse's best response is

A. "I am sure we can give you your medications enterally."
B. "We will monitor you for immunosuppression."
C. "Most antiretroviral medications are available in intravenous form."
D. "Because you are critically ill right now, you are at increased risk for pancreatitis if we continue your antiretroviral treatment."

3-42. The 12-lead ECG changes below are indicative of which of the following?

A. ST segment myocardial infarction (STEMI)
B. Age-indeterminate myocardial infarction
C. Left bundle branch block making myocardial injury difficult to determine
D. Myocardial ischemia

3-43. A trauma surgeon states that nurses do not know how to care for patients with chest tubes and requests that only two specific nurses be assigned to care for his patients when they are in the ICU. The unit's nursing staff can best manage this situation by

A. Suggesting that the surgeon meet with the nurse manager
B. Convening a task force to review unit standards of care for these patients
C. Discussing the surgeon's specific concerns with him
D. Scheduling a mandatory in-service for all unit nurses on care of these patients

3-44. A patient is recovering from an acute exacerbation of COPD. The physician requests that the patient start ambulating around his room. The nurse knows that this activity

A. Often triggers a relapse of bronchitis
B. Represents a key component of pulmonary rehabilitation
C. Requires support with supplemental oxygen
D. Should be preceded by premedication with bronchodilators

3-45. Biventricular pacemaker implantation is indicated for heart failure associated with which of the following?

A. Severe diastolic and systolic dysfunction
B. Severe systolic dysfunction with left ventricular hypertrophy
C. Atrial fibrillation refractory to pharmacologic therapy
D. Left ventricular hypertrophy and documented ventricular tachycardia

3-46. A patient in the ICU is experiencing insomnia and associated agitation. The patient prefers not to take a controlled substance as a sleep aid. In addition to reducing noise and interruptions, which of the following interventions has been shown to be both valuable and feasible in this situation?

A. Massage
B. Aromatherapy
C. Alternative sedatives
D. Progressive muscle relaxation

3-47. Cardiac catheterization reveals total occlusion of the left anterior descending artery and a filling defect resulting in right ventricular filling during left heart catheterization. Oxygen saturation of the right atrium is 80%, of the right ventricle is 96%, and of the left ventricle is 96%. Which of the following complications associated with acute myocardial infarction do these findings indicate?

A. Ventricular septal defect
B. Atrial septal defect

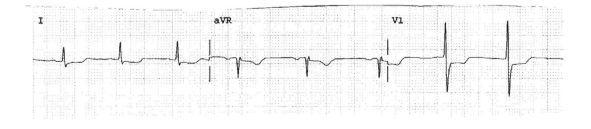

C. Papillary muscle rupture

D. Rupture of the ventricular free wall

3-48. An older patient is admitted after a fall that resulted in a momentary loss of consciousness. The patient's medications include atenolol, furosemide, digoxin, and paroxetine, and vital signs are BP 110/72 mm Hg, heart rate 56 beats/min, respiratory rate 18 breaths/min. During the nursing history, the patient describes yesterday's bowel movement as sticky and black in color. Based on these findings, the nurse would initiate interventions aimed at monitoring this patient's

A. Intracranial pressure and level of consciousness.

B. 12-lead ECG to evaluate the bradycardia

C. Diet and nutritional support systems in the home

D. Hemoglobin and hematocrit to evaluate blood loss

3-49. The echocardiogram of a patient with acute infectious endocarditis demonstrates tricuspid and pulmonary insufficiency. The patient is intubated and placed on mechanical ventilation and receives propofol and lorazepam for sedation as well as antibiotic therapy. Which of the following is potentially an immediate life-threatening problem for this patient?

A. Acute drug withdrawal and seizures

B. Abscess formation and septicemia

C. Pulmonary infarction

D. Stroke

3-50. A comatose patient of Gypsy culture is in the ICU and is at the end of life. The nurse should approach the request for organ donation based on which of the following?

A. This cultural group does not usually agree to organ donation unless a close family member is the intended recipient.

B. Although members of this cultural group generally prefer cremation, they may agree to organ donation under special circumstances.

C. Members of this cultural group believe that the soul remains active for 1 year after death, so the body must remain intact.

D. Persons in this cultural group typically agree to organ donation, but only for another member of their culture.

3-51. During an initial neurologic assessment, the nurse finds that the patient has a positive Brudzinski's sign and a positive Kernig's sign. Otherwise, the patient's examination is nonfocal. Since the lumbar puncture performed earlier showed high protein and low glucose in the CSF, the nurse's most appropriate action at this time is to

A. Prepare for brain MRI to rule out mass lesion

B. Arrange for initiation of plasmaphoresis

C. Prepare to administer intravenous antibiotics

D. Prepare the patient for a repeat LP to withdraw accumulating CSF

3-52. Which of the following findings best indicates that fluid resuscitation for hypovolemic shock has been appropriate?

A. SVO_2 45%, CO 3.0 L/min, SVR 800 dynes/sec/cm^{-5}

B. SVO_2 45%, CO 5.0 L/min, SVR 1900 dynes/sec/cm^{-5}

C. SVO_2 68%, CO 5.0 L/min, SVR 2100 dynes/sec/cm^{-5}

D. SVO_2 68%, CO 4.4 L/min, SVR 1100 dynes/sec/cm^{-5}

3-53. A patient has a feeding tube in place. Feedings have not yet been started. The nurse aspirates some contents from the feeding tube to check for placement and obtains a small amount of watery, straw-colored fluid with a pH of 7. Which of the following is indicated at this time?

A. Collaborate with the respiratory therapist to double-check correct feeding tube placement using the auscultatory method

B. Administer the feeding as prescribed, consulting with the dietitian if problems arise

C. Flush the tube with 30 mL of saline and notify the physician if respiratory distress occurs

D. Speak with the physician so a chest x-ray can be ordered for this purpose

3-54. Which of the following sets of arterial blood gas results indicates acute respiratory failure that requires immediate endotracheal intubation?

   A. pH 7.30, PaO_2 69 mm Hg, $PaCO_2$ 48 mm Hg
   B. pH 7.50, PaO_2 64 mm Hg, $PaCO_2$ 52 mm Hg
   C. pH 7.20, PaO_2 60 mm Hg, $PaCO_2$ 53 mm Hg
   D. pH 7.50, PaO_2 65 mm Hg, $PaCO_2$ 20 mm Hg

3-55. The patient with fulminating liver disease secondary to hepatitis B infection mentions to the nurse that he has been sharing needles with friends. Which of the following will help protect these people from developing an active hepatitis B infection?

   A. Acetaminophen administration to prevent inflammation
   B. Vaccination against hepatitis B to promote antibody development
   C. Gamma globulin to increase available antibodies
   D. Exchange transfusions to replace infected blood with noninfected blood

3-56. A patient with a traumatic brain injury (TBI) has just been admitted to the ICU after resuscitation in the emergency department. Which of the following initial studies should the nurse anticipate in this patient?

   A. Magnetic resonance imaging (MRI) of the brain
   B. Computed tomography (CT) scan of the head
   C. Lumbar puncture (LP)
   D. Cerebral angiography

3-57. A family has donated monies to support the redesign of an ICU. The intensivist has been working with the contractor on the unit design. The nurse on the design team reviews the plans and has concerns that they are not conducive to the comfort needs of visitors to the unit. Which of the following would be the best approach for the nurse to communicate these concerns to the design team?

   A. Speak with the nurse manager regarding these concerns
   B. Assemble a team of nurses to revise the plan

   C. Mention these concerns at the next scheduled team design meeting
   D. Gather data on the needs of family members who visit ICU

3-58. Coronary reperfusion after thrombolytic administration is best evidenced by

   A. An increase in CPK-MB and troponin levels in 1 hour
   B. A decrease in CPK-MB and troponin levels in 1 hour
   C. The development of dysrhythmias
   D. The resolution of ST segment elevation

3-59. An end-stage renal disease (ESRD) patient receiving hemodialysis three times per week is admitted to the CCU with an acute anterior wall myocardial infarction. The patient's BP is 108/46 mm Hg, HR is 62/min, and RR is 24/min. The critical care nurse should anticipate that this patient's dialysis will be managed by

   A. Slow continuous ultrafiltration
   B. Continuous venovenous hemodialysis
   C. Hemodialysis
   D. Peritoneal dialysis

3-60. An 81-year-old ICU patient injured in a motor vehicle crash has elevated intracranial pressure (ICP). In addition, the patient's serum glucose level is noted to be elevated. His wife is concerned because she claims her husband does not have a history of diabetes. Which of the following would the nurse state while providing teaching to the wife?

   A. "Your husband will likely need to take insulin once he is sent home."
   B. "It is common for older persons to develop decreased glucose tolerance."
   C. "It is likely due to an impaired ability to absorb nutrients that occurs in older adults, made worse by the trauma."
   D. "Your husband likely had diabetes prior to his hospitalization, but was not aware of it until laboratory tests were done."

3-61. ST and T wave abnormalities are of greatest concern for the nurse in patients with

   A. Dilated cardiomyopathy
   B. Arrhythmogenic right ventricular cardiomyopathy

C. Left bundle branch block

D. Pericarditis

3-62. A 56-year-old male with a history of diverticulitis is wheeled into the ICU with a diagnosis of acute abdomen and dehydration. On assessment, the nurse notes that he is complaining of sudden onset of severe (9/10) left lower quadrant abdominal pain with wall tenderness, diaphoresis, nausea, and pallor. He is becoming increasingly more agitated. His blood pressure has dropped from 135/86 mm Hg to 90/54 mm Hg, and his HR has risen from 92 beats/min to 135 beats/min, while his temperature is 101° F. Which of the following interventions should the nurse focus on at this point?

A. Restoring circulating volume

B. Completing an abdominal assessment

C. Instituting cooling measures

D. Obtaining the patient's medication list

3-63. A patient admitted with fever, dyspnea, and a cough productive of large amounts of rust-colored sputum now complains of severe pleuritic chest pain. His temperature is 39.5° C, heart rate is 120/min, respiratory rate is 40/min, SO_2 is 95% on 50% FiO_2, and BP is 100/40 mm Hg after 1 L of normal saline. His breath sounds are diminished bilaterally with fine, inspiratory crackles in both bases, and a chest x-ray is obtained. Which of the following interventions should the critical care nurse anticipate next?

A. Thoracentesis for a likely pulmonary effusion

B. Chest tube insertion for a pneumothorax

C. Administration of an analgesic agent

D. Administration of a diuretic

3-64. A major concern of the nurse caring for a patient receiving inhaled nitric oxide for pulmonary hypertension would be which of the following?

A. Rebound pulmonary hypertension when nitric oxide is discontinued

B. Hypotension caused by nitric oxide administration

C. Decreased oxygen saturation related to nitric oxide uptake

D. Pulmonary embolus related to nitric oxide effects on platelet aggregation

3-65. A patient is admitted to the ICU with the diagnosis of acute myocardial infarction related to cocaine abuse. Specific guidelines developed by the American College of Cardiology and the American Heart Association recommend prompt administration of medications once the diagnosis of acute MI is determined. Which of the following medications is not recommended for patients with a cocaine-induced myocardial infarction?

A. β-blocker

B. Morphine

C. Nitroglycerin

D. Aspirin

3-66. A pregnant woman (28 weeks' gestation) is admitted to the ICU after sustaining a head injury. The patient is receiving intracranial monitoring, is intubated, and is receiving mechanical ventilation. Intracranial pressure readings this hour range from 12-14 mm Hg. The nurse assigned to this patient is the most experienced ICU nurse on duty that evening but has not provided care to a critically ill obstetric patient before. Which of the following responses by this nurse will serve the patient best?

A. Contact the perinatal clinical nurse specialist for collaboration in providing care

B. Speak to the intensivist regarding setup and use of fetal monitoring equipment

C. Collabrate with the emergency department nursing staff regarding patient care needs

D. Contact the neurosurgical nurse practitioner for collaboration in patient monitoring

3-67. The 12-lead ECG for a patient with chest pain demonstrates sinus rhythm at a rate of 70/min. The QRS width in all leads is 0.14 seconds with a QS pattern and 1 mm ST segment elevation in leads V_1, V_2, and V_3 and ST segment depression in leads V_5 and V_6. Based on these findings, the nurse will plan care for a patient with

A. Acute anterior wall myocardial infarction

B. Acute posterior wall myocardial infarction

C. Acute anterolateral wall myocardial infarction

D. Inconclusive findings unless cardiac serum markers are elevated

3-68. A patient with end-stage renal failure is hypoglycemic and confused, but conversant and able to obey most commands. The patient's most recent capillary glucose measurement was 60 mg/dL. Which of the following nursing interventions is appropriate at this time?

A. Ensure the patient drinks ½ cup (120 mL) of orange juice
B. Provide ½ cup regular (not diet) soft drink with ice chips
C. Assist the patient in ingesting 10 jelly beans
D. Distribute some sugared breath mints to the patient for halitosis

3-69. A gay teenager involved in a motor vehicle crash is admitted to the ICU for observation. His partner visits frequently, and the couple hold hands during those visits. Visitors of other patients complain about this behavior and demand that the nurse "do something" about it. The ICU nurse can best resolve this situation by

A. Convening a multidisciplinary staff meeting to determine an approach to this issue
B. Explaining to the patient and his visitor that their behavior is upsetting to others and must cease
C. Listening to the visitors' concerns while clarifying that the behavior they describe is a comfort gesture
D. Moving the patient to another ICU cubicle where the occupants are less visible to others

3-70. A patient who has been healthy for 3 years since a liver transplant was admitted to the ICU somewhat lethargic and feverish, with an incidence of acute rejection suspected. Admission laboratory values reveal elevated liver function tests. Which of the following should the nurse do next?

A. Prepare the patient for transport for magnetic resonance imaging
B. Ensure the patient's bladder is empty in preparation for percutaneous liver biopsy
C. Gather supplies and equipment for placement of a central line and a pulmonary artery catheter.
D. Obtain baseline measurements of abdominal girth and intra-abdominal pressure

3-71. After being found on the floor at home, an 82-year-old patient is admitted to the ICU with diminished mental status and new onset seizures. The patient is lethargic, oriented to name only, and calling out for water. His BP is 86/40 mm Hg and his HR is 136 beats/min. Laboratory findings include: Na 150 mEq/L, K 3.4 mEq/L, Ca 8.7 mg/dL, Mg 1.5 mEq/L, serum osmolality 306 mOsm/kg, and urine specific gravity 1.036. Based on this clinical data, which of the following should the nurse anticipate administering first?

A. Magnesium
B. Free water
C. Potassium
D. Vitamin D

3-72. The rhythm strip below would best be described as which of the following?

A. Complete capture DDD pacemaker
B. Incomplete capture DDD pacemaker
C. Complete capture VVI pacemaker
D. Complete capture AAI pacemaker

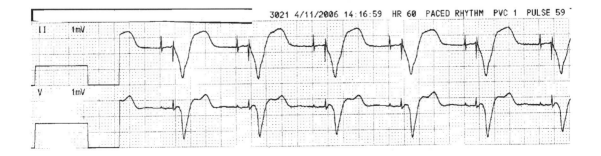

3021 4/11/2006 14:16:59 HR 60 PACED RHYTHM PVC 1 PULSE 59

3-73. During episodes of shock owing to acute blood loss, compensatory mechanisms attempt to increase oxygen delivery to vital organs. When the nurse provides care to a patient in hemorrhagic shock, which of the following is an anticipated finding attributable to such compensation?

    A. Widened pulse pressure
    B. Vasodilatation of arteries
    C. Decreased heart rate
    D. Decreased urine sodium

3-74. A 96-year-old man with a history of long-standing esophageal reflux is admitted to the surgical ICU post esophagogastrectomy. His vital signs are temperature 99.0° F, BP 146/76 mm Hg, pulse 122 beats/min. His incisional pain is 8/10. Which of the following interventions would be key to reducing this patient's risk of mortality and morbidity?

    A. Pulmonary care
    B. Pain management
    C. Administration of large amounts of IV fluids
    D. Immediate institution of tube feedings

3-75. A nurse has just admitted a patient diagnosed with an acute ischemic stroke to the ICU. Which of the following assessment findings should alert the nurse to a contraindication for rt-PA therapy?

    A. NIH Stroke Scale score of 1
    B. History of seizure disorder
    C. A mild traumatic brain injury from a motor vehicle collision 6 months ago
    D. INR greater than 1.3

3-76. A patient is intubated and mechanically ventilated. The FiO_2 is 100%, and a recently drawn arterial blood gas study shows a PaO_2 of 68 mm Hg. When the P/F ratio is calculated, which of the following conditions does the nurse now know needs to be managed in this patient?

    A. Acute respiratory distress syndrome
    B. Acute pulmonary embolism
    C. Acute pulmonary edema
    D. Pneumonia

3-77. A patient with pulmonary edema is receiving continuous infusions of nitroglycerin 5 mcg/min, nitroprusside (Nipride) 5 mcg/kg/ min, and dobutamine 5 mcg/kg/min. Hemodynamic values obtained include MAP 70 mm Hg, CVP 18 mm Hg, PCWP 14 mm Hg, and SVR 1200 dyne/sec/cm^{-5}. Which of the following nursing interventions is most appropriate at this time?

    A. Increase nitroglycerin infusion to 10 mcg/min
    B. Increase nitroprusside (Nipride) to 10 mcg/kg/min
    C. Increase dobutamine to 10 mcg/kg/min
    D. Discontinue dobutamine and start dopamine 5 mcg/kg/min

3-78. A critical care nurse is working a double shift with two assigned patients and the time is 1800 hours. One patient is a 15-year-old newly diagnosed with diabetic ketoacidosis requiring hourly blood glucose monitoring, and the other is a 20-year-old who needs hourly neurologic checks for a closed head injury and whose mother needs constant reassurance. A recently graduated nurse has asked this nurse to help her change a colostomy bag on a fresh postoperative patient; in addition, the nurse manager stops by the unit to ask the nurse to look over the staffing schedule for the next 6 weeks. As the nurse considers this work load, she realizes that some of the work will need to be delegated to ensure that that priority patient needs are met. Which of the following best reflects an appropriate and safe delegation strategy?

    A. Hourly glucose checks delegated to another RN
    B. Hourly neurological check delegated to the UAP
    C. Helping new nurse delegated to another RN
    D. Staffing schedule review delegated to the new nurse

3-79. A young man was admitted 3 days ago after a motorcycle accident in which he sustained a closed head injury and fracture of his right femur. The nurse notes on assessment a petechial skin rash over his chest and neck. The patient is now disoriented to both person and place, which is a change from the previous shift. His platelet count had dropped from 290,000/mm^3 to 49,580/mm^3. Which of the following is the most likely explanation for this patient's development of hypoxia?

A. Thrombus resulting from venous stasis obstructed pulmonary blood flow
B. Injury to the endothelial lining of pulmonary capillaries caused alveolar flooding
C. Bronchociliary clearance mechanisms are overwhelmed
D. Blood is being shunted through poorly ventilated areas of pulmonary consolidation

3-80. Dysrhythmias anticipated after atrial septal defect repair include which of the following?

A. Ventricular fibrillation and ventricular tachycardia
B. Second-degree and third-degree heart block
C. Atrial fibrillation and supraventricular dysrhythmias
D. Sinus arrest and sinus arrhythmia

3-81. Assessment parameters for a patient in septic shock reveal the following hemodynamic values: HR 90/min, BP 80/50 mm Hg, PAP 36/15 mm Hg, CVP 13 mm Hg, CO 2.5 L/min, CI 1.9 L/min/m², SVR 1000 dynes/sec/cm⁻⁵, SVO_2 60% Which of the following treatments should the nurse expect to administer to this patient?

A. Norepinephrine and dobutamine
B. Dopamine and 500 mL fluid bolus
C. Dobutamine and 500 mL fluid bolus
D. Norepinephrine and sodium bicarbonate

3-82. A patient has a pulmonary artery catheter in place. Which of the following interventions should be performed in order to assure accurate readings?

A. Perform a square wave test prior to obtaining each reading
B. Level the transducer to the left atrium
C. Maintain the patient in a flat supine position whenever measurements are taken
D. Obtain readings at the end of inhalation

3-83. Initial interventions to ensure tissue perfusion in vasogenic shock states include administration of

A. Norepinephrine (Levophed) to maintain SBP >90 mm Hg
B. Milrinone (Primacor) to maintain SBP >80 mm Hg
C. Crystalloid to achieve SBP >90 mm Hg
D. Dopamine to achieve SBP >80 mm Hg

3-84. A patient remains in ICU 1 week after undergoing thoracotomy for repair of a traumatic aortic tear. She has been extubated for 2 days and remains on an aero mask with FiO_2 .50. Her vitals are HR 88 beats/min, BP 130/82 mm Hg, O_2 sat 97%, temperature 37.9° C. Pain control has been an issue, but she is currently comfortable with a morphine PCA and long-acting narcotics. Over the past 3 hours, she has become increasingly agitated, and now complains of difficulty breathing. Her vitals now are HR 140 beats/min, BP 95/50 mm Hg, and O_2 sat 88%. The nurse telephones the physician and anticipates which of the following orders?

A. Increase the FiO_2, call anesthesia to intubate STAT, and alert the operating room
B. Administer an anxiolytic, change to a short-acting narcotic, and call for a STAT anesthesia consult
C. Increase the FiO_2, PA, and lateral chest x-ray, and prepare the patient for CT angiogram of the chest
D. PA and lateral chest x-ray, discontinue the PCA, and prepare the patient for emergent surgery

3-85. A patient admitted after a motor vehicle crash in which he was the driver now complains of severe left shoulder pain when lying supine. There are bruises across the abdomen and chest from the seat belts. Vital signs are BP 120/80 mm Hg, pulse 112 beats/min, and RR 18 breaths/min. The nurse is reassessing the patient. Which of the following findings should the nurse interpret as an emergency situation?

A. Epigastric pain with belching
B. Abdominal distention with absent bowel sounds
C. Decreased breath sounds bilaterally
D. Pain and burning with hematuria

3-86. A 28-year-old patient presents to the ICU confused, combative, and unable to report any personal information or medical history. Toxicology screen and blood alcohol levels are negative, and no focal deficits are apparent. If this patient has some type of encephalopathy, which of the following investigations should the nurse now anticipate for this patient?

A. Intracranial pressure monitoring
B. Serum osmolarity and ammonia testing
C. Lumbar puncture for immunoassay
D. Cerebral angiographic evaluation

3-87. In planning care for a patient with acute renal failure, the critical care nurse knows the patient is achieving outcome criteria when the patient's

A. CVP is 1 mm Hg
B. CI is 2.8 L/min/m²
C. MAP is 60 mm Hg
D. PAOP is 6 mm Hg

3-88. Nonparoxysmal junctional tachycardia with a rate of 110/min is best treated with which of the following?

A. Overdrive pacing
B. Withholding administration of digoxin
C. Administration of 0.25 mg of digoxin
D. Administration of 6 mg adenosine

3-89. Which of the following findings suggests that the pulmonary artery catheter is overwedged owing to migration of the catheter?

A. PCWP is lower than the RAP
B. PCWP is lower than the PAD
C. PCWP is 2 mm Hg higher than the PAD
D. The waveform does not pulsate

3-90. A patient's family requests the patient's withdrawal from mechanical ventilation. In order to prepare them for what to expect, the nurse should include

A. The name of the person who will be performing the procedure
B. The anticipated time frame to death
C. Manifestations the patient will likely exhibit
D. The need to insert an airway to remove secretions that cause a "death rattle"

3-91. The critical care nurse is reviewing orders for diagnostic tests for a patient with suspected hospital-acquired pneumonia. Which

of the following diagnostic tests should the nurse refrain from securing until the order can be verified with the physician?

A. PA and lateral chest x-ray
B. Blood cultures
C. Expectorated sputum for culture
D. Pan-cultures prior to antibiotics

3-92. A patient of Appalachian descent is admitted to ICU for acute myocardial infarction. The patient has a history of hypertension and diabetes and is a two-pack-per-day tobacco smoker. Which of the following nursing strategies would be most appropriate for teaching this patient about risk factors for heart disease and prudent heart living?

A. Teach the patient about the positive health effects of diet and exercise
B. Collaborate with the smoking cessation specialist to discuss various cessation methods with the patient
C. Determine ways that the patient's health can be improved by altering his environment
D. Speak with the patient's significant others to assist the patient with preventative measures.

3-93. Tumor necrosis factor-α (TNF) is a polypeptide secretory product of the monocyte-macrophage system that is released during SIRS. Nurses who work with critically ill patients need to be especially vigilant regarding clinical situations that may precipitate release of TNF because one of the most serious cellular responses to this mediator is

A. Microvascular vasodilation
B. Metabolic alkalosis
C. Decreased oxygen consumption
D. Increased capillary permeability

3-94. A new graduate orientee is providing care to a relatively stable patient who is recovering from thoracic trauma incurred from a motorcycle accident 10 days ago. During report, the orientee heard that this patient's recovery is being delayed by a persistent air leak, manifested by continuous bubbling in his chest tube. When the nurse preceptor arrives and explains the alternatives that could be employed for definitive treatment of a persistent air leak, which of the following would be the *least likely* treatment for this disorder?

A. Bronchoscopy
B. Instillation of antibiotics into the chest tube
C. Progressive advancement of the chest tube
D. Surgery

3-95. A 68-year-old end-stage renal disease (ESRD) patient who receives hemodialysis for 3 hours, three times per week, presents to the ED with a complaint of sharp, stabbing chest pain that increases on inspiration and dyspnea on exertion. The patient's vital signs are BP 110/68 mm Hg, HR 122/min, RR 28/min and labored, temperature 100.2° F. The patient has a pericardial friction rub. Management of this patient will now include

A. Four hours of hemodialysis three times per week
B. Four hours of hemodialysis done daily
C. Peritoneal dialysis, four exchanges per day
D. Peritoneal dialysis, five exchanges per day

3-96. The nurse is performing an admission assessment on a patient diagnosed with diabetes insipidus. Which of the following assessment findings would the nurse expect to see in a patient with that condition?

A. Elevated systolic blood pressure, tachycardia, decreased urinary output
B. Elevated serum potassium, bradycardia, numbness in hands
C. Polyuria, extreme thirst, decreased urinary specific gravity
D. Widened pulse pressures, dilated pupils, decerebrate posturing

3-97. For a patient in acute pulmonary edema, initial nursing interventions would include

A. Administering oxygen and obtaining arterial blood gas analysis
B. Obtaining a 12-lead ECG and initiating IV access
C. Obtaining a chest x-ray and an echocardiogram
D. Administering furosemide (Lasix) and nitroglycerin

3-98. A 5-year-old child is admitted to the adult ICU with a diagnosis of hemolytic uremic syndrome. In order to provide optimal nursing care for this child, which of the following should serve as the primary goal of care?

A. Protecting target organs from ischemic injury
B. Reducing uric acid levels through hydration
C. Replacing clotting factors by means of transfusion
D. Removing excess platelets through plasmaphoresis

3-99. A patient is on a ventilator in the ICU with the following vital signs: BP 96/50 mm Hg, HR 102 beats/min, RR 32/min, temperature 100.8° F (38.2° C). New onset urosepsis is suspected, and fluid resuscitation is in progress. Which therapeutic end points of fluid resuscitation are recommended for this situation?

A. CVP 12-15 mm Hg and mean arterial pressure $\geq$65 mm Hg
B. Urinary output equal to or greater than 30 mL/hr and improved mental status
C. Decreased serum lactate and systolic blood pressure >90 mm Hg
D. CVP 8-12 mm Hg and urinary output $\geq$30 mL/hr

3-100. Which of the following medications is the most rapid and effective agent to reduce preload in acute pulmonary edema?

A. Morphine sulfate
B. Furosemide (Lasix)
C. Nitroglycerin
D. Captopril (Capoten)

3-101. A 28-year-old woman is admitted to the ICU following a motorcycle accident in which she sustained a severe pelvic fracture and blunt trauma to her lower extremities. She is on bed rest and has been started on a clear liquid diet. Her hemoglobin continues to drift down over the last 36 hours from a high after transfusion of 11 g/dL to 9.3 g/dL. The physician has ordered continued monitoring of her hemoglobin and administration of 2 units of packed cells. Her BP is 110/72 mm Hg, pulse is 98 beats/min, and RR is 18 breaths/min. Her risks for development of pulmonary emboli are increased because of

A. Venous stasis, vein injury, and a hypercoagulable state
B. Intravascular cannulation, dehydration, and age
C. Hypoxia, interstitial edema, and right ventricular dysfunction
D. Pulmonary artery hypertension, atelectasis, and immobility

3-102. A patient is admitted with the dysrhythmia below. The onset of this dysrhythmia cannot be determined, and the patient complains of palpitations, fatigue, and moderate shortness of breath. Which of the following initial interventions should the nurse anticipate?

A. Cardioversion with 100 joules monophasic
B. Cardioversion with 50 joules biphasic
C. Administration of dofetilide 250 mg orally
D. Administration of diltiazem 15 mg intravenously over 2 minutes

3-103. A patient is admitted after exploratory laparotomy and debridement for severe necrosing pancreatitis. Intraoperative blood loss was 4000 mL. Upon return to ICU, the patient's BP is 76/45 mm Hg, pulse is 145 beats/min, respirations are 32 breaths/min, and urine output is 20 mL/hr for the last 2 hours. She receives 4 units of packed cells, 1 unit of fresh frozen plasma, and 2000 mL of crystalloid volume replacement. The patient's urine output remains 20 mL/hr, and vital signs are BP 100/67 mm Hg, pulse 128 beats/min, respirations 28 breaths/min. The physician decides to initiate continuous veno-venous hemofiltration (CVVH). The rationale for choosing CVVH is that this therapy

A. Provides ultrafiltration and solute removal by convection without significant hemodynamic consequences
B. Avoids complications such as clotting and infection associated with other forms of renal replacement
C. Is the optimal treatment for chronic renal failure
D. Will more effectively maintain the BUN level at less than 100 mg/dL

3-104. A 58-year-old man is admitted with shortness of breath, oxygen saturation of 82%, respirations 32/min, and moderate confusion. A chest x-ray shows the patient has a large pleural effusion. A thoracentesis is planned to remove the fluid. The patient is a newlywed of 4 months, and his wife, after signing the consent form, requests to be present during the procedure. Which of the following is the best response that the patient's nurse could make to the wife's request?

A. "Our unit policy states that during procedures family wait in the waiting room."
B. "Have you ever seen a thorocentesis before? The procedure uses needles."
C. "Because the procedure requires a sterile field, family must stay in the waiting room."
D. "Family members usually are not present during these procedures, but let me talk to the physician about your staying."

3-105. A sodium nitroprusside (Nipride) infusion is to be used for a patient in hypertensive crisis with a blood pressure of 240/140 mm Hg.

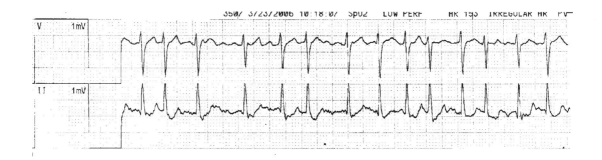

The nurse should titrate the nitroprusside (Nipride) drip to achieve a systolic BP of

A. 140 mm Hg within 1 hour
B. 150 mm Hg within 2 hours
C. 170 mm Hg within 2 hours
D. 120 mm Hg within 3 hours

3-106. A 70 kg patient with acute respiratory distress syndrome is mechanically ventilated on the following settings: FiO_2 70%, tidal volume 450 mL, rate 10/min, PEEP 20 cm H_2O. On these settings, the patient's PaO_2 is 76 mm Hg. The patient currently has a core temperature of 37 ° C, heart rate of 116/min, and blood pressure of 78/58 mm Hg. Which of the following interventions should the nurse now anticipate?

A. Decrease PEEP to decrease intrathoracic pressure
B. Administer 500 mL fluid bolus of normal saline
C. Initiate a norepinephrine infusion to maintain systolic BP at least 80 mm Hg
D. Increase tidal volume to 700 mL

3-107. A 70-year-old woman is directly admitted to the ICU following an exploratory laparotomy and Hartman's procedure for a perforated colon. The patient is mechanically ventilated and is currently receiving PRBCs for anemia and FFP for an elevated prothrombin time. Initial hemodynamic parameters are as follows: temperature 35.8° C, HR 100 beats/min atrial fibrillation, BP 120/70 mm Hg, PAP 40/18 mm Hg, CVP 15 mm Hg, SVO_2 85%, CO 3.0 L/min, SVR 1600 dynes/sec/cm^{-5}, CI 1.5 L/min. Laboratory data is as follows: WBC 25,000/mm³, Hb 9.0 g/dL, platelets 200,000/mm³, HCT 27.2%. Based on these findings, the nurse determines that the most likely explanation for the patient's SVO_2 value is

A. Hypothermia
B. Anemia
C. Low cardiac output
D. Atrial fibrillation

3-108. The purpose for administration of continuous nitroglycerin infusion in a coronary artery bypass patient in whom the radial artery was utilized as a conduit is to

A. Maintain the systolic blood pressure below 140 mm Hg

B. Prevent myocardial ischemia
C. Lower systemic vascular resistance
D. Prevent graft spasm

3-109. An older patient with longstanding obstructive pulmonary disease is admitted to the hospital with an exacerbation of COPD. His initial ABGs are pH 7.35, pO_2 75 mm Hg, pCO_2 70 mm Hg, HCO_3 35 mEq/L. Which of the following represents the primary goal for nursing management of patients with an acute exacerbation of COPD?

A. Optimize arterial blood gases based on patient baseline values
B. Identify triggers of the exacerbation so these can be avoided
C. Administer broad-spectrum antibiotics early based on WBC count
D. Administer bronchodilators only if necessary to avoid cardiovascular effects

3-110. A patient was just intubated and placed on mechanical ventilation for respiratory failure. Which of the following interventions should the nurse provide in order to reduce the incidence of ventilator-associated pneumonia?

A. Maintain the head of bed at 30 to 45 degrees unless medically contraindicated
B. Use closed (versus open) suctioning methods
C. Place the patient on a kinetic bed
D. Collaborate with respiratory therapist to ensure routine changing of ventilator circuitry

3-111. The nurse is caring for a patient who had a coronary artery bypass graft 2 days ago. The patient has become increasingly anxious and irritable over the past 2 to 3 hours. He sometimes holds his head and says it hurts but is unable to grade the pain on a scale of 1 to 10. He is oriented to person but believes he is in a bus station and needs to leave. Which of the following interventions should the nurse perform first?

A. Dipstick urine for specific gravity
B. Medicate with oral acetaminophen
C. Measure capillary glucose levels
D. Apply soft limb restraints to wrists

3-112. A patient with neutropenia has been placed in protective isolation. When providing care for this patient, it is important the nurse keeps in mind that the most common source of infection in immunocompromised patients is

A. Hospital equipment contaminated with pathogens
B. Poorly cleansed hands of health care workers
C. Normal flora and fauna from the patient's body
D. Family members coughing or sneezing on the patient

3-113. Which of the following is the most life-threatening complication of radiofrequency ablation of cardiac accessory pathways?

A. Development of second-degree heart block type II
B. Pericardial tamponade
C. Cardiac valve damage
D. Dislodgement of microemboli

3-114. A female patient of Asian descent has sepsis. She is hemodynamically unstable, is receiving aggressive fluid therapy and vasopressors, and is intubated and receiving full ventilatory support. For the past 2 days, her renal function has steadily declined and she has remained unresponsive to painful stimuli. The patient's husband has been at her bedside each day for several hours. As the ICU nurse updates the husband on his wife's status, his eyes are directed down and away from the nurse. Which of the following would be the most appropriate nursing response to the husband's behavior?

A. Collaborate with the social worker to assist in delivering the update
B. Continue to provide the husband with the update
C. Request that the husband make eye contact so the nurse can be assured he is listening
D. Speak louder to be sure he can hear you

3-115. Acute treatment for non–ST segment (NSTEMI) myocardial infarction includes which of the following?

A. Administration of thrombolytics within 30 minutes
B. Administration of thrombolytics within 60 minutes

C. Percutaneous coronary intervention (PCI) within 24 hours
D. Percutaneous coronary intervention (PCI) within 72 hours

3-116. Upon admission to the ICU, a patient has a respiratory rate of 32 breaths/min shallow, with coarse crackles and a heart rate of 130 beats/min. SpO_2 is 88% on 100% non-rebreather mask. Test results for this patient include WBC 9 mm^3, RBC 4.0×10^6, Hgb 9 g/100 mL. Chest x-ray demonstrates patchy infiltrates in the right middle lobe. Immediate interventions that the nurse needs to anticipate for this patient include

A. Administration of one unit of packed red blood cells
B. Administration of triple antibiotic coverage
C. Administration of furosemide (Lasix) 40 mg intravenous
D. Immediate intubation

3-117. An end-stage renal disease (ESRD) patient presents to the ED with complaints of nausea, vomiting, and abdominal cramps. While waiting to be seen by the ED physician, the patient becomes unresponsive, with no detectable blood pressure, and the cardiac monitor shows pulseless electrical activity (PEA). Which of the following will the nurse now need to administer for initial management of this patient?

A. Insulin and glucose
B. Lidocaine
C. Polystyrene sulfonate (Kayexalate)
D. Amiodarone

3-118. In a patient with acute coronary artery syndrome, the physical examination findings

A. May be normal or non-specific
B. Usually include pulmonary rales
C. Typically include mitral regurgitation murmur
D. Include tachycardia and hypotension

3-119. While performing ST segment monitoring, which of the following patient positions is recommended for accurate monitoring?

A. Side lying with any head elevation
B. Supine with head of bed <45°
C. Flat
D. High Fowler's

3-120. Endotracheal intubation puts patients at risk for developing ventilator-associated pneumonia (VAP). The critical care nurse can help minimize this risk by interventions such as

A. Keeping the patient's head of bed elevated above 30 degrees

B. Keeping the patient totally sedated to minimize the basal metabolic rate

C. Avoiding aggressive oral care because it can cause bleeding of the oral mucosa

D. Instituting parenteral rather than enteral nutrition

3-121. A patient with aortic valve stenosis undergoes aortic valve replacement. Postoperatively, the following hemodynamic values are obtained: BP 130/70 mm Hg, MAP 90 mm Hg, PCWP 12 mm Hg, CO 3.0 L/min, HR 70/min 100% paced. For this patient, the nurse anticipates

A. Initiating a nitroglycerin infusion to maintain MAP 70-80 mm Hg

B. Administering a fluid bolus of 250 mL normal saline to increase PCWP

C. Administering dobutamine to increase cardiac output

D. Performing no interventions and continuing routine postoperative monitoring

3-122. A 78-year-old resident of a skilled nursing facility receives enteral feedings via a gastrostomy tube. This morning his regular caregivers noticed a decrease in his level of consciousness that may have begun the day before, with shallow, rapid respirations; a blood pressure of 98/38 mm Hg; and continual incontinence of urine. The nurse's assessment finds no visible signs of head or other trauma from a possible unreported fall, so the nurse suspects this patient is experiencing

A. Diabetic ketoacidosis

B. Syndrome of inappropriate antidiuretic hormone

C. Hyperglycemic, hyperosmolar non-ketotic coma

D. Diabetes insipidus

3-123. In heart failure, afterload reduction is best accomplished by diuretics as well as

A. Digoxin and beta-blockers

B. Low-sodium diet and fluid restriction

C. Nitrates and ACE inhibitors

D. Nesiritide (Natrecor) and digoxin

3-124. Which of the following leads is suggested to help distinguish ventricular tachycardia from supraventricular tachycardia with aberrant conduction?

A. II

B. aVL

C. I

D. V_1

3-125. A patient with colorectal cancer was admitted to the ICU 1 week after the last chemotherapy treatment. On admission 90 minutes ago, the patient complained of fatigue and was pale with a blood pressure of 110/72 mm Hg and a pulse of 88 beats/min. The BP is now 130/84 mm Hg, the pulse is 110 beats/min, and the patient is passing dark, tarry stools. The nurse's plan of care will center on this patient's most immediate needs related to

A. Malnutrition

B. Gastrointestinal bleeding

C. Anemia

D. Immunosuppression

3-126. In a patient with hypercapnic acute respiratory failure, oxygen administration at an FiO_2 of 40% may increase $PaCO_2$ levels because

A. FiO_2 of 100% is needed to replace CO_2 with O_2

B. Alveolar hypoventilation is not corrected by oxygen administration

C. Increased ventilation in anemia does not lower $PaCO_2$

D. In patients with a decreased A-a gradient, carbon dioxide does not diffuse

3-127. Which of the following indicates that a stable atherosclerotic lesion has progressed to a thrombus or embolus in a coronary artery?

A. Chest pain relieved by rest

B. Chest pain relieved by nitroglycerin

C. Chest pain occurring with deep inspiration

D. Chest pain unrelieved by nitroglycerin or rest

3-128. When providing nursing care for a patient with suspected stroke, the most important factor related to the use of fibrinolytic therapy is to

A. Begin the therapy within 90 minutes of the patient's arrival
B. Obtain a detailed history of the patient's allergies
C. Establish the nature and time of symptom commencement
D. Start a large-bore central IV line

3-129. Which of the following clinical findings indicates to the nurse that a patient is entering the late period of decompensated shock?

A. Tachycardia greater than 120 beats/min
B. Urine output less than 30 mL/hr
C. Capillary refill time greater than 3 seconds
D. Peripheral edema

3-130. A patient is admitted after a 75-foot fall off a roof. The patient is in respiratory distress, on 100% high-flow mask with a respiratory rate of 34/min using accessory muscles, BP 100/60 mm Hg, pulse 134 beats/min. ABGs are pH 7.33, PCO$_2$ 55 mm Hg, PaO$_2$ 54 mm Hg. The nurse notes asymmetrical chest wall motion, with the left greater than the right. Respirations are shallow, and lung sounds are diminished bilaterally. The nurse palpates crepitus over the right chest wall and notes paradoxical movement of a segment of ribs on the right lateral chest. Which of the following interventions have the highest priority?

A. Pain management, position patient injured side up, and stabilize floating rib segment
B. Rapid administration of fluid bolus, position patient in Trendelenberg, and prepare for chest tube insertion
C. Administration of inotropic medications, apply CPAP mask, and stabilize flail chest with pronation
D. Position patient injured side down, pain management, and prepare for intubation

3-131. An older patient in the ICU has had an extended stay related to difficulty weaning from mechanical ventilation. Once extubated, which of the following is the most essential initial consult that will be required?

A. Nutritionist to evaluate nutritional status
B. Physical therapist to assist with progressive activity tolerance
C. Endoscopy department to evaluate the patient's ability to swallow
D. Respiratory therapy to evaluate for laryngeal edema

3-132. After a patient undergoes aortic valve replacement for aortic regurgitation, the following hemodynamic values are obtained: HR 70 beats/min 100% paced, BP 90/40 mm Hg, MAP 56 mm Hg, PCWP 18 mm Hg. Urine output is 100 mL/hr. Which of the following interventions is most appropriate to increase the patient's blood pressure?

A. Administering 250 mL normal saline bolus
B. Initiating a dobutamine infusion
C. Initiating an infusion of norepinephrine
D. Increasing the pacing rate to 80/min

3-133. Approximately 48 hours after admission to the ICU following a surgical procedure, a patient with a known history of ETOH abuse begins to exhibit signs and symptoms of alcohol withdrawal syndrome: anxiety, disorientation, tremors, and irritability. Knowing that delirium tremens (DTs) is a life-threatening emergency, the initial intervention that the critical care nurse should provide to prevent DTs is to

A. Administer Haldol®
B. Apply restraints for patient safety
C. Turn on the televsion to distract the patient
D. Administer benzodiazepines

3-134. When performing patient teaching with a heart failure patient, the nurse should instruct the patient to immediately contact the health care provider for which of the following?

A. Weight gain greater than 2 kg in 24 hours
B. Development of cough
C. Leg edema
D. Increased fatigue and exercise intolerance for 24 hours

3-135. A patient in the ICU with sepsis and respiratory failure secondary to acute respiratory distress syndrome has been unstable for several days despite receiving maximal mechanical ventilator support. The family, who seems to understand the patient's condition, refuses to sign a do-not-resuscitate order at a family meeting with the multidisciplinary team. The patient's SpO_2 acutely drops to 84%, and the physician orders the FIO_2 to be decreased to 21%. Which of the following should the nurse do at this time?

  A. Call respiratory therapy to reduce the FIO_2
  B. Request that the family speak with the physician
  C. Ask the physician to provide a rationale for the change
  D. Administer doses of sedation and pain medication to avoid discomfort

3-136. A patient was admitted last night with a COPD exacerbation. He has been receiving bronchodilators, mucolytics, and steroid therapy. His most recent vital signs are temperature 38.1° C, HR 115 beats/min, BP 134/80 mm Hg, SpO_2 88% on 35% and CPAP mask +10, RR 42 breaths/min and labored. His most recent ABGs are as follows: ABGs pH 7.27, $PaCO_2$ 65 mm Hg, PaO_2 55 mm Hg, SaO_2 87%, HCO_3 35 mEq/L. Which of the following interventions does the nurse need to anticipate based on these findings?

  A. Intubation for respiratory compromise
  B. Initiation of helium/oxygen (Heliox) therapy
  C. Increasing to a 100% non-rebreather mask
  D. Increasing the CPAP level

3-137. A patient in the ICU is noted to have a cool, blue great toe on his right foot. Dorsalis pedis and posterior tibial pulses are not palpable. Which of the following interventions is *contraindicated* for this patient?

  A. Elevation of the right foot on pillows to decrease edema
  B. Placing the bed in reverse Trendelenberg position
  C. Administration of heparin
  D. Administration of vasodilators

3-138. A patient visiting the United States from Holland is intubated and mechanically ventilated for respiratory failure and requires frequent pulmonary toileting, turning, and repositioning. Whenever the nurse initiates this care, the patient becomes restless and attempts to push the nurse's hands away. Which of the following is a likely cause of this response?

  A. The patient is communicating that she does not want to be taken care of at that time
  B. The patient requires administration of analgesics prior to these therapies
  C. The patient may be trying to withdraw from unwanted touching
  D. The patient may prefer someone of her own gender to provide care

3-139. A new trauma patient is being turned during a bath when the nurse notices a small wound approximately 2 cm on the left posterolateral chest wall with bubbles around the site. Upon closer examination of the wound, the nurse can hear a faint sucking sound. The patient's BP is 100/70 mm Hg, pulse is 120 beats/min, RR is 24 breaths/min. The nurse's next intervention should be to

  A. Continue with the bath
  B. Apply an occlusive dressing to the wound
  C. Notify the physician and prepare for a chest tube insertion
  D. Notify the physician and prepare for intubation

3-140. A 42-year-old is admitted to the ICU following a 35 mph motor vehicle crash, in which he was the unrestrained driver. The patient has right flank ecchymosis and fractures of the right 10th, 11th, and 12th ribs. Which of the following initial diagnostic examinations will most likely be needed to assist in determining the location and extent of this patient's renal injuries?

  A. Ultrasound
  B. CT scan
  C. Renal scan
  D. Renal angiography

3-141. A patient recovering from a gastric resection for a bleeding peptic ulcer is taking pain medication, ambulating, and advancing to a regular diet. The patient now complains of abdominal distention and pain, and the nurse's assessment elicits hyperactive bowel sounds and a tender abdomen. Vital signs are BP 118/66 mm Hg, pulse 94 beats/min, respirations 20 breaths/min, and temperature 99° F with diaphoresis. The WBC is 5.4 c/mm³, and Hgb is 10.9 mg/dL; both of these have been stable. The last bowel movement was 2 days ago. The most likely cause of this patient's discomfort is development of

- A. Intra-abdominal infection
- B. Surgical wound infection
- C. Postoperative ileus
- D. Intra-abdominal hemorrhage

3-142. Which of the following interventions would the nurse anticipate for effective management of a patient who exhibited the rhythm strip below?

- A. Initiate transcutaneous pacing at a rate of 70/min
- B. Administer atropine 0.5 mg IV
- C. Prepare for insertion of transvenous pacemaker
- D. Continue to monitor the patient

3-143. Hemoperfusion is the most effective treatment option for patients who have ingested toxic quantities of

- A. Phenytoin
- B. Lithium
- C. Salicylate
- D. Ethanol

3-144. Approximately 30% of ICU patients develop hospital-acquired infections (HAIs). When a nurse's hands are soiled, what should be used to decontaminate hands between patient contacts?

- A. Alcohol-based hand rub
- B. Donning gloves
- C. Soap and water
- D. 10-minute scrub time

3-145. A patient is admitted to the ICU after stab wound to the left chest at the level of the 5ᵗʰ rib. Treatment received in the ED included a bolus of 500 mL normal saline and chest tube placement. 75 mL of bloody drainage is present in the chest tube collection chamber, and the patient has a minimal air leak. The anterior chest wound dressing is dry and intact. Upon arrival in the ICU, the patient's vital signs are heart rate 120 beats/min, BP 98/76 mm Hg, and RR 24 breaths/min on a 100% non-rebreather mask. SpO_2 is 100%. A follow-up chest x-ray obtained on arrival in the ICU shows an enlarged cardiac silhouette and 10% pneumothorax despite chest tube placement. The most likely cause of the patient's low blood pressure is which of the following?

- A. Pericardial tamponade
- B. Tension pneumothorax
- C. Hemothorax
- D. Hypovolemia

3-146. The nurse is explaining treatment priorities for a mechanically ventilated patient with emphysema to a group of senior nursing students. Which of the following concepts should be emphasized to the students regarding adjustments to mechanical ventilation for these patients?

- A. Airway pressure changes must be closely monitored due to greater risk for barotrauma

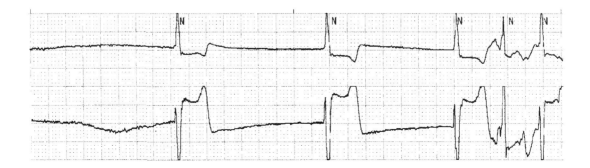

B. Changes in FiO_2 are not likely to improve their PaO_2

C. Tidal volumes will need to be increased to 12 mL/kg to prevent atelectasis

D. The ventilatory mode will need to be changed to pressure-targeted ventilation

3-147. The respiratory status of a patient with chronic obstructive pulmonary disease has improved, and she is using 2 L/min of oxygen via cannula. She has been receiving steroid therapy to decrease inflammation. This morning the patient's previously normal laboratory results reveal a serum glucose of 280 mg/dL and the following arterial blood gas results: pH 7.22, PCO_2 46 mm Hg, PO_2 91 mm Hg, and HCO_3 21 mEq/L. Which of the following interventions is warranted to manage these findings?

A. IV fluid and electrolyte replacement

B. Administration of 6 units of regular insulin IV bolus

C. Low-dose insulin in normal saline drip

D. 50 mL bicarbonate solution bolus

3-148. After thoracic aortic repair, a motor vehicle crash victim is on continuous cardiac and hemodynamic pressure monitoring, as well as CSF pressure monitoring. Which of the following interventions is contraindicated in the care of this patient?

A. Administration of 200 mL/hr of normal saline

B. Administration of nitroglycerin to maintain SBP less than 170 mm Hg

C. Drainage of 100 mL of CSF to maintain CSF pressure less than 10 mm Hg

D. Administration of fresh frozen plasma (FFP) and platelets at 75 mL/hr

3-149. Use of noninvasive, positive pressure ventilation (NPPV) in exacerbations of chronic obstructive pulmonary disease (COPD) may augment treatment by

A. Decreasing air trapping by dropping resistance to exhalation

B. Maximizing ventilation and perfusion matching

C. Increasing alveolar recruitment

D. Resolving mucous plugging in the distal airways

3-150. Age-related changes found in older patients that may affect oxygenation and ventilation include which of the following?

A. Increased chest wall compliance

B. Decreased residual lung volumes

C. Increased alveolar surface area

D. Decreased FEV_1

3-1. **(A)** Extra heart sounds are heard in both right and left ventricular failure due to filling patterns in a noncompliant ventricle. Basilar crackles, orthopnea, and elevated pulmonary artery pressures are found in patients with left ventricular failure.

> **Reference:** Woods, S. L., Froelicher, E. S., Motzer, S. U., Bridges, E. J. *Cardiac Nursing,* 5th ed. Philadelphia, Lippincott Williams & Wilkins, 2005.

3-2. **(C)** The patient appears to be in status epilepticus. *Status epilepticus* is defined as seizure activity lasting longer than 5 to 10 minutes or repetitive seizures occurring without full recovery between ictal episodes. These may be generalized convulsive, nonconvulsive (without visible movement), or focal motor seizures. Benzodiazepines are commonly given to stop acute seizures (usually concurrently with an anticonvulsant drug such as phenytoin) and may be repeated after ten minutes if seizure activity persists. While an EEG (Option A) is helpful in diagnosis and treatment planning for patients with seizure disorders, a STAT EEG would not provide any additional information during the acute period. Although some electrolyte disturbances can cause seizures, the description of patient activity is characteristic for status epilepticus, so STAT labs (Option B) are not as high a priority as stopping the seizure activity. The longer a seizure lasts, the more difficult it is to control. Most commonly, seizures refractory to these treatments are stopped with barbiturate infusion. However, the above measures are attempted prior to treatment with barbiturates (Option D). Additionally, the barbiturate dose is twice the recommended dosing (10 mg/kg over 30 minutes followed by a continuous infusion at a lower rate).

> **Reference:** Alspach, J. G. (ed.). *Core Curriculum for Critical Care Nursing,* 6th ed. St. Louis, Elsevier, 2006, pp 510-517.

3-3. **(D)** Up to 70% of houses built before 1960 have surfaces covered in lead-based paint. Lead poisoning does not produce a classic toxidrome that facilitates easy diagnosis. Lead is compartmentalized into three main areas: bones, soft tissue (including the brain), and blood. Organic lead is assimilated rapidly by the CNS and can produce a host of neuropsychiatric manifestations as described. Cyanide poisoning presents with signs and symptoms that are primarily cardiopulmonary in nature: dysrhythmias, asystole, hypotension, and cardiovascular collapse. Carbon monoxide (CO) exposure results in tissue hypoxia and cellular toxicity. CO binds with hemoglobin in place of oxygen. The organs with the greatest sensitivity to hypoxia—the CNS and cardiovascular system—are affected the most. In addition to neuropsychiatric manifestations, patients with CO poisoning will present with dyspnea, tachycardia, and cardiac ischemia. Pesticide exposure produces a cholinergic crisis. Signs and symptoms would include sweating, pupillary constriction, excessive salivation, bradycardia, and blurred vision.

Reference: Newberry, L., Criddle, L. M. (eds.). *Sheehy's Manual of Emergency Care,* 6th ed. Philadelphia, Elsevier, 2006, pp 476-477.

Urden, L. D., Stacy, K. M., Lough, M. E. *Thelan's Critical Care Nursing: Diagnosis and Management,* 5th ed. St. Louis, Elsevier, 2006, p 1057.

3-4. **(D)** The left anterior descending coronary artery supplies the left ventricle (LV) and septum, including the bundle of His and bundle branches. Occlusion of the left anterior descending artery may cause LV failure, resulting in heart failure, pulmonary edema, and heart block. Bradycardia is associated with occlusion of the right coronary artery which supplies the SA and AV nodes. Left ventricular aneurysm is associated with circumflex artery occlusion and posterior myocardial infarction. Mitral regurgitation and papillary muscle dysfunction are associated with right coronary artery and circumflex artery occlusions.

Reference: Chulay, M., Burns, S. M. *AACN Essentials of Critical Care Nursing.* New York, McGraw-Hill, 2006.

3-5. **(A)** Many Mediterranean males have a glucose-6-phosphate dehydrogenase enzyme (G6PD) deficiency. This genetic variation increases the risk for hemolysis if the patient receives aspirin. Options B, C, and D are incorrect because the metabolism of these medications is not altered with G6PD deficiency.

Reference: Glucose-6-phosphate dehydrogenase deficiency. Available at www.nlm.nih.gov/medlineplus/ency/article/000528.htm. Retrieved on July 1, 2006.

3-6. **(D)** The incision in abdominal aortic aneurysm extends from thorax to umbilicus. Pain control is the most urgent problem for the hemodynamically stable patient in the immediate postoperative period. Return of circulation to the extremities after aneurysm repair is dependent upon the preoperative circulatory status. Coughing and deep breathing and use of incentive spirometry are required after extubation and may require premedication with analgesics to prevent incisional pain. The patient is usually extubated within 24 hours unless pre-existing pulmonary disease is present. Because the patient is NPO and may have had a preoperative bowel prep, a bowel protocol is usually instituted after 2 or more days after surgery.

Reference: Fahey, V. A. *Vascular Nursing,* 4th ed. St. Louis, Elsevier, 2004.

3-7. **(B)** Because this patient is minimally responsive, endotracheal intubation is indicated for acute respiratory failure. The diagnosis of acute respiratory failure is supported by the ABG findings of respiratory acidosis and hypoxemia. BiPAP may be used in respiratory failure patients who are responsive. Although low flow oxygen is frequently used in COPD, this patient is in acute respiratory failure, and the low flow delivery would not be beneficial in correcting the $PaCO_2$. Correction of pH is best accomplished by decreasing the $PaCO_2$. If the pH was lower than 7.20, sodium bicarbonate might also be indicated.

Reference: Markou, N. K., Myrianthefs, P. M., Baltopoulos, G. J. Respiratory failure: an overview. *Crit Care Nurs Q,* 27, 2004, 353-379.

3-8. **(B)** Hepatitis B infections are prevalent in persons of Asian descent. Many individuals are infected at birth and remain unaware of the infection until they develop symptoms. Acute presentation includes jaundice, elevated transaminases, positive HBVsAg, and positive HBV DNA quantititive level of virus. Hepatitis A (Option A) would be the diagnosis if the HAV IgM was positive and the HAV IgG was negative. This would indicate an acute infection with hepatitis A virus. The HAV IgG being positive in this case indicates a past infection with hepatitis A. Hepatitis C infection (Option C) is usually asymptomatic and noted in a lab result of HCV ab (antibody) that is positive. In this case, the antibody result is negative. Hepatitis D (Option D) is associated with hepatitis B but is not reflected in the laboratory results shown in the table on the next page.

References: McMahon, B. J. Epidemiology and natural history of hepatitis B. *Semin Liver Dis,* 25(Suppl 1), 3-8, 2005.

Radovich, P. Gastrointestinal system. In J. G. Alspach (ed.). *Core Curriculum for Critical Care Nursing,* 6th ed. St. Louis, Elsevier, 2006, pp 739-743.

Table 3-1.

Hepatitis A Virus (HAV)	
HAV Total Antibody	Presence in serum confers lifelong immunity.
HAV IgM	Rises early during infection (detectable at 3-4 weeks after exposure and just before liver tests elevate); indicates acute infection; returns to normal in approximately 8 weeks.
HAV IgG	Rises slowly during infection (detectable at 6-12 weeks after exposure and persists for more than 10 years after infection).
Hepatitis B Virus (HBV)	
HBsAg	HBV *surface* antigen; most commonly used marker for HBV infection; detectable within 30 days of exposure and persists up to 3 months after jaundice unless a carrier state develops, in which case it will persist longer; presence in serum (seropositivity) indicates active hepatitis B infection.
HBsAb	Antibody to HBsAg; presence in serum (seropositivity) indicates HBV immunity due to HBV infection or vaccination; detectable 4-12 weeks after HBsAg disappears.
HBeAg	HBV *e* antigen; found only in sera positive for HBsAg; presence in serum (seropositivity) indicates high titer of HBV (extensive viral replication) and increased infectiousness (ongoing viral replication); detectable 4-6 weeks after exposure. Persistence of this marker in the blood predicts the development of chronic HBV infection.
HbeAb	HBV e antibody; indicates that an acute phase of HBV infection is over or almost over with reduced infectability. Appears at 4-6 weeks.
HBcAg	HBV *core* antigen; not detectable in serum, detectable only in hepatocytes.
HbcAb Total	Antibody to HBcAg; detectable 3-12 weeks after exposure during what is referred to as the "window phase" (after HBsAg disappears but before HBsAb appears).

3-9. **(D)** Left ventricular strain pattern on the ECG indicates that myocardial end organ dysfunction has occurred. Blurred vision may be caused by vitreal hemorrhages or cotton-wool patches common in hypertensive crisis. These are usually reversible when hypertension is controlled. The BUN is normal and does not indicate renal end organ dysfunction. It is anticipated that patients will feel lethargic following blood pressure reduction for hypertensive crisis.

Reference: Baird, M. S., Keen, J. H., Swearingen, D. L. *Manual of Critical Care Nursing: Nursing Interventions and Collaborative Management.* St: Louis, Elsevier, 2005.

3-10. **(D)** Contralateral symptoms in the lower extremity usually relate to anterior cerebral artery circulation problems. All of these findings can occur after aneurysmal subarachnoid hemorrhage, but the clinical signs described are most commonly associated with vasospasm of the right anterior cerebral artery. Hyponatremia (Option A) does occur in this patient population but is not a likely cause of a focal deficit or acute change. Rebleed (Option B) as well as hydrocephalus (Option C) would likely cause deficits of a more global nature.

References: Greenberg, M. S. (ed.). *Handbook of Neurosurgery,* 6th ed. New York, Thieme Medical Publishers, 2006.

Hickey, J. V. (ed.). *The Clinical Practice of Neurological and Neurosurgical Nursing,* 5th ed. Philadelphia, Lippincott Williams & Wilkins, 2002.

3-11. **(A)** Because the patient must undergo cardiopulmonary bypass and hypothermia, as well as receive multiple transfusions, this patient is at high risk for coagulopathy. Aneurysm development is associated with smoking and hypertension. Presence of an aneurysm may contribute to traumatic rupture but need not be present for rupture to occur. If the patient had a history of both hypertension and smoking, he may be at risk of difficulty in the weaning process. The large surgical incision could place the patient at risk of pain interference with weaning, but this may be controlled with adequate analgesic measures. Since hemodynamic instability is anticipated in the early postoperative period, weaning is generally deferred at that time. Postoperative myocardial infarction is associated with the presence of cardiac risk factors and may be related to the original cause of the motor vehicle crash. Cross-clamping of the aorta places the patient at high risk of spinal cord injury, but not stroke.

Reference: Leung, J. M. *Cardiac and Vascular Anesthesia.* Philadelphia, Elsevier, 2004.

3-12. **(C)** COPD patients can demonstrate isolated elevations in PA pressures because of compensatory hypoxemic vasoconstriction, which increases pressures in the pulmonary circulation. Option A shows elevation across all hemodynamic variables, a finding often associated with pericardial tamponade. Option B shows uniformly low hemodynamic pressures, a pattern that may be observed in patients with hypovolemia. Option D shows an isolated elevation in the PAOP, a finding associated with left ventricular failure.

Reference: Darovic, G. O. *Hemodynamic Monitoring: Invasive and Noninvasive Clinical Applications,* 3rd ed. Philadelphia, Elsevier, 2002.

3-13. **(B)** Ventricular septal rupture and papillary muscle rupture may occur abruptly after acute MI and are associated with loud systolic murmurs and left ventricular (LV) failure. Immediate treatment is aimed at reducing LV afterload using vasodilators and IABP therapy. If surgery was performed for this patient, CABG would not be the appropriate procedure because patency of the coronary arteries is not responsible for the clinical findings. PCI is ineffective to treat either ventricular septal rupture or papillary muscle rupture. Emergency valve or septal surgery is indicated in this case. Endovascular repair of septal defects may be performed. Administration of vasoconstricting agents may worsen failure.

Reference: Woods, S. L., Froelicher, E. S., Motzer, S. U., Bridges, E. J. *Cardiac Nursing,* 5th ed. Philadelphia, Lippincott Williams & Wilkins, 2005.

3-14. **(C)** This patient has low levels in ability to participate in care related to her vision impairment. Data support that case management planning and coordination of care has the potential to reduce patient readmission rates. Option A is not correct at this time as all other options should be explored prior to removing the patient from her home. Option B is incorrect as it does not address the patient's visual problem, though it would have been part of the solution if the patient were lacking understanding of how to administer insulin. Option D is not correct as there is no indication that family members can be relocated to care for the patient at home.

Reference: Ko, H. C., Pai, Y. C., Chu, K. M. Promoting the efficacy of discharge planning through the case management model. *Hu Li Za Zhi,* 52(4), 40-50, 2005.

3-15. **(D)** Identification and treatment of the underlying source of inflammation or infection is the most important element in reducing mortality associated with SIRS/MODS. Medical and surgical interventions to remove sources of infection or contamination may limit the inflammatory response and improve the patient's chances of recovery. Pain and associated anxiety can increase the patient's oxygen consumption. For patients who are exhibiting signs of low tissue perfusion, pain management needs to be addressed. Maintenance of tissue oxygenation by focusing on interventions that decrease oxygen demand and increase oxygen delivery will preserve organ function until the underlying problem (infectious process or inflammatory condition) is corrected or re-solved. Hypermetabolism in SIRS/MODS results in profound weight loss, cachexia, and loss of organ function. The goal of nu-tritional/metabolic support is to preserve organ structure and function. Nutrition will prevent generalized nutritional deficiencies and preserve gut integrity.

Reference: Urden, L. D., Stacy, K. M., Lough, M. E. *Thelan's Critical Care Nursing: Diagnosis and Management,* 5th ed. St. Louis, Elsevier, 2006, p 1042-1045.

3-16. **(A)** If the balloon catheter advances too far caudally, it obstructs the subclavian artery, resulting in pallor and decreased pulses in the left upper extremity. If the balloon were obstructing the renal artery, urine output would decrease. Balloon timing is assessed by placing the patient on 1:2 timing and ob-serving the balloon assisted systolic and di-astolic waveforms with the patient's arterial waveform and ECG. The patient described here does not evidence problems related to timing (e.g., suboptimal hemodynamics). Pulses in the lower balloon insertion ex-tremity would be decreased when compared with the unaffected extremity if the balloon catheter was impeding flow to the insertion extremity.

Reference: Chulay, M., Burns, S. M. *AACN Essen-tials of Critical Care Nursing.* New York, Mc-Graw-Hill, 2006.

3-17. **(A)** When providing care for bariatric pa-tients, the nurse should expect to find a high incidence of low self-esteem. This popula-tion will likely benefit from clear and fea-sible goals established frequently with considerable amounts of encouragement distributed generously during the postop-erative period. Although some bariatric pa-tients may have needs related to dependence versus independence, personal autonomy, and trusting others, these have not been identified in the literature as characteristic of the bariatric patient.

References: Barth, M. M., Jenson, C. E. Postopera-tive nursing care of gastric bypass patients. *Am J Crit Care*, 2006, 15(4), 378-388.

Mulligan, A., Young, L. S., Randall, S., et al. Best practices for perioperative nursing care for weight loss surgery patients. *Obes Res,* 13(2), 267-273, 2005.

3-18. **(C)** COPD is characterized by perma-nent impairment in airflow, so cessation of smoking will not restore "normal lungs" to this patient. Stopping smoking will, how-ever, slow continuing COPD damage to the lungs, reduce the likelihood of exacerba-tions of COPD, and diminish the patient's risk of developing both lung cancer and coronary heart disease. Smoking cessation is a major component in preventing progres-sion and exacerbation of COPD. Alpha-1 related emphysema is caused by an inher-ited lack of the protective protein, alpha-1 antitrypsin. Cessation of smoking in pa-tients with this disorder accrues comparable benefits as those with emphysema from other causes and, similarly, does not restore normal lungs.

References: Anthonisen, N. R., Skeans, M. A., Wise, R. A., et al. The effects of a smoking ces-sation intervention on 14.5-year mortality: a ran-domized clinical trial. *Ann Intern Med,* 142(4), 233-239, 2005.

Calverley, P. Chronic obstructive pulmonary dis-eases. In M. P. Fink, E. Abraham, J. L. Vincent, P. M. Kochanek (eds.). *Textbook of Critical Care,* 5th ed. Philadelphia, Elsevier, 2005.

Nici, L., Donner, C., Wouters, E., et al. American Thoracic Society/ European Respiratory Soci-ety statement on pulmonary rehabilitation. *Am J Respir Crit Care Med,* 173, 1390-1413, 2006.

3-19. **(B)** Hypovolemia is common in paralytic ileus due to fluid shifts from the distended bowel segments into the interstitial space. Sepsis would be associated with a subnor-mal or elevated temperature. GI hemorrhage would likely present as hemetemesis or me-lena. An SpO_2 of 94% does not indicate im-pending respiratory failure.

Reference: Baird, M. S., Keen, J. H., Swearingen, P. L. *Manual of Critical Care Nursing.* St. Louis, Elsevier, 2005.

3-20. **(C)** When contrast dye will be administered, it is recommended that administration of metformin be temporarily halted because it has been associated with nephrotoxicity and lactic acidosis. N-Acetylcysteine works di-rectly in the kidney to vasodilate the tubule and scavenge oxygen free radicals; how-ever, studies are inconclusive as to whether administration will prevent nephrotoxicity. All diuretics should be held on the day of the procedure to prevent volume depletion.

Current literature cites that renal dose dopamine does not prevent the onset of acute renal failure, decrease the need for dialysis, or reduce mortality.

References: Mitchell, J. G. Renal disorders and therapeutic management. In L. D. Urden, K. M. Stacy, M. E. Lough (eds.). *Priorities in Critical Care Nursing,* 4th ed. St. Louis, Elsevier, 2004, pp 333-356.

Schera, M. Renal assessment and diagnostic procedures. In L. D. Urden, K. M. Stacy, M. E. Lough (eds.). *Priorities in Critical Care Nursing,* 4th ed. St. Louis, Elsevier, 2004, pp 323-332.

Stark, J. L. The renal system. In J. G. Alspach (ed.). *Core Curriculum for Critical Care Nursing,* 6th ed. St. Louis, Elsevier, 2006, pp 525-607.

3-21. **(B)** The nurse is demonstrating caring practices with concern over adequacy of comfort measures. One of the main concerns of family members when a patient is at end of life is the comfort of their loved one. Assessing comfort can be challenging in an unresponsive patient. The Bispectral (BIS) Index Monitor can assist in the assessment and management of analgesic effectiveness. BIS monitoring provides information about the effects of pain medication and sedation. It involves placing an external sensor on a patient's forehead. No internal wires are required. Option A is incorrect since BIS monitoring does not alarm when the patient is brain dead. Option C is incorrect as BIS monitoring does not measure ICP. Option D is incorrect as BIS monitoring is not used on all comatose patients.

Reference: Olson, D. M., Chioffi, S. M., Macy, G. E., et al: Potential benefits of bispectral index monitoring in critical care: a case study. *Crit Care Nurse,* 23(4), 45-5, 2003.

3-22. **(C)** Pericardial effusion with friction rub predisposes the patient to development of pericardial tamponade. Chronic renal failure with delayed hemodialysis places the patient at risk of developing pericardial tamponade owing to uremic deposits in the pericardium. When renal failure is treated promptly with hemodialysis, this does not occur. Acute MI and thrombolytic therapy predispose to intracranial, genitourinary, and gastrointestinal bleeding, as well as oozing from gums and puncture sites, but not within the pericardium. Insertion of the aortic balloon pump does not cause cardiac

tamponade; however, if the reason for insertion is to treat conditions such as myocarditis, the patient may be at risk of development of tamponade related to the underlying condition and administration of heparin.

References: Stone, C. K., Humphries, R. L. *Current Emergency Diagnosis and Treatment,* 5th ed. New York, Lange Medical Books, 2004.

Woods, S. L., Froelicher, E. S., Motzer, S. U., Bridges, E. J. *Cardiac Nursing,* 5th ed. Philadelphia, Lippincott Williams & Wilkins, 2005.

3-23. **(B)** A number of different systems have been developed to help determine the severity and prognosis for patients with acute pancreatitis. Current consensus is that the 11 Ranson's signs system should now be replaced by the more useful and predictive indicators afforded by the patient's (Acute Physiology and Chronic Health Evaluation-II) APACHE-II score and C-reactive protein (CRP). An APACHE-II score of 24 or higher predicts a mortality of at least 80%. Neither serum amylase nor arterial oxygen is used as a prognostic indicator for pancreatitis. CRP is a highly sensitive but not specific marker for the inflammatory processes associated with acute pancreatitis.

References: Baillie, J. The importance of anatomic severity classifications in predicting complications. In AGA clinical symposium: problems and pitfalls of Atlanta Classification for Acute Pancreatitis. AGA, APA and IAP to revisit. Program and abstracts of *Digestive Disease Week,* May 20-25, 2006, Los Angeles. Accessed at Baillie, J. Emerging Issues in Pancreatic Disease: A Clinical Update. http://www.medscape.com/viewprogram/5452.

Imamura, T., Tanaka, S., Yoshida, H., et al. Significance of measurement of high-sensitivity C-reactive protein in acute pancreatitis. *J Gastroenterol,* 37(11), 935-938, 2002.

Parker, M. Acute pancreatitis. *Emerg Nurse,* 11(10), 28, 2004.

3-24. **(C)** Higher levels of PEEP can elevate pulmonary pressures and escalate the risk for additional pneumothorax or air leaks, especially in single-lung ventilation. Prompt ventilator weaning and aggressive pulmonary toilet are essential for reducing the risk of ventilator-associated pneumonia and baro-/volutrauma. Adequate pain management enhances the patient's ability to perform coughing, deep breathing, and incentive spirometry.

References: Alspach, J. G. (ed.). *Core Curriculum for Critical Care Nursing,* 6th ed. St. Louis, Elsevier, 2006.

Smeltzer, S. C., Bare, B. G. (eds.). *Brunner & Suddarth's Textbook of Medical-Surgical Nursing,* 10th ed. Philadelphia, Lippincott Williams & Wilkins, 2004.

3-25. **(C)** Continuous arterial venous hemofiltration (CAVH) uses the patient's blood pressure to force fluid through a filter where it is removed. When diuretics fail to cause diuresis, either a change of diuretic or the use of CAVH, CVVH, or hemodialysis may be used to remove fluid and decrease pulmonary vascular congestion. Since furosemide (Lasix) and bumetanide (Bumex) did not produce diuresis, an alternate diuretic or hemofiltration is needed. Spironolactone (Aldactone) or thiazide diuretics may be tried. Dopamine infusion is not indicated in a hypertensive patient. Low- dose dopamine (below 5 mcg/kg/min) may improve renal perfusion and assist with diuresis.

Reference: Baird, M. S., Keen, J. H., Swearingen, D. L. *Manual of Critical Care Nursing: Nursing Interventions and Collaborative Management.* St. Louis, Elsevier, 2005.

3-26. **(A)** Disseminated intravascular coagulation (DIC) is a complex, consumptive coagulopathy that occurs in patients with a variety of disorders. It manifests as an overstimulation of the normal coagulation process and results in microvascular clotting and hemorrhage in organ systems that lead to thrombosis and fibrinolysis. Clotting factor derangements precipitate further inflammation and thrombosis and microvascular damage leads to additional organ injury. Cell injury and damage to the endothelium activate the intrinsic and extrinsic coagulation pathways. Low platelet counts and elevated D-dimer concentrations and fibrin degradation products are clinical indicators of DIC. A prothrombin time (PT) >12.5 seconds and an activated partial thromboplastin time (aPTT) >40 seconds are also key laboratory findings with DIC.

Reference: Urden, L. D., Stacy, K. M., Lough, M. E. *Thelan's Critical Care Nursing: Diagnosis and Management,* 5th ed. St. Louis, Elsevier, 2006, pp 1042, 1132.

3-27. **(D)** The aPTT is approximately twice the normal value. Removal of the epicardial pacing wires with an elevated aPTT would place the patient at risk for bleeding and pericardial tamponade. Therefore, the nurse should obtain an order to defer removal of the epicardial pacing wires until the aPTT is within normal values. The patient does not have symptomatic bradycardia as indicated by the stable BP and therefore does not require pacing. Low-molecular-weight heparin has a longer half-life than unfractionated heparin, but it is generally accepted that a delay of 12 hours or more after administration of the last dose provides a safe margin for invasive interventions. The INR is within normal range so it would be appropriate to remove epidural pacing wires.

Reference: Davis, L. *Cardiovascular Nursing Secrets.* St. Louis, Elsevier, 2004.

3-28. **(C)** Ventricular assist devices are treatments, not cures. The mortality on device support is high. While most devices are used as a bridge to transplant, there is a portable VAD on the market that can be inserted so patients may then be discharged home. The pump is placed in the upper part of the abdomen. Another tube attached to the pump is brought out of the abdominal wall to the outside of the body and attached to the pump's battery and control system. Patients with LVADs can be discharged from the hospital and have an acceptable quality of life while waiting for a donor heart to become available.

References: American Heart Association: Left ventricular assist device. Available at www.americanheart.org/presenter.jhtml?identifier=4599. Retrieved on September 2, 2006.

MacIver, J., Ross, H. J. Withdrawal of ventricular assist device support. *J Palliat Care,* 21(3), 151-156, 2005.

3-29. **(C)** In ethanol ablation, the septal perforator arteries are ablated, causing shrinkage of the tissues and decreased outflow obstruction in hypertrophic cardiomyopathy. Septal ablation may result in conduction problems such as heart blocks, so patients may require temporary or permanent pacing after the procedure. Although supraventricular dysrhythmias including atrial fibrillation are commonly seen in cardiomyopathy, their incidence is not increased by the ablation procedure. Medications for these dysrhythmias may be used, but only if the patient was on the medication prior to the procedure. Since ablation affects the myocardial tissues, elevation of cardiac biomarkers is anticipated.

Reference: Woods, S. L., Froelicher, E. S., Motzer, S. U., Bridges, E. J. *Cardiac Nursing,* 5th ed. Philadelphia, Lippincott Williams & Wilkins, 2005.

3-30. **(C)** ITP is a deficiency of platelets with measurable amounts of antiplatelet antibodies resulting in bleeding into the skin and other organs. Acute ITP is generally a disease that affects children, while chronic ITP is generally experienced by adolescents and adults. Because of blood loss, replacing circulating blood volume is the primary goal when managing patients with idiopathic thrombocytopenic purpura. Changes in the airway and respiratory function arise only when volume replacement is not adequate and shock occurs. While coping with the bruises and purpura is a challenge for the patient, this is not a major focus of nursing interventions.

References: Nettina, S. M. *The Lippincott Manual of Nursing Practice,* 7th ed. Philadelphia, Lippincott Williams & Wilkins, 2000, pp 886-888

Urden, L. D., Stacy, K. M., Lough, M. E. *Thelan's Critical Care Nursing: Diagnosis and Management,* 5th ed. St. Louis, Elsevier, 2006, pp 1135-1136.

3-31. **(C)** Current guidelines for the prevention and management of CVC infection include effective handwashing, maximum sterile precautions during catheter insertion, skin prep antisepsis with 2% chlorhexidine, avoidance of routine replacement of CVCs, insertion of antiseptic/antibiotic-impregnated short-term catheter if infection rate is high, culture of blood and catheter to confirm clinical suspicion of infection, treatment of intravascular catheter infection with IV antimicrobial therapy, removal of CVC if infected, and adequate education of staff who insert and maintain CVCs. Prevention is the best defense against complications resulting from infections. Migration of skin organisms at the insertion site into the cutaneous catheter tract with colonization of the catheter tip has been designated as the primary mechanism in the pathogenesis of catheter-related infections. Current recommendations for insertion of a CVC include effective handwashing and use of sterile precautions and technique by the physician and staff during insertion of the catheter. Routine replacement of CVCs after a period of time to prevent infection showed no significant difference in rate of infection so the practice is no longer recommended. There is potential to promote fungal infections and antimicrobial resistance with the use of antibiotic ointment or cream at the insertion site. Use of *either* transparent dressing alone or gauze dressing with tape is recommended. If the patient is diaphoretic or if there is bleeding at the site, a gauze dressing is preferred. Otherwise, a transparent dressing is indicated to allow visual inspection of insertion site. Do not use multiple types of dressings simultaneously. A gauze dressing covered with a transparent dressing can harbor moisture and provide an environment for bacterial growth.

References: Lynn-McHale Wiegand, D. J., Carlson, K. K., (eds.) *AACN Procedure Manual for Critical Care,* 5th ed. St. Louis, Elsevier, 2005, pp 502-505.

Urden, L. D., Stacy, K. M., Lough, M. E. *Thelan's Critical Care Nursing, Diagnosis and Management,* 5th ed. St. Louis, Elsevier, 2006, pp 397-400.

3-32. **(B)** The patient has pulmonary hemorrhage, which requires a return to the operating room for exploration and definitive treatment. Insertion of a second chest tube would help evacuate the blood, but stopping the hemorrhage is a higher priority than removing the blood from the pleural space and could add more trauma to the area. Dopamine is not needed at this time as this patient requires fluid resuscitation. Using a positively inotropic agent can increase myocardial workload and cause myocardial ischemia in patients with reduced preload. A bronchoscopy will not likely be helpful in identifying the source of this rapid bleeding, as it may exist outside the tracheobroncheal tree.

References: Ellstrom, K. Pulmonary system. *Core Curriculum for Critical Care Nursing,* 6th ed. St. Louis, Elsevier, 2006, p 149.

Yamamoto, L., Schroeder, C., Morely, D., Beiveau, C. Thoracic trauma: the deadly dozen. *Crit Care Nurse Q,* (28)1, 22-40, 2005.

3-33. **(C)** Cerebral arterial vasospasm is the most common cause of neurologic deterioration 4 to 7 days after SAH in both operated and nonoperated patients. It can be definitively diagnosed with either CT or traditional angiography as well as by clinical examination and transcranial doppler ultrasonography. Transluminal balloon angioplasty (TBA) of the major affected intracerebral arteries can be performed during the same procedure as the diagnostic angiogram. It has led to successful resolution of refractory, angiographically demonstrated vasospasm and to successful reversal of delayed neurologic deficits. Nimodipine is the only medication shown to prevent vasospasm and improve patient outcome after aneurysmal SAH. Administration of this calcium channel blocking agent has become a standard practice for vasospasm prevention. Occasionally, the usual dose of 60 mg every 4 hours is changed to 30 mg every 2 hours if patients become relatively hypotensive with standard dosing. Increasing the dose to 60 mg every 2 hours (Option A), however, is not appropriate. Because of nimodipine's vasodilator effect, BP should be carefully monitored. Triple-H therapy (hypertensive-hypervolemic hemodilution [HHH]) increases cardiac output and BP with aggressive intravascular volume loading and vasopressor medications. Fluid loading usually leads to hemodilution. Vasoactive drugs are administered to increase BP if intravascular volume expansion alone is inadequate. Filling pressures (CVP or PCWP) are also monitored to guide volume dosing. Fluid restriction (Option B) is contraindicated in this patient population. Lumbar puncture (Option D) is not indicated at this time, since cerebral vasospasm is the most likely cause of the patient's symptoms. If the patient had other signs and/or symptoms of meningitis, then LP would be indicated.

> **Reference:** Bader, M. K., Littlejohns, L. R. (eds.). *AANN Core Curriculum for Neuroscience Nursing,* 4th ed. St. Louis, Elsevier, 2004.

3-34. **(B)** The process of weaning from mechanical ventilation can be challenging and complex, especially for older patients with numerous chronic comorbidities. Data suggest that improved outcomes can result when collaborative decision-making processes are used (e.g., by ventilator teams who focus on patients such as this who need extra support). Discharge to a long-term care facility may not be appropriate, particularly for a patient with compromised pulmonary status. The patient is not sufficiently strong for discharge home, and no family members are mentioned to provide this care. Although optimizing the patient's nutritional status will surely benefit him, it does not afford a promising avenue for any near-term solution to the weaning problem.

> **Reference:** Salipante, D. M. Developing a multidisciplinary weaning unit through collaboration. *Crit Care Nurse,* 22, 30-39, 2002.

3-35. **(A)** Stroke may occur during left heart catheterization as emboli are released from the left heart and travel to the aorta and cerebral arteries. Catheterization of the right heart releases thrombi to the pulmonary artery, causing pulmonary embolus. Right heart catheterization may irritate vagus nerve endings in the SA or AV node, causing vagal stimulation that results in bradycardia or hypotension. Flushing and nausea are side effects of contrast administration and are self limiting.

> **Reference:** Zipes, D. P., Libby, P., Bonow, R. O., Braunwald, E. (eds.). *Braunwald's Heart Disease: A Textbook of Cardiovascular Medicine,* 7th ed. Philadelphia, Elsevier, 2005.

3-36. **(D)** Replacement of bicarbonate is the most appropriate intervention for the patient with diabetic ketoacidosis and a pH below 7.0 and should be repeated every 2 hours until the pH exceeds 7.0. Even though the patient's admitting glucose is only 200 mg/dL, the patient is experiencing dehydration and an anion gap to have been admitted with a diagnosis of diabetic ketoacidosis, so administration of NPH insulin will not provide a timely reduction of serum glucose. Absorption of insulin via the subcutaneous route would be impaired owing to diminished circulation associated with hypovolemia. Oral fluids should also be discouraged, as they are unlikely to be absorbed and may result in nausea and emesis. Delaying treatment for a period of hours while a specimen is obtained and sent to the laboratory and the results reported could have potentially lethal consequences for this patient.

References: Morton, P. G, Fontaine, D. K, Hudak, C. M, Gallo, B. M. *Critical Care Nursing: A Holistic Approach,* 8th ed. Philadelphia, Lippincott Williams & Wilkins, 2005, p 1044.

Newberry, L., Criddle, L. *Sheehy's Manual of Emergency Care,* 6th ed. Philadelphia, Elsevier, 2006, pp 426-431.

3-37. **(A)** An endotracheal tube cuff leak allows oral secretions above the cuff to leak into the bronchial tree, placing the patient at high risk of developing ventilator-associated pneumonia. Enteral feedings place the patient at risk of VAP if a semirecumbent position is not maintained or if residual volumes are increased. A diminished level of consciousness and obtundation are risk factors for hospital-acquired pneumonia (HAP) in a nonintubated patient. Nasogastric tubes place the nonintubated patient at risk of HAP.

Reference: Napolitano, L. M. Hospital acquired and ventilator associated pneumonia. *Am J Surg,* 186, 4S-14S, 2003.

3-38. **(D)** In the 12-lead ECG, QRS width greater than 0.12 seconds is indicative of both bundle branch block and ventricular initiated rhythms. Negative QRS concordance, or presence of QS complexes in all precordial leads, is a distinguishing feature of ventricular tachycardia. In bundle branch blocks, leads V_1 and V_6 are helpful to determine if LBBB or RBBB is present. In RBBB, the QS complex is seen in lead V_6, while an upright rSR′ may be seen in lead V_1. In LBBB, the QS complex is seen in lead V_1 and an upright RS in lead V_6. Pericarditis may present on ECG as ST segment elevation in precordial leads.

Reference: Woods, S. L., Froelicher, E. S., Motzer, S. U., Bridges, E. J. *Cardiac Nursing,* 5th ed. Philadelphia, Lippincott Williams & Wilkins, 2005.

3-39. **(D)** Patients with the best outcome following a traumatic arrest are those who are promptly transported to a trauma care facility where appropriate interventions can be initiated. The focus of prehospital/hospital resuscitation should be to safely extricate and stabilize the patient and to minimize interventions that will delay transport to definitive care at a trauma center. The primary

and secondary surveys, including exposure of the patient to determine the extent of injury, are performed within minutes of the patient arriving at the tertiary care facility. Aggressive fluid resuscitation is now recommended only for patients with isolated head or extremity trauma, either blunt or penetrating. It is not recommended for penetrating trauma, especially in the urban setting, because it is likely to increase blood pressure and accelerate the rate of blood loss.

References: Alspach, J. G. (ed.). *Core Curriculum for Critical Care Nursing,* 6th ed. St. Louis, Elsevier, 2006, pp 907-911.

Hazinski, M. F., Chameides, L., Elling, B., Hemphill, R. (eds.). 2005 American Heart Association Guidelines for Cardiopulmonary Resuscitation and Emergency Cardiovascular Care. *Circulation* 112(24 Suppl), IV-146-149, December 2005.

3-40. **(A)** Troponins are specific to cardiac tissue and are not affected by skeletal muscle injury. Creatinine kinase is found in skeletal muscle and is therefore a nonspecific indicator of MI in the surgical patient. C-reactive protein is synthesized in the liver in response to inflammation and is used to determine risk of cardiovascular disease. C-reactive protein levels less than 1.0 mg/L indicate a patient has a low risk of developing cardiovascular disease, whereas a level higher than 3.0 mg/L identifies a patient at high risk of cardiovascular disease. Myoglobin levels increase in skeletal muscle injury and are therefore unreliable indicators of myocardial infarction in the surgical patient.

Reference: Rajappa, M., Sharma, A. Biomarkers of cardiac injury: an update. *Angiography,* 56, 677-691, 2005.

3-41. **(B)** Withholding antiretroviral treatment may result in increased resistance and increased immunosuppression owing to viral load rebound. When patients are admitted to the ICU and intubated, oftentimes oral medications are held. Many antiretroviral therapies are not available in intravenous form. Some medications, when given enterally, may be inadequately absorbed. This may lead to drug resistance. ICU nurses must also observe for serious toxicities of the agents prescribed, such as pancreatitis. Option D does not exhibit sensitivity to the patient's concerns. Antiretroviral therapy has resulted in rare but potentially life-threatening toxic effects, such as hypersensitivity reactions, pancreatitis, and lactic acidosis, but these conditions are not related to the onset of critical illness, but rather to the medications themselves.

Reference: Huang, L., Quartin, A., Jones, D., Havlir, D. Intensive care of patients with HIV infection. *New Engl J Med,* 355(2), 173-181, 2006.

3-42. **(D)** ST segment depression indicates myocardial ischemia and is evident in lead I and lead V_1. ST segment elevation indicates myocardial injury or ST segment elevation myocardial infarction (STEMI). Q waves indicate that myocardial necrosis has occurred and may resolve or persist as permanent ECG changes. New onset left bundle branch block suggests acute myocardial infarction, but is not evident in the ECG because the QRS duration is less than 0.12 seconds and lead V_1 does not demonstrate the deep S waves commonly seen in LBBB.

Reference: Chulay, M., Burns, S. M. *AACN Essentials of Critical Care Nursing.* New York, McGraw-Hill, 2006.

3-43. **(C)** There are many approaches to problem solving, depending on the nature of the problem and the people involved, but most approaches involve clarifying the nature and extent of the problem, analyzing causes, identifying alternatives, assessing each alternative, choosing one, implementing it, and evaluating whether the problem was solved. The most effective approach to defuse this situation is to begin problem identification by asking the surgeon to explain what happened and describe the reason(s) underlying his comments. This fact finding will help to isolate the problem(s) and lend clarity to determining its possible causes and appropriate solutions. Option A delays dealing with the physician's displeasure and defers problem solving to the nurse manager. Option B is inappropriate as there is no basis currently established to question the efficacy of existing unit standards. Option D applies an instructional solution to a problem yet to be identified.

References: Lehwaldt, D. Timmins, F. Nurses' knowledge of chest drain care: an exploratory descriptive survey. *Nurs Crit Care,* 10(4), 192-200, 2005.
McNamara, C. Problem solving. Available at www.managementhelp.org/prsn_prd/prob_slv.htm. Retrieved September 2, 2006.

3-44. **(B)** Maintaining activity levels is a key component of pulmonary rehabilitation because it prevents many of the physical and psychological complications common to patients with COPD. Bronchitis exacerbations may be associated with many environmental factors, only one of which is increased physical activity. Supplemental oxygen and bronchodilators are interventions that may make resumption of physical activity easier for the patient and should be considered, but only if indicated.

Reference: Nici, L., Donner, C., Wouters, E., et al. American Thoracic Society/ European Respiratory Society statement on pulmonary rehabilitation. *Am J Resp Crit Care Med,* 173, 1390-1413, 2006.

3-45. **(A)** Patients with severe diastolic dysfunction may benefit from resynchronization therapy achieved via implantation of a biventricular pacemaker. Synchronized right and left ventricular pacing with a programmed atrial rate provides adequate time for ventricular filling and preserves "atrial kick," which enhances cardiac output. Biventricular pacing is not helpful in the patient with systolic dysfunction because there is no problem with diastolic filling. Atrial fibrillation refractory to pharmacologic therapy may be treated with radiofrequency ablation, cardioversion, or dual chamber (DVI/VVI) pacing. Patients with systolic dysfunction may present with tachydysrhythmias or heart blocks. If the patient has heart block, a dual chamber pacemaker may be implanted. If the patient has tachydysrhythmias, a combination ICD/pacemaker may be implanted.

Reference: Woods, S. L., Froelicher, E. S., Motzer, S. U., Bridges, E. J. *Cardiac Nursing,* 5th ed. Philadelphia, Lippincott Williams & Wilkins, 2005.

3-46. **(A)** Studies have demonstrated that massage, music therapy, and therapeutic touch promote relaxation and comfort in critically ill patients. Environmental interventions are safe and logical interventions to use to help patients sleep. Options B and C are not recommended for sleep promotion in critically ill patients because the safety data related to aromatherapy and alternative sedatives (e.g., valerian, melatonin) are unclear. Progressive muscle relaxation has been extensively studied and shown to be effective in enhancing sleep in persons with insomnia, but it requires that patients consciously relax specific muscle groups and practice these techniques. This may be challenging for many critically ill patients and impossible for others.

Reference: Richards, K., Nagel, C., Markie, M., et al. Use of complementary and alternative therapies to promote sleep in critically ill patients. *Crit Care Nurs Clin North Am,* 15(3), 329-340, 2003.

3-47. **(A)** Ventricular septal rupture causes a left to right shunt of oxygenated blood from the left ventricle into the right ventricle as indicated by the flow of contrast from the left ventricle to the right ventricle and equal oxygen saturation levels in the ventricles. An atrial septal defect would cause flow from the left atrium to the right atrium and a step-up oxygen saturation in the right atrium. Papillary muscle rupture is a complication of acute myocardial infarction, which causes left ventricular failure and mitral valve regurgitation. Rupture of the free ventricular wall would cause signs of pericarditis, cardiogenic shock, and pulseless electrical activity.

References: Kamran, M., Attari, M., Webber, G. Ventricular septal defect complicating an acute myocardial infarction. *Circulation,* 112, e337-e338, 2005.

Woods, S. L., Froelicher, E. S., Motzer, S. U., Bridges, E. J. *Cardiac Nursing,* 5th ed. Philadelphia, Lippincott Williams & Wilkins, 2005.

3-48. **(D)** Selective serotonin reuptake inhibitors (SSRIs) are frequently prescribed to elderly patients for depression. Gastrointestinal bleeding has been described in patients taking these medications and may result in hospitalization. The patient's hemoglobin and hematocrit values will afford a good initial estimate of possible bleeding. Because the patient is taking digoxin, the heart rate may not increase as a compensatory response to the bleeding. Signs of increased intracra-

nial pressure include a widening pulse pressure and bradycardia. The patient's pulse pressure is not widened, and the bradycardia is more likely attributable to taking digoxin. Since the bradycardia is medication induced, it does not require intervention. While the patient's diet and nutritional support may need attention at some point, this is not currently a pressing need.

References: Maher, A. B. Serotonergic antidepressants and need for blood transfusions. *Orthop Nurs,* 23, 20, 2004.

Mansour, A., Pearce, M., Johnson, B., et. al. Which patients taking SSRIs are at greatest risk of bleeding? *J Fam Pract,* 55, 206-209, 2006.

3-49. **(C)** Both the tricuspid and pulmonary valves are right heart structures. Emboli released from diseased valves would lodge in the pulmonary tree and cause ventilation/perfusion mismatch and potentially prevent adequate oxygenation. Endocarditis associated with right heart valves is frequently associated with intravenous drug abuse, but this patient is at low risk for seizures owing to administration of lorazepam. Antibiotic therapy reduces the risk of septicemia. Stroke would be a potential complication of endocarditis affecting left heart valves.

Reference: Woods, S. L., Froelicher, E. S., Motzer, S. U., Bridges, E. J. *Cardiac Nursing,* 5th ed. Philadelphia, Lippincott Williams & Wilkins, 2005.

3-50. **(C)** Members of the Gypsy culture are usually not agreeable to organ donation because they believe the person's soul remains active for a year following death, so the body must remain intact during that time. Option A is true for African American families, Option B is true for patients of Vietnamese descent, and Option D is true among Filipino families.

References: American Red Cross: Tissue donation. Statements from various religions. Available at www.redcross.org/donate/tissue/relgstmt.html. Retrieved July 10, 2006.

Glanville, C. L. People of African American heritage. In L. D. Purnell, B. J. Baulanka (eds.). *Transcultural Health Care. A Culturally Competent Approach,* 2nd ed. Philadelphia, F. A. Davis, 2005, pp 40-53.

Nowak, T. T. People of Vietnamese heritage. In L. D. Purnell, B. J. Baulanka (eds.). *Transcultural Health Care. A Culturally Competent Approach,* 2nd ed. Philadelphia, F. A. Davis, 2005, pp 327-343.

Pacquiao, D. F. People of Filipino heritage. In L. D. Purnell, B. J. Baulanka (eds.). *Transcultural Health Care. A Culturally Competent Approach,* 2nd ed. Philadelphia, F. A. Davis, 2005, pp 138-59.

3-51. **(C)** The patient is exhibiting signs of meningitis, which include headache, chills, fever, nausea, vomiting, photophobia, back pain, and generalized seizures. Signs of meningeal irritation may include stiff neck (nuchal rigidity), Brudzinski's sign (adduction/flexion of legs as examiner flexes neck), and Kernig's sign (after examiner adducts thigh against abdomen, examiner's attempts to extend the leg are met with resistance). Common CSF findings in meningitis include high protein, low glucose, and elevated white blood cell count. Bacterial meningitis is most commonly caused by Staphylococcus and is most appropriately treated with antibiotics. Meningitis is diagnosed with lumbar puncture for CSF evaluation after head CT scan is obtained. CT is the preferred scan in this population and MRI (Option A) to rule out any intracranial pathology such as a mass lesion (e.g., brain tumor) is not indicated. Plasmaphoresis (Option B) is indicated for patients with Guillain-Barré syndrome when IV immune globulin (IVIG) is not used. It is generally used every other day for 10 to 15 days and works by removing detrimental immune factors. There is no basis for serial LPs (Option D) in this scenario. Typically, CSF findings for patients with meningitis include elevated protein and low glucose. Another population with clinical findings of meningeal irritation are patients who have had a subarachnoid hemorrhage (SAH). LP is typically done only if SAH is suspected but head CT is negative. LP in SAH commonly includes elevated cell count (particularly RBCs) and xanthochromia, but neither elevated protein nor low glucose.

References: Alspach, J. G. (ed.). *Core Curriculum for Critical Care Nursing,* 6th ed. St. Louis, Elsevier, 2006, pp 474, 477.

Bader, M. K., Littlejohns, L. R. (eds.). *AANN Core Curriculum for Neuroscience Nursing,* 4th ed. St. Louis, Elsevier, 2004.

3-52. **(D)** Normal cardiac output is 4-8 L/min but is dependent on multiple factors such as stroke volume and heart rate. The normal mixed venous oxygen saturation (SVO_2) is 60% to 80%. Decreased SVO_2 indicates hypovolemia, decreased hemoglobin, or increased oxygen consumption by the tissues. Normal systemic vascular resistance (SVR) is 800 to 1200 dynes/sec/cm^{-5}. Increased SVR indicates that peripheral vasoconstriction is occurring to support cardiac output, an indication that fluid resuscitation is not adequate. Increased SVR indicates the patient needs more volume to maintain cardiac output.

Reference: Baird, M. S., Keen, J. H., Swearingen, P. L. *Manual of Critical Care Nursing.* St. Louis, Elsevier, 2005.

3-53. **(D)** Radiographic confirmation is the only reliable method to date of confirming enteral tube placement. An aspirate from a gastric tube often has a pH of 5 or less and is usually grass-green or clear and colorless, with off-white to tan mucus shreds. An aspirate from a small bowel tube often has a pH of 6 or greater and is usually bile stained (ranging in color from light to golden yellow or brownish-green). An aspirate from a tube inadvertently positioned in the tracheobronchial tree or the pleural space typically has a pH of 6 or greater. An aspirate from a tube in the pleural space is usually straw-colored and watery, possibly tinged with bright-red blood from perforation of the pleura by the tube. Option A is incorrect because there are numerous reports of tubes entering the respiratory tract undetected. In most of these cases, the auscultatory method falsely ensured that the tube was correctly positioned in the stomach. Options B and C are incorrect as they can cause harm to the patient if they provide a false-negative result despite incorrect positioning of the tube.

Reference: AACN Practice Alert. Verification of Feeding Tube Placement. Available at www.aacn.org/AACN/practiceAlert.nsf/Files/FTP/$file/Verification%20of%20Feeding%20Tube%20Placement.pdf Retrieved on July 1, 2006.

3-54. **(C)** Acute respiratory failure is defined by a PaO_2 lower than 60 mm Hg and/or a $PaCO_2$ higher than 50 mm Hg. The additional finding of respiratory acidosis indicates an acute respiratory condition. Patients with chronic respiratory conditions may compensate for their chronically low PaO_2 and/or elevated $PaCO_2$ with a pH greater than 7.45. These patients may benefit from low flow oxygen or noninvasive modes of ventilation. Metabolic acidosis is indicated by a low pH and low $PaCO_2$.

Reference: Markou, N. K., Myrianthefs, P. M., Baltopoulos, G. J. Respiratory failure: an overview. *Crit Care Nurs Q,* 27, 353-379, 2004.

3-55. **(C)** When administered within 2 weeks of exposure, gamma globulin will help provide antibodies to prevent active hepatitis B infection. Acetaminophin administration will stress the liver and, in large enough quantities, can produce chemical hepatitis or liver failure. It is too late for those contacts to build antibodies through the vaccination process, but vaccination would afford immunity to future exposures. Transfusions would not be useful, as the infected person would not acquire immunity, and transfusion would subject the recipient to unnecessary risks, including contracting viruses, circulatory overload, or even hemolytic reactions related to clerical and patient identity errors.

References: Durston, S. Cirrhosis, scarred for life. In *Nursing Made Incredibly Easy,* Philadelphia, Lippincott Williams & Wilkins, 2004, pp 14-24.

Newberry, L., Criddle, L. *Sheehy's Manual of Emergency Care,* 6th ed. Philadelphia, Elsevier, 2006, p 916.

Urden, L. D., Stacy, K. M., Lough, M. E. (eds.). *Thelan's Critical Care Nursing: Diagnosis and Management,* 5th ed. St. Louis, Elsevier, 2006, pp 881-885, 1142.

3-56. **(B)** CT scan of the head is useful for looking at bone and blood and is the best imaging study to view most intracranial processes, including trauma, intracerebral hemorrhage, and hydrocephalus. MRI (Option A) is useful for evaluating tumors, spinal pathology, spinal cord injury, and other processes. It is most helpful for looking at tissue, structures, and perfusion. MRI may also be used after the acute period following TBI has passed, when it can help identify injuries such as diffuse axonal injury and shearing injuries. An LP (Option C) is contraindicated until intracranial pathology has been ruled out and is not useful in the initial evaluation of TBI. An LP assists in detection of infection or increased ICP. Option D, cerebral angiog-

raphy, is valuable for evaluating and managing cerebral aneurysms, arteriovenous malformations, and cerebral vasospasm. Angiography may also be used to identify carotid artery dissection in some traumatic cases.

Reference: Bader, M. K., Littlejohns, L. R. (eds.). *AANN Core Curriculum for Neuroscience Nursing,* 4th ed. St. Louis, Elsevier, 2004.

3-57. **(D)** Reviewing relevant research findings related to the nature and scope of support that family members of ICU patients need can afford a sound and evidence-based approach to identifying family- and visitor-friendly features that should be incorporated into waiting areas. The nurse member of the design team can provide valuable input by gathering, compiling, and summarizing the findings of this research. Facilitating visitor comfort can then operate in conjunction with open visitation policies to provide additional elements in the patient support system. Summarizing these findings is well within the capability of a single nurse, so involvement of the nurse manager or another group of nurses is not necessary. Waiting until the next meeting to mention these concerns unnecessarily delays addressing the problem.

Reference: Berwick, D. M., Kotagel, M. Restricted visiting hours in ICUs. Time to change. *J Am Med Assoc,* 292, 736-737, 2004.

3-58. **(D)** Return of ST segments to baseline signifies return of coronary artery perfusion. CPK-MB and troponin levels may increase with evolving and extending acute MI. Serum troponin levels remain elevated for 7 to 10 days after myocardial injury. Dysrhythmias may be associated with reperfusion, but may also occur as a complication of acute MI.

Reference: Woods, S. L., Froelicher, E. S., Motzer, S. U., Bridges, E. J. *Cardiac Nursing,* 5th ed. Philadelphia, Lippincott Williams & Wilkins, 2005.

3-59. **(C)** The patient is currently on hemodialysis, and it would be continued. Hemodialysis is the most effective of all of the renal replacement therapies and is considered the "gold standard" for the treatment of acute and chronic renal failure. Hemodialysis is contraindicated in patients with hemodynamic instability, hypovolemia, coagulation disorders, or vascular access problems. Slow continuous ultrafiltration is used for patients with fluid volume excess and some degree of renal function. It has minimal impact on urea and creatinine levels. Continuous venovenous hemodialysis is used for patients who are hemodynamically unstable and unable to tolerate the rapid fluid and electrolyte shifts that occur with hemodialysis. Peritoneal dialysis is slower and less effective than hemodialysis.

Reference: ANNA. *Continuous Renal Replacement Therapy.* Pitman, NJ, American Nephrology Nurses Association, 2005, pp 1-12.

Hinkle, C. Renal system. In Chulay, M., Burns, S. M. (ed.). *AACN Essentials of Critical Care Nursing.* New York, McGraw-Hill, 2006, pp 341-355.

3-60. **(B)** Several changes in GI function normally occur in older adults and include a decrease in glucose tolerance, which is partly associated with an increase in insulin resistance. This may be modified with diet and exercise and does not require insulin (Option A). The incidence of diabetes increases by 0.5% to 1% in individuals age 65 years and older. Although motility, secretory function, and absorption capabilities may decrease with age, there is no significant impairment of function within the GI tract in healthy older adults, so Option C is not correct. Option A is not a true statement based on the information provided in the case; his hyperglycemia can be managed and resolved well before discharge. Option D is incorrect because there is no evidence of pre-existing diabetes, and the patient would very likely have manifested signs and symptoms of that disorder if it had existed.

Reference: Kane, R. L., Ouslander J. G., Abrass, I. B. *Essentials of Clinical Geriatrics,* 5th ed. New York, McGraw-Hill, 2003.

3-61. **(A)** ST and T wave changes indicate myocardial ischemia. ST and T wave changes occur in dilated, restrictive, and hypertrophic cardiomyopathies that affect the left ventricle and are associated with inadequate coronary filling during diastole resulting in ischemia. Arrhythmogenic right ventricular cardiomyopathy causes right ventricular dilation and signs of right ventricular failure and is associated with right bundle branch block and ventricular tachycardia. Bundle branch blocks are associated with QRS, ST and T wave abnormalities that reflect altered conduction rather than ischemia. ST segment elevation in the precordial leads occurs in pericarditis, but does not reflect the severity of this disorder.

Reference: Bruce, J. Getting to the heart of cardiomyopathies. *Nursing 2005,* 35, 44-47, 2005.

3-62. **(A)** The focus should be on restoring circulating volume and preventing the complications of hypovolemia. Signs and symptoms of early hypovolemic shock include diminished level of consciousness, which can manifest as agitation or restlessness; cool, clammy skin; tachycardia; and vasoconstriction. The patient is having an acute deterioration in his cardiovascular status. After fluid resuscitation is instituted, the nurse can complete the abdominal assessment. Although the patient's fever may be contributing to his tachycardia and vasodilation, it is not the cause of this acute change, so is of lesser importance now. Initiation of fluid resuscitation should be the first intervention with cultures and cooling measures following. It is important to identify the patient's current medications; however, this can be delegated to another member of the nursing staff until cardiovascular stabilization is achieved.

Reference: Kelley, D. M. Hypovolemic shock: an overview. *Critical Care Nurse Q,* 28, 2-19, 2005.

3-63. **(C)** Pleuritic chest pain is a common occurrence with pneumococcal pneumonia (Option C) and needs to be treated in order to improve the patient's ventilation. Pleural effusions, pneumothoraces, and pulmonary edema are not consistent with the patient's clinical presentation (Options A, B, and D).

References: American Thoracic Society. Guidelines for the management of adults with hospital-acquired, ventilator-associated and healthcare-associated pneumonia. *Am J Respir Crit Care Med,* 171, 388-416, 2005.

Ellstrom, K. The pulmonary system. In J. G. Alspach (ed.). *Core Curriculum for Critical Care Nursing,* 6th ed. St. Louis, Elsevier, 2006, pp 45-184.

3-64. **(A)** Rebound pulmonary hypertension may occur when nitric oxide is discontinued. Patients on nitric oxide may develop methemoglobinemia, which prevents release of oxygen to tissues, falsely elevating SpO$_2$ and thus making SpO$_2$ an unreliable indicator of oxygenation status. Although hypotension is common with the administration of nitric oxide (since it causes vasodilation), it can be readily treated with vasopressors or by titration of nitric oxide delivery rates, so is not a major concern. Nitric oxide may cause coagulation defects, including thrombocytopenia and bleeding disorders.

Reference: Raja, S. G., Basu, D. Pulmonary hypertension in congenital heart disease. *Nursing Standard,* 19, 41-49, 2005.

3-65. **(A)** β-Blockers help to reduce mortality in acute myocardial ischemia and infarction owing to atherosclerosis. There are two contraindications, however, to the use of β-blockers in myocardial ischemia: one is when the ischemia is related to Prinzmetal's angina, and the other is when it is due to cocaine. Cocaine stimulates both the α- and β- peripheral receptors. The administration of a β-blocker would leave the α- activity unopposed. This would enhance coronary vasoconstriction, systemic hypertension, and heart rate. For that reason, β-blockers are contraindicated in the management of MI related to cocaine use. Morphine is indicated to manage chest pain and anxiety, both of which could increase heart rate and myocardial oxygen consumption. Nitroglycerin is a vasodilator and reverses the cocaine-induced coronary artery vasospasm. Aspirin reduces clotting activity and is recommended to prevent the formation of thrombi.

References: Buchanan Keller, K. The cocaine-abused heart. *Am J Crit Care* 12(6), 562-566, 2003. Website: http://www.acc.org/clinical/guidelines/stemi/Guideline1/index.pdf. Accessed May 7, 2006.

3-66. **(A)** The approach that will best serve this patient's needs is for the ICU team to collaborate with the perinatal team, with the perinatal CNS serving as the initial bridge between those patient care areas by providing immediate support in establishing priorities of care, particularly for aspects of maternal and fetal monitoring unfamiliar to the ICU nurse. Once the basic plan of care is developed and procedures are reviewed, the perinatal team may continue their consult-

ing involvement less directly, on a more as-needed basis. Collaboration between perinatal and ICU teams in caring for critically ill pregnant women works best to promote the best possible outcomes for mothers and babies. Option B is not optimal because the ICU nurse likely does not have competency to initiate and manage fetal heart monitoring without more direct assistance and needs to know much more about this patient's care than just fetal monitoring. Although both ED nurses and neurosurgical CNSs could lend some support to the ICU nurse, neither has the unique expertise and skills required for optimal care of this patient that the prenatal CNS has.

Reference: Simpson, K. R. Critical illness during pregnancy: considerations for evaluation and treatment of the fetus as the second patient. *Crit Care Nurs Q,* 29(1), 20-31, 2006.

3-67. **(D)** ECG characteristics of left bundle branch block (LBB) include QRS duration greater than 0.12 seconds and a QS pattern in V$_1$ and V$_2$ with ST segment orientation opposite to the QRS deflection. LBBB is an indicator of acute MI if the block is new or if it is associated with elevated cardiac serum markers such as CPK-MB, myoglobin, or troponin. Since LBBB alters repolarization, ST segment elevation is commonly seen. Some studies indicate that markedly elevated ST segments may indicate acute MI in patients with LBBB; however, a diagnosis of acute MI in patients with LBBB by ECG alone is not conclusive. Acute anterior wall MI is indicated by ST segment elevation or Q waves in leads V$_3$ and V$_4$. Posterior wall MI is indicated by large R waves in leads V$_1$ and V$_2$. Anterolateral MI shows ST segment elevation in leads V$_3$-V$_4$ and V$_5$-V$_6$. In the presence of LBBB, ST segment elevation is not a reliable indicator of acute ischemia.

Reference: Brady, W. J., Lentz, B., Barlotta, K., et al: ECG patterns confounding the ECG diagnosis of acute coronary syndrome: left bundle branch block, right ventricular paced rhythms, and left ventricular hypertrophy. *Emerg Med Clin North Am,* 23, 999-1025, 2005.

3-68. **(C)** Ten jelly beans provide 15 grams of simple carbohydrate with a minimal fluid volume. While the orange juice and soft drink provide approximately 15 grams of carbohydrate, they also provide fluid and electrolytes that may affect the patient's clinical findings related to renal failure. The breath mints contain simple sugars, but it is unlikely the patient will consume enough of them to increase the circulating glucose level.

References: Newberry, L., Criddle, L. *Sheehy's Manual of Emergency Care,* 6th ed. Philadelphia, Elsevier, 2006, pp 428-432.

Urden, L. D., Stacy, K. M., Lough, M. E. *Thelan's Critical Care Nursing: Diagnosis and Management,* 5th ed. St. Louis, Elsevier, 2006, pp 926.

3-69. **(C)** The behavior described in the visitors' complaints is a comfort gesture between two people. Although some visitors may not personally like the gesture, there is nothing inherent in the behavior that warrants convening a team conference or moving the patient to a different cubicle. Option B puts visitors' needs and preferences above those of a patient and does not support caring practices (i.e., creating a compassionate and therapeutic environment) toward that patient.

Reference: Molter, N. Professional caring and ethical practice. In J. G. Alspach (ed.). *Core Curriculum for Critical Care Nursing,* 6th ed. St. Louis, Elsevier, 2006, pp 1-44.

3-70. **(B)** In order to determine if this patient is experiencing acute rejection, preparation for liver biopsy is essential, as this provides definitive diagnosis of rejection. Later in the course of treatment, should rejection be ruled out, magnetic resonance imaging or a CT scan may be employed in an effort to detect lesions. Cardiovascular instability unresponsive to less invasive treatment is not mentioned, so neither a central nor a PA line requires insertion at this point. Abdominal girth measurement should have been performed with the admission assessment. There is no indication that this patient has ascites or other basis for intra-abdominal pressure monitoring.

References: Morton, P. G., Fontaine, D. K., Hudak, C. M., Gallo, B. M. *Critical Care Nursing: A Holistic Approach,* 8th ed. Philadelphia, Lippincott Williams & Wilkins, 2005, pp 1114-1115.

Schell, H., Puntillo, K. A. *Critical Care Nursing Secrets,* 2nd ed. St. Louis, Elsevier, 2006, pp 587-589.

3-71. **(B)** The critical care nurse should first administer free water because the patient is in a hyperosmolar state, as evidenced by his serum sodium and osmolality and urine SG values. The goal is to gradually normalize the serum sodium level over 48 to 72 hours. Older patients are at very high risk for osmolality disorders because with advanced age, the hypothalamus becomes less sensitive to changes in osmolality and less able to produce the physiologic adjustments necessary for maintaining a normal range of osmolality. In older patients, neurologic signs such as a change in mental status, disorientation, lethargy, and delusions, indicative of osmolality disorders, may be erroneously attributed to advanced age rather than osmolality imbalances. Hyperosmolar disorders can be caused by inadequate intake of water, excessive water loss, or conditions that cause an inhibition of antidiuretic hormone. The patient's magnesium level is within normal limits. Potassium may be administered at a later time for the slightly low potassium level. The patient's calcium level is within normal limits, and vitamin D is not indicated.

References: Hinkle, C. Renal system. In M. Chulay, S. M. Burns (eds.). *AACN Essentials of Critical Care Nursing.* New York, McGraw-Hill, 2006, pp 341-355.

Mitchell, J. K. Renal disorders and therapeutic management. In L. D. Urden, K. M. Stacy, M. E. Lough (eds.). *Priorities in Critical Care Nursing,* 4th ed. St. Louis, Elsevier, 2005, pp 333-356.

Stark, J. L. The renal system. In J. G. Alspach (ed.). *Core Curriculum for Critical Care Nursing,* 6th ed. St. Louis, Elsevier, 2006, pp 525-607.

3-72. **(A)** The rhythm strip indicates a DDD pacemaker because atrial contraction is sensed and, when not sensed within the set limits, an atrial pacemaker spike is initiated. The ventricular pacemaker follows within the timeframe associated with a normal PR interval (0.20 sec or less). Complete capture is evidenced by the presence of P waves in the MCL_1 strip below the lead II strip, even though the pacemaker spike is not evident. A VVI pacemaker would not sense or pace the atria. An AAI pacemaker would not pace the ventricles.

Reference: Woods, S. L., Froelicher, E. S., Motzer, S. U., Bridges, E. J. *Cardiac Nursing,* 5th ed. Philadelphia, Lippincott Williams & Wilkins, 2005.

3-73. **(D)** Acute blood loss results in the development of hypovolemic shock, which occurs as a result of inadequate fluid volume in the intravascular space. When this occurs, the kidneys will increase retention of sodium, thereby conserving both sodium and body water and increasing circulating volume. The pulse pressure narrows when systolic pressure is low and the diastolic blood pressure is rising because of compensatory vasoconstriction. Arterial vasodilation would worsen the shock state and diminish oxygen delivery to tissues, while vasoconstriction increases systemic vascular resistance and systolic blood pressure, thereby improving tissue perfusion. The heart rate increases in response to increased sympathetic nervous system stimulation.

Reference: Urden, L. D., Stacy, K. M., Lough, M. E. *Thelan's Critical Care Nursing: Diagnosis and Management,* 5th ed. St. Louis, Elsevier, 2006, pp 1012-1014.

3-74. **(B)** Although pulmonary complications are a significant risk after esophageal surgery, pain control is essential in ensuring good pulmonary toilet. Pain control is key in the patient who has undergone an esophageal surgical procedure. Without optimal pain control, many of the other interventions to prevent complications (e.g., pulmonary toilet) cannot be performed effectively. Patients who undergo esophageal surgical procedures are susceptible to noncardiogenic pulmonary edema. Major fluid shifts occur in the first few days after surgery, however; because of the reduced clearance of lymph, patients are predisposed to interstitial pulmonary edema, so large volumes of IV fluid would not be appropriate. While a feeding tube is placed during surgery, these patients may not receive tube feedings for 2 to 3 days after surgery to allow sufficient time for peristalsis to redevelop.

References: Bacak, B. S., Tweed, E. What is the best way to manage GERD symptoms in the elderly? *J Fam Pract,* 55, 251-254, 2006.

Mackenzie, D. J. Care of patients after esophagectomy. *Crit Care Nurse,* 16-29, Feb 2004.

3-75. **(A)** Isolated, mild deficits (NIH Stroke Scale score of 1 or less) represent a contraindication to rt-PA therapy. While a seizure at the onset of stroke is a contraindication, a history of epilepsy or seizure disorder (Option B), in itself, would not constitute a contraindication. Another stroke, intracranial surgery, or serious head trauma within the past 3 months would exclude a patient from rt-PA use, but not a mild TBI 6 months prior (Option C). Current use of anticoagulants or an INR greater than 1.7 would qualify as a contraindication, but an INR of 1.3 (Option D) would be acceptable.

References: Adams, H., Adams, R., Del Zoppo, G., Goldstein, L. B. Guidelines for the early management of patients with ischemic stroke: 2005 guidelines update. A scientific statement from the Stroke Council of the American Heart Association/American Stroke Association. *Stroke,* 36, 916-923, 2005.

Brott, T., Bogousslavsky, D. Treatment of acute ischemic stroke. *New Engl J Med,* 343(10), 710-722, 2000.

Chuang, Y. M., et al. Use of CT angiography in patient selection for thrombolytic therapy. *Am J Emerg Med,* 21(3), 167-172, 2003.

3-76. **(A)** The P/F ratio is obtained by dividing the PaO_2 by the FiO_2. For this patient, the P/F ratio is $68 \div 1.00$, or 68. The P/F ratio is used to distinguish whether the patient has an acute lung injury or ARDS. A P/F ratio of less than 300 indicates acute lung injury, whereas a P/F ratio of 200 or less indicates ARDS.

Reference: Diepenbrock, N. H. *Quick Reference to Critical Care.* Philadelphia, Lippincott Williams & Wilkins, 2004.

3-77. **(A)** The MAP, PCWP, and SVR indicate afterload reduction is optimized for this patient. The primary effect of nitroglycerin infusion is to decrease preload. The CVP is elevated, and the patient would benefit from preload reduction to reduce pulmonary congestion and improve coronary artery perfusion. Option B, nitroprusside (Nipride), reduces preload but also reduces afterload. Dobutamine is an inotropic agent; increasing contractility (Option C) would increase cardiac workload and may worsen ischemia. Dopamine at low doses (Option D) may increase renal perfusion and myocardial contractility, but also contributes to tachycardia, which would increase myocardial work.

Reference: Woods, S. L., Froelicher, E. S., Motzer, S. U., Bridges, E. J. *Cardiac Nursing,* 5th ed. Philadelphia, Lippincott Williams & Wilkins, 2005.

3-78. **(C)** The nurse should delegate tasks to ensure that priority patient care needs are met in a timely fashion and that staff needs for instruction are accommodated in accordance with patient care priorities. A nurse who must devote full attention to patient care needs to seek a colleague who may be in a better position to lend support to the new nurse. In deciding the best course of action, the nurse should consider that both patients would benefit from assessments performed by the same provider to ensure continuity of care. Hourly glucose checks on a young patient with DKA reflect a patient whose care requires close and frequent nursing supervision that should not be disrupted unnecessarily. Hourly neurological checks should be performed only by a skilled RN. A new nurse should not be asked to review a staffing schedule, as this requires considerable experience and knowledge of other staff members' competency.

Reference: Molter, N. Professional caring and ethical practice. In J. G. Alspach (ed.). *Core Curriculum for Critical Care Nursing,* 6th ed. St. Louis, Elsevier, 2006, pp 1-44.

3-79. **(B)** The presence of fat in the pulmonary circulation injures the endothelial lining of the capillary, increasing capillary permeability and resulting in alveolar flooding. The skin rash, diminished level of consciousness, and reduction in platelet count are indications of fat emboli most likely associated with the femur fracture. A thrombus resulting from venous stasis or deep vein thrombosis is more likely to cause a pulmonary embolus. The bronchociliary clearance mechanisms are protective mechanisms usually affected in cases of aspiration or pneumonia. Although they could be affected in this patient, there is no evidence of this in the scenario described. The shunting of blood through poorly ventilated areas of pulmonary consolidation can produce hypoxia, but this scenario does not describe a patient who has aspirated or developed pneumonia.

References: Chulay, M Respiratory system. In Chulay, M., S. Burns. *AACN Essentials of Critical Care Nursing*. New York, McGraw-Hill, 2006, p 260.
O'Steen, D. Orthopedic and neurovascular trauma. In *Sheehy's Emergency Nursing Principles and Practice,* 5th ed. Philadelphia, Elsevier, p 325.

3-80. **(C)** Surgery for atrial septal defect involves surgical incisions and scar development in the atrial septum leading to development of re-entry dysrhythmias and atrial fibrillation. These dysrhythmias are frequently successfully treated with radiofrequency ablation.

References: Butera, G., Carminati, M., Chessa, M., et al. Percutaneous versus surgical closure of secundum atrial septal defect: comparison of early results and complications. *Am Heart J,* 151, 228-234, 2005.
Elahi, M. M., Belcher, P. R., Pollock, J. C. Closure of secundum atrial septal defect in adults. *J.C.P.S.P,* 13, 127-129, 2003.

3-81. **(A)** Intravenous infusions of norepinephrine and dobutamine are indicated for this patient based on the provided hemodynamic parameters. Norepinephrine will increase the patient's mean arterial pressure. Dobutamine is an inotropic agent that will increase myocardial contractility, cardiac output, and cardiac index. Both agents will increase tissue perfusion and subsequent oxygen delivery. Fluid administration with intravenous dopamine is not warranted for this patient because both the pulmonary artery pressure and the central venous pressure indicate adequate intravascular volume. There is no evidence that the patient is in metabolic acidosis, so sodium bicarbonate does not appear to be indicated.

Reference: Dellinger, R. P., Carlet, J. M., Masur, H., et al. Surviving Sepsis Campaign guidelines for management of severe sepsis and septic shock. *Crit Care Med,* 32(3), 858-873, 2004.

3-82. **(B)** Leveling the transducer air-fluid interface to the left atrium corrects for changes in hydrostatic pressure in vessels above and below the heart. Data suggest that in the supine position, the external landmark for the left atrium is the phlebostatic axis (fourth ICS/half AP diameter of the chest). Option A is incorrect because a square wave test is only performed on the initial system setup, then at least once each shift, after opening the catheter system (e.g., for rezeroing, drawing blood, or changing tubing), and whenever the PAP waveform appears to be damped or distorted. Option C is not a requirement because data support that the head of the bed elevation can be at any angle from 0° (flat) to 60° for measurement. Accurate measurements require reading pressure waveforms during end expiration, so Option D is incorrect.

Reference: AACN Practice Alert. Pulmonary Artery Pressure Measurements. Available at www. aacn.org//AACN/practiceAlert.nsf/Files/PAP-Monitoring4-7-04/$file/PAPMonitoring.pdf. Retrieved on July 1, 2006.

3-83. **(C)** In vasogenic shock, vasodilation may lead to a relative hypovolemia that causes hypotension. If the status of circulating volume is not known with certainty, crystalloids may be administered to support BP and correct hypovolemia. If circulating volume is adequate, vasopressor therapy such as norepinephrine may then be initiated and guided by CVP or PCWP pressures. Norepinephrine (Levophed) is an alpha stimulant that restores circulating volume via vasoconstriction. Milrinone (Primacor) causes vasodilation and increased myocardial contractility. Since the patient in vasogenic shock is already vasodilated, further vasodilation is contraindicated At high doses, dopamine exhibits alpha effects similar to norepinephrine and is also indicated after volume deficits have been corrected.

Reference: Lewis, S. M., Heitkemper, M. M., Dirksen, S. R. *Medical-Surgical Nursing*, 6ᵗʰ ed. St. Louis, Elsevier, 2004.

3-84. **(C)** Diagnostic studies are needed to evaluate for pulmonary embolism or bleeding from the aorta. Although the patient's clinical picture has deteriorated, neither intubation (Option A) nor emergency surgery (Option D) is indicated without diagnostic evaluation. The patient may require sedation and analgesia (Option B), but further workup needs to precede administration of those agents so the cause of her acute decompensation can be determined.

References: Alspach, J. G. (ed.). *Core Curriculum for Critical Care Nursing,* 6ᵗʰ ed. St. Louis, Elsevier, 2006.

McQuillan, K. A., et al. (eds.). *Trauma Nursing,* 3ʳᵈ ed. St. Louis, Elsevier, 2002.

3-85. **(B)** The Kehr sign is characterized by severe left shoulder pain when in a supine position and is caused by diaphragmatic irritation typically owing to phrenic nerve irritation from the presence of intraperitoneal blood and air. The clinical significance of Kehr's sign is its association with splenic injuries such as splenic laceration with bleeding, which will result in a reduction in bowel sounds and increased abdominal girth. Epigastric pain with belching is symptomatic of esophageal reflux. This is not an emergency condition. Decreased breath sounds bilaterally indicate atelectasis or consolidation. While over time this may adversely affect the patient's condition, this is not an emergent condition. Pain and burning with hematuria are symptomatic of a urinary tract infection. Urinary tract infections can lead to septicemia; however, at this time this is not an emergent condition.

Reference: Eckert, K. L. Penetrating and blunt abdominal trauma. *Crit Care Nurse Q*, 28(1), 41-59, 2005.

3-86. **(B)** Encephalopathy is not a disease itself but always occurs as the end result of another disease process. Evaluation for these disease processes—often infectious or metabolic—should be considered first. For example, diabetic ketoacidosis may precipitate encephalopathy and be evidenced by headache and lethargy, which suggest cerebral edema. A second disorder, water intoxication, may be ruled out by checking serum osmolarity, and a third, hepatic encephalopathy, can be determined by checking serum ammonia. Level of consciousness is most important in monitoring these patients. The nurse should look for signs of increased ICP (e.g., hypertension, increased muscle tone in extremities, hyperventilation, dilated pupils). ICP monitoring (Option A) would be indicated in stage III hepatic encephalopathy but would not be a first-line action in this patient. Lumbar puncture (LP) (Option C) is not indicated in this patient. If ICP were elevated, LP could be harmful. Immunoassay is not indicated for this patient, and a CT of the head would be a more appropriate diagnostic study than (Option D) cerebral angiography.

Reference: Alspach, J. G. (ed.). *Core Curriculum for Critical Care Nursing,* 6ᵗʰ ed. St. Louis, Elsevier, 2006, p 724.

Bader, M. K., Littlejohns, L. R. (eds.). *AANN Core Curriculum for Neuroscience Nursing,* 4ᵗʰ ed. St. Louis, Elsevier, 2004.

Greenberg, M. S. (ed.). *Handbook of Neurosurgery,* 6ᵗʰ ed. New York, Thieme, 2006.

3-87. **(B)** Increasing the cardiac index to greater than 2.2 L /min/m² will increase renal blood flow and enhance renal tissue perfusion. If MAP, PAOP, PAD, and CVP are within normal limits, then the patient has achieved outcome criteria. Other outcome criteria include electrolytes within normal limits, normalization of acid-base balance, lungs clear on auscultation, normal level of consciousness, BUN and creatinine within normal limits, urine output within normal limits or patient stable on dialysis, stable hemoglobin and hematocrit values. In Options A, C, and D, the patient's CVP, MAP, and PAOP are low, indicating decreased renal blood flow and tissue perfusion.

> **References:** Schera, M. Renal assessment and diagnostic procedures. In L. D. Urden, K. M. Stacy, M E. Lough (eds.). *Priorities in Critical Care Nursing,* 4th ed. St. Louis, Elsevier, 2004, pp 323-332.
> Stacy, K. M. Nursing management plans. In L. D. Urden, K. M. Stacy, M E. Lough (eds.). *Thelan's Critical Care Nursing: Diagnosis and Management,* 5th ed. St. Louis, Elsevier, 2006, pp 1147-1200.
> Stark, J. L. The renal system. In J. G. Alspach (ed.). *Core Curriculum for Critical Care Nursing,* 6th ed. St. Louis, Elsevier, 2006, pp 525-607.

3-88. **(B)** Junctional tachycardia is a non–life-threatening dysrhythmia often associated with digoxin toxicity. Withholding digoxin until sinus rhythm is restored is often the only treatment necessary. Overdrive pacing is not effective in junctional tachycardia due to enhanced AV nodal conduction. Administration of digoxin is contraindicated in heart block. Adenosine is not indicated for a tachycardia of only 110/min.

> **Reference:** Blomstrom-Lundqvist, C., Scheinman, M. M., Aliot, E. M., et al. ACC/AHA/ESC guidelines for the management of patients with supraventricular arrhythmias: a report of the American College of Cardiology/American Heart Association Task Force on practice guidelines and the European Society of Cardiology Committee for Practice Guidelines and the European Society of Cardiology Committee. 2003: http://www.acc.org/clinical/guidelines/arrythmias/sva_index.pdf.

3-89. **(D)** Overwedging is usually caused by migration of the PA catheter forward into the pulmonary capillaries. When that situation occurs, the waveform no longer pulsates with pulmonary artery pressure variations because the catheter tip is now obstructed in a small branch of the pulmonary artery. If the catheter is overwedged, the PCWP will be much higher than the RAP and the PAD.

> **Reference:** Fawcett, J. A. *Hemodynamic Monitoring Made Easy.* St. Louis, Elsevier, 2006.

3-90. **(C)** By providing correct and appropriate information, the nurse is helping to promote a caring environment for the family during a potentially stressful time. A number of physiologic changes will likely be manifested by the patient following withdrawal of mechanical ventilation, some of which may be distressing to the family unless they know about them beforehand. The anticipated time frame to death is variable and cannot be predicted with any confidence. The name of the person performing the procedure will not likely be relevant to the family or contribute to promoting a caring environment to the family. Secretions associated with a "death rattle" do not cause discomfort to the patient. This fluid should not be suctioned, as suctioning can cause discomfort to the patient.

> **References**: Bickel, K., Arnold, R. Fast fact and concept #109: death rattle and oral secretions. Available at www.eperc.mcw.edu/fastFact/ff_109.htm. Retrieved on September 2, 2006.
> Kirchhoff, K. T., Conradt, K.L., Anumandla, P. R. ICU nurses' preparation of families for death of patients following withdrawal of ventilator support. *Appl Nurs Res,* 16(2), 85-92, 2003.

3-91. **(C)** Sputum aspirate with quantitative or semiquantitative cultures is a more sensitive test for diagnosing HAP than expectorated samples with Gram's stain. Chest x-rays are useful in determining the location of a pneumonia (Option A). Blood cultures are a key component of distinguishing primary from secondary infections, particularly in pneumococcal pneumonia (Option B). All cultures should be drawn prior to antibiotic administration to avoid masking organisms (Option D).

> **References:** American Thoracic Society. Guidelines for the management of adults with hospital-acquired, ventilator-associated and healthcare-associated pneumonia. *Am J Respir Crit Care Med,* 171, 388-416, 2005.
> Ellstrom, K. The pulmonary system. In J. G. Alspach (ed.). *Core Curriculum for Critical Care Nursing,* 6th ed. St. Louis, Elsevier, 2006.

3-92. **(C)** Some Hispanics, Appalachians, and Puerto Ricans believe that health is externally controlled and, as a result, are less likely to take personal responsibility for preventive actions. If the patient does not assume personal responsibility for his own health, teaching him about managing risk factors will not likely have any effect. Each of the other choices involves the patient taking measures to prevent a future cardiac event, which is inconsistent with this patient's health beliefs.

Reference: Giger, J., Davidhizar, R. *Transcultural Nursing: Assessment and Intervention,* 4th ed. St. Louis, Elsevier, 2004.

3-93. **(D)** Tumor necrosis factor-α is released from macrophages and lymphocytes in response to endotoxin, tissue injury, viral agents, and interleukins. Cellular responses to TNF include increased formation of oxygen radicals; recruitment and activation of neutrophils, macrophages, and lymphocytes; increased cytokine production; initial hyperglycemia followed by hypoglycemia, hypotension, metabolic acidosis, and coagulopathy; fever and increased oxygen consumption; increased capillary permeability, vasodilation, microvascular vasoconstriction, and noncardiac pulmonary edema; activation of the coagulation cascade; and production of nitric oxide.

Reference: Alspach, J. G. (ed.). *Core Curriculum for Critical Care Nursing,* 6th ed. St. Louis, Elsevier, 2006, pp 760-761.

3-94. **(C)** Definitive treatment for a persistent air leak can include bronchoscopy to introduce endobronchial glue, obliteration of the pleural space with chemical irritants such as antibiotics, or surgical decortication with removal of the pleural lining. Progressive advancement of the chest tube would not be included among the treatments for air leak; that intervention is used to treat empyemas.

Reference: Lois, M., Noppen, M. Bronchopleural fistulas: an overview of the problem with special attention to endoscopic management. *Chest,* 128, 3955-3965, 2005.

3-95. **(B)** Four hours of hemodialysis needs to be done daily because the patient is manifesting symptoms of uremic pericarditis. Management of this disorder includes increasing the duration and frequency of hemodialysis. Peritoneal dialysis would not be considered for management in this case, as the patient is already on hemodialysis.

References: Lessig, M. L. The cardiovascular system. In J. G. Alspach (ed.). *Core Curriculum for Critical Care Nursing,* 6th ed. St. Louis, Elsevier,2006, pp 185-380.

Mitchell, J. K. Renal disorders and therapeutic management. In L. D. Urden, K. M. Stacy, M. E. Lough (eds.). *Priorities in Critical Care Nursing,* 4th ed. St. Louis, Elsevier, 2005, pp 333-356.

Stark, J. L. The renal system. In J. G. Alspach (ed.). *Core Curriculum for Critical Care Nursing,* 6th ed. St. Louis, Elsevier, 2006, pp 525-607.

3-96. **(C)** Patients with diabetes insipidus would be expected to be thirsty and produce large volumes of dilute urine. They will usually exhibit a decrease in blood pressure and increase in heart rate related to hypovolemia secondary to an increased urinary output. Alterations in potassium level will occur as electrolytes are lost in the urine; however, tachycardia is expected with hypovolemia, and numbness and tingling in the extremities would be expected with a magnesium imbalance. Widened pulse pressure, pupillary changes, and posturing are symptoms produced by elevated intracranial pressure, not diabetes insipidus.

References: Newberry, L., Criddle, L. *Sheehy's Manual of Emergency Care,* 6th ed. Philadelphia, Elsevier, 2006, pp 433-434.

Urden, L. D., Stacy, K. M., Lough, M. E. *Thelan's Critical Care Nursing: Diagnosis and Management,* 5th ed. St. Louis, Elsevier, 2006, pp 952-953.

3-97. **(A)** Initial management of pulmonary edema should follow the ABCs of resuscitation. Airway adequacy should be assessed and treated first. Oxygen should be administered and an arterial blood gas obtained to determine whether the patient requires intubation. When the airway is secure, further testing, intravenous access, and medications may be administered.

Reference: Matta, A., Martinez, J. P., Kelly, B. S. Modern management of cardiogenic pulmonary edema. *Emerg Med Clin North Am,* 23, 1105-1125, 2005.

3-98. **(A)** Hemolytic uremic syndrome is a renal disorder with kidney failure, microangiopathic hemolytic anemia, and a platelet deficiency. Most children recover with dialysis and supportive care, while prognosis in adults varies with the patient's health status. Because irreversible organ damage and death can occur from clots, the primary goal is to prevent ischemia through frequent repositioning and maintaining the airway while providing dialysis as needed. Hydration and platelet removal may be employed as treatments, but the goal of these interventions is to minimize the amount of ischemic damage that occurs from a clotted microvasculature. These medical interventions are secondary to vigilant nursing care. Since this syndrome generally involves an inadequate number of platelets, removal of platelets is contraindicated.

References: Morton, P., Fontaine, D. K., Hudak, C., Gallo, B. M. *Critical Care Nursing: A Holistic Approach,* 8th ed. Philadelphia, Lippincott Williams & Wilkins, 2005, pp 1175-1177.

Urden, L. D., Stacy, K. M., Lough, M. E. Thelan's *Critical Care Nursing: Diagnosis and Management*, 5th ed. St. Louis, Elsevier, 2006, p 1042.

3-99. **(A)** According to the Surviving Sepsis Campaign guidelines, during the first 6 hours of treatment, the goal is to achieve and maintain a CVP of 8 to 12 mm Hg, or 12 to 15 mm Hg for patients receiving mechanical ventilation and a MAP of at least 65 mm Hg with fluid resuscitation. Options B, C, and D are inconsistent with the current evidence-based guidelines.

Reference: AACN Practice Alert. Severe Sepsis. Available at www.aacn.org/AACN/practiceAlert.nsf/Files/ss/$file/Severe%20Sepsis.pdf Retrieved on July 1, 2006

3-100. **(C)** Nitroglycerin may be administered orally, intravenously, transdermally, or topically to reduce both preload and afterload in the patient with pulmonary edema. Furosemide (Lasix), morphine sulfate, and captopril (Capoten) are weaker agents. Morphine sulfate has not been found to consistently decrease PCWP in patients with pulmonary edema, but it is effective in decreasing anxiety. Furosemide (Lasix) is not as rapid as nitroglycerin in decreasing preload as effects take longer than 30 minutes to produce diuresis. ACE inhibitors such as captopril (Capoten) reduce afterload and are weak diuretics.

Reference: Matta, A., Martinez, J. P., Kelly, B. S. Modern management of cardiogenic pulmonary edema. *Emerg Med Clin North Am,* 23, 1105-1125, 2005.

3-101. **(A)** Rudolf Virchow described the triad of venous stasis, vein injury, and a hypercoagulable state as risk factors for the development of pulmonary emboli. Pelvic fractures require immobility; lower extremity trauma that results in swelling reduces blood flow, and the need for blood replacement products heightens this patient's risk for thrombi. Recognition of these risks provides the greatest opportunity for prevention of the complication of pulmonary embolism. Intravascular cannulation can lead to vein injury, and dehydration can result in venous stasis, but this patient's age is not a factor in the triad. Hypoxia and intersitital edema result from rather than cause development of pulmonary embolus. Right ventricular dysfunction, pulmonary artery hypertension, and atelectasis are complications seen in the critically ill patient but do not increase a patient's risk for pulmonary embolism

References: Ellstrom, K. Pulmonary system. In J. G. Alspach (ed). *Core Curriculum for Critical Care Nursing,* 6th ed. St. Louis, Elsevier, 2006, p 146.

Yang, J. C. Prevention and treatment of deep vein thrombosis and pulmonary embolism in critically ill patients. *Crit Care Nurse Q,* 28(1), 72-79, 2005.

3-102. **(D)** When the onset of atrial fibrillation cannot be determined, it is possible that a thrombus has developed. Rate control is an immediate concern, and diltiazem is the drug of choice to decrease the ventricular rate in atrial fibrillation. Cardioversion is performed if the patient is unstable or has failed to respond to chemical cardioversion with diltiazem or ibutelide. Dofetilide is used for atrial fibrillation that is refractory to other medical therapies and is not a first-line medication. In addition, dofetilide requires close assessment of the QT interval and creatinine clearance to determine dosage.

Reference: Baird, M. S., Keen, J. H., Swearingen, D. L. *Manual of Critical Care Nursing: Nursing Interventions and Collaborative Management.* St. Louis, Elsevier, 2005.

3-103. **(A)** The patient already demonstrates hypotension and tachycardia related to hypovolemia, so attaining the primary goal of replacing renal function via ultrafiltration while obtaining solute removal via convection that will not further compromise hypotension represents the rationale for selecting this mode of renal replacement therapy. Patients treated with CVVH are not less vulnerable to developing complications such as clotting and infection. This patient would be expected to benefit from CVVH because she is experiencing acute (rather than chronic) renal failure owing to perioperative hypotension associated with hypovolemia related to operative blood loss. In acute renal failure, the BUN level does not elevate to the same level as it does in chronic renal failure, when BUN is over 100 mg/dL.

References: Stark, J. Renal system. In J. G. Alspach (ed.). *Core Curriculum for Critical Care Nursing,* 6th ed. St. Louis, Elsevier, pp 565-569.

Radovich, P. Gastrointestinal system. In J. G. Alspach (ed.). *Core Curriculum for Critical Care Nursing,* 6th ed. St. Louis, Elsevier, pp 739-743.

3-104. **(D)** The nurse will advocate for the family by facilitating the wife's request with the physician and then identifying the best location for the wife. The advantage to the wife's staying is consistent with a holistic family-centered approach to care that sees the patient and family as the unit of care. Denying the request owing to unit policy (Option A) does not advocate for the family. Option B seems to approach refusal by attempting to intimidate the wife. Option C fails to advocate for the family and attempts to harness the notion of sterility as the reason the family should not stay.

References: Molter, N. Professional caring and ethical practice. In J. G. Alspach (ed.). *Core Curriculum for Critical Care Nursing*, 6th ed. St. Louis, Elsevier, 2006, pp 39-40.

Stannard, D., Hardin S. R. Advocacy and moral agency. In S. R. Hardin, K. Kaplow (eds.). *Synergy for Clinical Excellence*. Sudbury, Jones & Bartlett, 2005, pp 63-68.

3-105. **(C)** Decreasing the blood pressure too quickly can overwhelm the cerebral autoregulatory system. Blood pressure should be reduced by 25% to 30% each 2 hours to enable the cerebral autoregulation mechanisms to remain intact.

Reference: Baird, M. S., Keen, J. H., Swearingen, D. L. *Manual of Critical Care Nursing: Nursing Interventions and Collaborative Management.* St. Louis, Elsevier, 2005.

3-106. **(B)** Hypotension in the mechanically ventilated patient may be related to increased intrathoracic pressure from high PEEP levels that decrease venous return. Administration of fluid bolus is indicated to treat hypotension. High PEEP levels are indicated in ARDS to improve oxygenation, and lowering PEEP would likely cause a further decrease in PaO_2. Norepinephrine may be administered if volume replacement is insufficient to increase blood pressure to acceptable levels but would not be given prior to the volume replenishment. Tidal volumes for patients with ARDS should be maintained at 5 to 8 mL/kg.

Reference: Chulay, M., Burns, S. M. *AACN Essentials of Critical Care Nursing.* New York, McGraw-Hill, 2006.

3-107. **(A)** Hypothermia decreases oxygen consumption due to reduced tissue metabolism as a result of the low body temperature. Therefore, the SVO_2 would be higher than normal (60% to 80%). Continuous SVO_2 monitoring allows the health care team to make a determination of the patient's oxygen balance by looking at oxygen supply and demand at the tissue level. The four factors that determine this balance are cardiac output, hemoglobin, arterial saturation, and tissue metabolism. Cardiac output, hemoglobin, and arterial saturation all contribute to oxygen supply. Tissue metabolism is a major determinant of oxygen consumption at the tissue level. Both anemia and a low cardiac output would contribute to a lower SVO_2 because both conditions reduce the supply of oxygen delivered to the tissues; as a result, the tissues would continue to extract oxygen despite its diminished supply. Atrial fibrillation would not have a specific bearing on the SVO_2 unless it altered the patient's cardiac output.

References: Bridges, E. J., Dukes, M. S. Cardiovascular aspects of septic shock: pathophysiology, monitoring and treatment. *Crit Care Nurse,* 25(2), 14-42, 2005.

Urden, L. D., Stacy, K. M., Lough, M. E. *Thelan's Critical Care Nursing: Diagnosis and Manage-

ment, 5th ed. St. Louis, Elsevier, 2006, pp 414-422.

3-108. **(D)** Nitroglycerin is routinely used when the radial artery is utilized for the graft in coronary artery bypass surgery to prevent spasm in the graft. The purpose of coronary bypass surgery is to revascularize the myocardium and resolve ischemia. Nitroglycerin may be used to decrease systemic vascular resistance or systolic blood pressure, but other agents such as nitroprusside may be utilized for these purposes.

Reference: Bojar, R. M. *Manual of Perioperative Care in Adult Cardiac Surgery*, 4th ed. Berlin, VT, Blackwell, 2005.

3-109. **(A)** For patients with COPD, goals of care related to ABGs are based on the patient's baseline values, not on textbook definitions of normal values. Some environmental or situational triggers that lead to exacerbations may be identifiable but not avoidable, and others may be unknown. Antibiotics may be used for these patients but would not be arbitrarily based on WBC counts since these are less reliable indicators in older patients. Bronchodilators are commonly used early in the care of these patients to relax the airways and reduce the work of breathing.

References: Ellstrom, K. The pulmonary system. In J. G. Alspach (ed.). *Core Curriculum for Critical Care Nursing,* 6th ed. St. Louis, Elsevier, 2006.

Gronkiewicz, C., Borkgren-Okonek, M.Acute exacerbation of COPD: nursing application of evidence based guidelines. *Crit Care Nurs Q,* 27, 336-352, 2004.

3-110. **(A)** Data suggest that maintaining the head-of-bed elevation at 30 to 45 degrees decreases the risk of ventilator-associated pneumonia. There are no supportive data to suggest that any of the other interventions decreases the risk of this complication.

Reference: AACN Practice Alert. Ventilator Associated Pneumonia. Available at www.aacn. org/AACN/practiceAlert.nsf/Files/VAPPP/ Retrieved on July 1, 2006.

3-111. **(C)** The patient is exhibiting anxiousness, irritability, and confusion, all of which could be a sign of hypoglycemia; therefore, assessment of capillary glucose levels would be the first intervention the nurse should perform. Assessing for the concentration of

urine may help distinguish between hyperglycemia and diabetes insipidus, but there is no mention of polyuria in this scenario. Medication with an analgesic is inappropriate before the reason for the pain and confusion is established. Use of restraints without thoroughly assessing the patient would delay appropriate treatment and could increase the patient's agitation.

References: Newberry, L., Criddle, L. *Sheehy's Manual of Emergency Care,* 6th ed. Philadelphia, Elsevier, 2006, pp 428-432.

Urden, L. D., Stacy, K. M., Lough, M *Thelan's Critical Care Nursing: Diagnosis and Management,* 5th ed. St. Louis, Elsevier, 2006, p 926.

3-112. **(C)** As the patient's natural immunity declines, his or her own normal body flora and fauna become the major source of opportunistic infections. While all of the other choices may contribute to the development of illness, they pose danger to the patient transiently and episodically rather than continually.

References: Newberry, L., Criddle, L. *Sheehy's Manual of Emergency Care,* 6th ed. Philadelphia, Elsevier, 2006, pp 527-529.

Urden, L. D., Stacy, K. M., Lough, M. E. *Thelan's Critical Care Nursing: Diagnosis and Management,* 5th ed. St. Louis, Elsevier, 2006, pp 237-238.

3-113. **(B)** Pericardial tamponade may occur in radiofrequency ablation from coronary artery perforation or dissection. Pericardial tamponade restricts myocardial pumping and may result in cardiogenic shock or pulseless electrical activity. Second-degree AV block is not life threatening unless the rate is so slow it is considered to be symptomatic bradycardia. Second-degree block may become life threatening if it progresses to third-degree AV block. Cardiac valve damage is generally not severe enough from the ablation catheter to cause immediate threat to life. Microemboli may cause TIA or CVA.

Reference: Blomstrom-Lundqvist, C., Scheinman, M. M., Aliot, E. M., et al. ACC/AHA/ESC guidelines for the management of patients with supraventricular arrhythmias: a report of the American College of Cardiology/American Heart Association Task Force on practice guidelines and the European Society of Cardiology Committee for Practice Guidelines and the European Society of Cardiology Committee. 2003: http://www.acc. org/clinical/guidelines/arrythmias/sva_index. pdf.

3-114. **(B)** This question illustrates the nurse's competency for response to diversity. Members of some cultures, such as Native Americans and Asians, look down when they are thinking or paying attention. They believe that it is rude to have prolonged eye contact. Since Asians often speak in a soft voice, nurses may be viewed as rude if they speak too loudly. Option A fails to recognize the nature of the communication problem at issue here. Options C and D appear to either neglect or disregard the cultural implications operating in this situation. Option D, in particular, demonstrates a lack of respect for cultural differences when this behavior is in direct opposition to the husband's cultural background.

Reference: Giger, J., Davidhizar, R. *Transcultural Nursing: Assessment and Intervention,* 4th ed. St. Louis, Elsevier, 2004.

3-115. **(C)** Initial treatment for non–ST segment myocardial infarction (NSTEMI) includes administration of aspirin, nitroglycerin, and oxygen. Percutaneous intervention is performed within 24 hours for NSTEMI and within 90 minutes for acute myocardial infarction. Thrombolytics are administered within 30 minutes for acute ST segment elevation myocardial infarction. Delay of percutaneous intervention for NSTEMI greater than 24 hours is associated with poor outcomes.

Reference: Chulay, M., Burns, S. M. *AACN Essentials of Critical Care Nursing.* New York, Mc-Graw-Hill, 2006.

3-116. **(D)** Immediate intubation is warranted for this patient due to the low SpO_2 on high-flow oxygen. The WBC level is within normal limits, indicating that there is no infectious process warranting antibiotic coverage. The RBC and Hgb levels are low but not sufficiently low to warrant administration of blood products or to produce the patient's low SpO_2. Patchy infiltrates in one lobe do not warrant administration of a diuretic and do not reflect pneumonia that requires antibiotic coverage.

Reference: Markou, N. K., Myrianthefs, P. M., Baltopoulos, G. J. Respiratory failure: an overview. *Crit Care Nurs Q,* 27, 353-379, 2004.

3-117. **(A)** The patient needs an immediate IV administration of insulin and glucose because he is demonstrating clinical signs of acute hyperkalemia. Clinical manifestations of hyperkalemia include irritability, restlessness, anxiety, nausea, vomiting, abdominal cramps, weakness, numbness, tingling, and cardiac irregularities. The presence of insulin forces potassium out of the serum and into the cells on a temporary basis, thereby protecting the heart from the effects of elevated serum potassium. In the patient with ESRD, potassium levels rise quickly owing to the complete loss of kidney function. Sodium polystyrene sulfonate (Kayexalate) is an ion resin that exchanges sodium for potassium in the bowel so that excessive amounts of potassium can be excreted via the feces. Although this is an effective means of ridding the body of excess potassium, its effects take longer to produce, making it a later option for management of hyperkalemia. Lidocaine and amiodarone are used to treat ventricular dysrhythmias and play no role in treating hyperkalemia.

References: Lough, M. E. Renal disorders and therapeutic management. In L. D. Urden, K. M. Stacy, M E. Lough (eds.). *Thelan's Critical Care Nursing: Diagnosis and Management,* 5th ed. St. Louis, Elsevier, 2006, pp 813-846.
Mitchell, J. K. Renal disorders and therapeutic management. In L. D. Urden, K. M. Stacy, M E. Lough (eds.). *Priorities in Critical Care Nursing,* 4th ed. St. Louis, Elsevier, 2005, pp 333-356.
Stark, J. L. The renal system. In J. G. Alspach (ed.). *Core Curriculum for Critical Care Nursing,* 6th ed. St. Louis, Elsevier, 2006, pp 525-607.

3-118. **(A)** Acute coronary syndrome encompasses both non ST segment elevation MI (NSTEMI) and unstable angina. Physical findings may be normal or nonspecific. ECG findings may be nonspecific. Pulmonary rales, mitral regurgitation murmur, tachycardia, and hypotension may reflect heart failure or acute myocardial infarction. Patients with pain of any kind may have tachycardia. Hypotension may result from use of diuretics or use of nitrates to relieve chest pain.

Reference: Achar, S. A., Kundu, S., Norcross, W. A. Diagnosis of acute coronary syndromes. *Am Fam Phys,* 72, 119-126, 2005.

3-119. **(B)** Data suggest that the patient must be in a supine position with the head of the bed (HOB) elevated no more than 30 to 45 degrees when ST segment analysis is performed. Option A is incorrect because if the ST alarm sounds and the patient is in a side-lying position, the patient should be returned to the supine position; only if the ST segment deviation persists with the patient supine should this finding be considered indicative of myocardial ischemia. Neither the completely flat (Option C) nor high Fowler's position (Option D) affords ST segment monitoring as accurately as the supine position with HOB elevated.

Reference: AACN Practice Alert. ST Segment Monitoring. Available at www.aacn.org//AACN/practiceAlert.nsf/Files/ECG%20ST%20Segment/ Retrieved on July 1, 2006.

3-120. **(A)** HOB elevation of 30-45 degrees is associated with a lower incidence of aspiration of gastric contents. The current best practices for preventing VAP call for daily sedation vacations to avoid oversedation (Option B), frequent oral care (Option C), and early enteral rather than parenteral nutrition (Option D).

References: American Thoracic Society. Guidelines for the management of adults with hospital-acquired, ventilator-associated and healthcare-associated pneumonia. *Am J Respir Crit Care Med,* 171, 388-416, 2005.

Ellstrom, K. The pulmonary system. In J. G. Alspach (ed.). *Core Curriculum for Critical Care Nursing,* 6th ed. St. Louis, Elsevier, 2006.

3-121. **(B)** In aortic stenosis, the left ventricle hypertrophies and requires higher filling pressures postoperatively to maintain adequate cardiac output. The filling pressure is demonstrated by the PCWP, which is generally maintained at 15 mm Hg or greater, so this patient needs the fluid bolus to raise filling pressure. Since nitroglycerin decreases preload, it would prevent adequate filling of the LV in the patient with aortic valve repair. Dobutamine is an inotropic agent, which would not be beneficial in this patient unless the volume status of the left ventricle was adequate. The patient requires nursing intervention to optimize cardiac output.

Reference: Bojar, R. M. *Manual of Perioperative Care in Adult Cardiac Surgery,* 4th ed. Berlin, VT, Blackwell, 2005.

3-122. **(C)** Persons receiving enteral nutrition are at increased risk for developing hyperglycemic, hyperosmolar, non-ketotic coma because these solutions provide high carbohydrate nourishment. Assessment findings indicate polyuria resulting in dehydration. Without a history of diabetes, it is unlikely the patient has developed ketoacidosis. No bruising or other signs of trauma have been found, so there is little possibility the patient has developed diabetes insipidus.

References: Newberry, L., Criddle, L. *Sheehy's Manual of Emergency Care,* 6th ed. Philadelphia, Elsevier, 2006, pp 431-433.

Urden, L. D., Stacy, K. M., Lough, M. E. (eds.). *Thelan's Critical Care Nursing: Diagnosis and Management,* 5th ed. St. Louis, Elsevier, 2006, p 934.

3-123. **(C)** Vasodilators such as nitrates and ACE inhibitors decrease vasoconstriction, which decreases afterload. In addition, ACE inhibitors have a mild diuretic effect that is beneficial in congestive failure. Beta-blockers control atrial dysrhythmias and improve diastolic filling but do not decrease afterload. Digoxin improves myocardial contractility and controls atrial fibrillation but does not affect afterload. Nesiritide vasodilates to decrease afterload and promote diuresis.

Reference: Chulay, M., Burns, S. M. *AACN Essentials of Critical Care Nursing.* New York, McGraw-Hill, 2006.

3-124. **(D)** Data suggest that the two leads of choice for distinguishing ventricular tachycardia from supraventricular tachycardia with aberrant conduction are V_1 and V_6. Either lead II (Option A) or lead III is recommended to monitor atrial activity. Neither Option B nor Option C is recommended for specific monitoring purposes. Other data suggest that nurses use a standard monitoring lead irrespective of patient diagnosis.

Reference: AACN Practice Alert. Dysrhythmia Monitoring. Available at www.aacn.org/AACN/practiceAlert.nsf/Files/ECG%20Dysrhythmia/ $file/ECG%20Dysrhythmia.pdf Retrieved on July 1, 2006.

3-125. **(B)** Chemotherapy regimens for colorectal cancer can have the side effect of gastrointestinal bleeding. Gastrointestinal perforation can occur. Dark-colored stools, fatigue, and the development of hypotension are sympyomatic of a gastrointestinal bleed. While malnutrition is a possibility in patients receiving chemotherapy, this patient does not exhibit evidence of that condition. The patient experiencing bleeding may well experience anemia, but stopping this patient's bleeding is a higher priority need than treating the anemia. Patients on chemotherapy will incur immunosuppression, but that is not a pressing concern at this time.

Reference: Hurwitz, H., Kabbinaavar, F. Bevacizumab combined with standard fluoropyrimidine based chemotherapy regimens to treat colorectal cancer. *Oncology,* 3(Suppl),17-24, 2005.

3-126. **(B)** A patient who is breathing shallowly does not move air effectively in and out of the lungs. Diminished ventilation increases the volume of dead space, or air that does not contribute to gas exchange. The patient with increased dead space effectively re-breathes carbon dioxide, causing a rise in $PaCO_2$. The amount of dead space affects the $PaCO_2$ value. Administration of oxygen to a hypercapneic patient may actually increase $PaCO_2$ because the higher amount of oxygen diminishes respiratory drive, thereby slowing the respiratory rate, which increases the $PaCO_2$. Oxygen administration does not increase the work of breathing, but administration of 100% oxygen in a patient relying on hypoxia for respiratory drive should be avoided. Not all hypercapneic patients require hypoxia to stimulate ventilation; that response pattern is usually seen in patients with chronic rather than acute pulmonary disease. Decreased hemoglobin levels in anemia do not change the ratio of oxygen to carbon dioxide and therefore will not affect $PaCO_2$. The A-a gradient is the difference in partial pressure of oxygen between arterial and alveolar blood. The normal value is 5 to 25 mm Hg or (age + 10) ÷ 4. High A-a gradients result from impaired diffusion or the presence of shunting. The higher the A-a gradient, the worse the diffusion defect. The A-a gradient reflects oxygenation and is independent of CO_2 levels.

Reference: Markou, N. K., Myrianthefs, P. M., Baltopoulos, G. J. Respiratory failure: an overview. *Crit Care Nurs Q,* 27, 353-379, 2004.

3-127. **(D)** Chest pain unrelieved by nitroglycerin or rest suggests that an atherosclerotic plaque has ruptured and embolized, causing occlusion of a coronary artery. Chest pain relieved by nitroglycerin or rest indicates that an atherosclerotic placque is stable and has not ruptured, causing distal occlusion. Chest pain associated with deep inspiration is characterized as pleuritic in nature.

Reference: Pope, J. H., Selker, H.P. Acute coronary syndromes in the emergency department: diagnostic characteristics. *Cardiol Clin,* 23, 423-452, 2005.

3-128. **(C)** Patients with sudden-onset neurologic deficiencies and persistent focal neurologic deficits should be considered for rt-PA therapy. Patients with persistent symptoms after 1 hour have an 85% risk of stroke with only a 15% chance of full recovery. Patients whose symptoms resolve rapidly are most likely having a TIA and should not receive rt-PA. It is essential to identify the time of the onset of symptoms or at least the last time the patient was seen without deficits. For therapy to be effective, it must begin within 3 hours of symptom onset, not arrival to the hospital (Option A). Patient allergies are important to identify (Option B) but are not the most important factor. The time window of treatment options is the primary limiting factor in treatment of these patients. Bleeding at a noncompressible site such as a central vein (Option D) should be avoided, so a peripheral IV line is preferred to a central line.

References: Adams, H., Adams, R., Del Zoppo, G., Goldstein, L. B. Guidelines for the early management of patients with ischemic stroke: 2005 guidelines update. A scientific statement from the Stroke Council of the American Heart Association/American Stroke Association. *Stroke,* 36, 916-923, 2005.
Braimah, J., Kongable, G., Rapp, K., et al. Nursing care of acute stroke patients after receiving rt-PA therapy. *J Neurosci Nurs,* 29(6), 373-383, 1997.
Brott, T., Bogousslavsky, F. Treatment of acute ischemic stroke. *New Engl J Med,* 343(10), 710-722, 2000.

3-129. **(D)** Signs of peripheral edema occur when shock has progressed and compensatory mechanisms are failing Peripheral edema, especially in dependent regions, occurs when increased capillary permeability allows plasma proteins to move from the vascular tree into the interstitial space. Tachycardia greater than 120 beats/min reflects progressive shock with cardiac compensation. Urine output less than 30 mL/hr may indicate early shock when renal vasoconstriction occurs. Increased capillary refill time occurs with vasoconstriction and may be present in early and progressive shock as well as during late shock.

Reference: Lewis, S. M., Heitkemper, M. M., Dirksen, S. R. *Medical-Surgical Nursing*, 6th ed. St. Louis, Elsevier, 2004.

3-130. **(D)** Positioning the patient with the injured side down and administering pain medication in the form of intercostal nerve blocks may be temporarily beneficial. The patient's ABG results indicate that the high-flow mask in ineffective in providing adequate ventilation and oxygenation, so intubation with mechanical ventilation is needed. Positioning the patient with the uninjured side up helps to improve the ratio of ventilation to perfusion. Care must be taken in administration of IV fluids owing to this patient's pulmonary contusion and the potential development of acute respiratory distress syndrome. The blood pressure is stable at this time, so inotropic support is unnecessary and would further compound existing significant tachycardia. The use of a CPAP mask would be less effective than intubation and pronation will increase the difficulty in management of the airway which is critically needed at this time. Trendelenberg positioning may impair ventilation without stabilization of the floating rib segment. Without a chest x-ray, it is difficult to know the extent of injury or whether a chest tube is warranted.

References: Peavey, A. A., Newberry, L. Thoracic trauma. *Sheehy's Emergency Nursing Principles and Practice,* 5th ed. Philadelphia, Elsevier, 2003, p 284.

Yamamoto, L., Schroeder, C., Morely, D., Beiveau, C. Thoracic trauma: The deadly dozen. *Crit Care Nurse Q,* 28(1), 22-40, 2005.

3-131. **(C)** Critically ill older patients exhibit delayed resolution of swallowing impairment post extubation. A fiberoptic endoscopic evaluation of swallowing should be considered in older patients following prolonged endotracheal intubation. While other consults (Options A and B) may be required,

they can be delayed until the patient's respiratory status is assured. Option D is incorrect because presence of laryngeal edema will be assessed prior to extubating the patient. Evaluation of the patient's ability to swallow is essential to help prevent post-extubation aspiration.

Reference: El Solh, A., Okada, M., Bhat, A., Pietrantoni, C. Swallowing disorders post orotracheal intubation in the elderly. *Intensive Care Med,* 29(9), 1451-1455, 2003.

3-132. **(C)** Aortic regurgitation results in dilation and noncompliance of the left ventricle. Vasopressor support with alpha-adrenergic agents such as norepinephrine (Levophed) increases the force of contraction and compliance of the left ventricle and constricts peripheral vessels to improve blood pressure. Volume boluses are often insufficient to improve BP and CO in a dilated, noncompliant left ventricle. In addition, PCWP and urine output indicate intravascular volume is adequate. Although dobutamine's beta-adrenergic effects on the myocardium would increase LV contractility and heart rate, its beta-2 effects may dilate the peripheral vasculature, thereby lowering BP. Increasing the pacing rate without enhancing circulating volume would add further myocardial work.

Reference: Bojar, R. M. *Manual of Perioperative Care in Adult Cardiac Surgery*, 4th ed. Berlin, VT, Blackwell, 2005.

3-133. **(D)** Most signs and symptoms of alcohol withdrawal are caused by rapid removal of the depressant effects of alcohol in the central nervous system. Alcohol withdrawal syndrome (AWS) usually occurs within 24 hours of the last drink and results in autonomic hyperreactivity (tremors, nausea, vomiting, sweating) and neuropsychiatric alterations (agitation, anxiety, auditory disturbances, clouding of sensorium, disturbances in visual or tactile senses). The worst form of AWS is called alcohol withdrawal delirium or delirium tremens, a life-threatening medical emergency that typically occurs 48 to 72 hours after the last drink. The autonomic hypersensitivity symptoms of delirium include hypertension, tachycardia, tachypnea, and tremors. Neuropsychiatric indications of delirium include hallucination, disorientation, and impaired attention. The cornerstone of pharmacologic management to halt progression of AWS and prevent DTs is administration of benzodiazepines, which provide CNS depression. Haldol is not indicated for the management of neuropsychiatric alterations associated with AWS. Restraints should not be applied, as they may intensify the neuropsychiatric alterations. The visual and auditory images associated with television may contribute to a patient's confusion and hallucinations.

References: McKinley, M. G. Alcohol withdrawal syndrome. Overlooked and mismanaged? *Crit Care Nurse,* 25(3), 40-49, 2005.

Newberry, L., Criddle, L. M. (eds.). *Sheehy's Manual of Emergency Care,* 6th ed. Philadelphia, Elsevier, 2005, pp 452-453.

3-134. **(A)** Weight gain greater than 2 kg or 5 lb in 24 hours indicates failure of diuretic therapy and potential to develop pulmonary edema in the heart failure patient. This requires immediate contact to the primary care provider to adjust diuretic therapy or other lifestyle changes such as diet or fluid intake. Cough is a common side effect seen with ACE inhibitors and may be irritating but is not as life threatening as pulmonary edema. Leg edema is a common sign of right heart failure and may be diminished by leg elevation. Increased fatigue and exercise intolerance are signs of worsening heart failure or the development of co-existing problems such as flu or infection. Exercise tolerance in patients with heart failure waxes and wanes and does not warrant immediate physician notification.

Reference: Woods, S. L., Froelicher, E. S., Motzer, S. U., Bridges, E. J. *Cardiac Nursing,* 5th ed. Philadelphia, Lippincott Williams & Wilkins, 2005.

3-135. **(C)** By seeking clarification and not readily implementing the order, the nurse is acting as an advocate for the patient. This is indicated as the patient's family has not agreed to a do-not-resuscitate order and the ordered ventilator change is not clinically indicated. Option B could place the family in the middle between the patient and the physician and does not reflect caring practices. The nurse should recognize that to change a patient from receiving maximal ventilator support to a room-air level of oxygen support

(Option A) when the patient's oxygen saturation is low is not physiologically sound and could cause discomfort to the patient. The nurse will need to perform an ongoing patient assessment for presence of pain and discomfort and administer the medications based on that assessment. Administration of medications, as suggested in Option D, is not indicated until an assessment is made.

Reference: Molter, N. Professional caring and ethical practice. In J. G. Alspach (ed.). *Core Curriculum for Critical Care Nursing,* 6th ed. St. Louis, Elsevier, 2006, pp 1-44.

3-136. **(A)** This patient shows evidence of severe respiratory compromise, including respiratory acidosis, significant hypoxemia, and desaturation. This degree of pulmonary deterioration warrants intubation and mechanical ventilation (i.e., treatment considerably more aggressive than NIV or raising the FiO_2). Although Heliox has been suggested for use in COPD as an adjunct to NIV, it is primarily used in treatment of status asthmaticus.

Reference: Calverley, P. Chronic obstructive pulmonary diseases. In M. P. Fink, E. Abraham, J. L. Vincent, P. M. Kochanek (eds.). *Textbook of Critical Care,* 5th ed. Philadelphia, Elsevier, 2005.

3-137. **(A)** Elevation of a pulseless extremity will decrease perfusion and is therefore contraindicated. Reverse Trendelenberg places the foot in a dependent position that would increase blood flow. Heparin could aid in resolving a clot which could be causing occlusion. Vasodilator medications would assist in promoting circulation to the foot and toe.

Reference: Fahey, V. A. *Vascular Nursing,* 4th ed. St. Louis, Elsevier, 2004.

3-138. **(C)**. In general, southern Europeans (e.g., Spain) find frequent touching to be reassuring and comforting. Conversely, northern Europeans and Asians prefer little or no touching. This patient may be exhibiting restlessness and resistance to treatments because of the touching that is involved.

Reference: Giger, J., Davidhizar, R. *Transcultural Nursing: Assessment and Intervention,* 4th ed. St. Louis, Elsevier, 2004.

3-139. **(C)** The most likely cause of these findings is a pneumothorax, and the physician will assess the situation and probably insert a chest tube. To do nothing and continue with the bath will delay management of a recognizable condition that requires treatment and could pose some risk to the patient. Application of an occlusive dressing could convert this pneumothorax into a potential tension pneumothorax, a serious and possibly lethal problem that could result in cardiac arrest. At this time, the patient does not appear to be in any pulmonary distress, so intubation is not warranted.

References: Ellstrom, K. Pulmonary system. In J. G. Alspach (ed.). *Core Curriculum for Critical Care Nursing,* 6th ed. St. Louis, Elsevier, 2006, p 149.

Yamamoto, L., Schroeder, C., Morely, D., Beiveau, C. Thoracic trauma: the deadly dozen. *Crit Care Nurse Q,* 28(1), 22-40, 2005.

3-140. **(B)** CT scan is used for patients with non-penetrating trauma to determine the location and extent of renal parenchymal damage. A CT scan can assess the extent of parenchymal laceration, urine extravasation, surrounding hemorrhage, and presence of vascular injury. Ultrasound has minimal value for nonpenetrating injury, although it can help evaluate renal parenchymal injury and locate a hematoma. Renal scan is used to evaluate renal blood flow and possible parenchymal injury. Renal angiography is done if the injury is not clearly defined by other radiologic studies.

Reference: Adams, K., Johnson, K. Trauma. In L. D. Urden, K. M. Stacy, M. E. Lough (eds.). *Thelan's Critical Care Nursing: Diagnosis and Management,* 5th ed. St. Louis, Elsevier, 2006, pp 969-1008.

Stark, J. L. The renal system. In J. G. Alspach (ed.). *Core Curriculum for Critical Care Nursing*, 6th ed. St. Louis, Elsevier, 2006, pp 525-607.

3-141. **(C)** Patients who have undergone major open abdominal procedures and are receiving postoperative opioids can develop a postoperative ileus. The complication is usually transient, and early recognition is key to expedient and effective management. Although the patient has a low-grade fever, no other signs of an intra-abdominal infection or wound infection are present, and the elevated white blood cell count that would be expected with infection is not evident. There is no evidence of an intra-abdominal

hemorrhage, as the patient's hemoglobin and vital signs are stable.

References: Carter, S. The surgical team and outcomes management: focus on postoperative ileus. *J Perianesth Nurs,* 21(2A), s2-s6, 2006.

Radovich, P. Gastrointestinal system. In J. G. Alspach (ed.). *Core Curriculum for Critical Care Nursing,* 6th ed. St. Louis, Elsevier, 2006, pp 739-743.

3-142. **(C)** This patient has pauses reflecting a heart rate of 19 beats/min followed by tachycardia. This is indicative of sick sinus syndrome and indicates need for a permanent pacemaker. A transcutaneous pacemaker could be used when the heart rate slows, but would not be effective when tachycardia appears. Atropine is not an appropriate treatment for a dysrhythmia which alternates between bradycardia and tachycardia. Continuous monitoring is indicated for this patient but is not sufficient for management and places the patient at risk for syncopal episodes which may result in patient injury.

Reference: Woods, S. L., Froelicher, E. S., Motzer, S. U., Bridges, E. J. *Cardiac Nursing,* 5th ed. Philadelphia, Lippincott Williams & Wilkins, 2005.

3-143. **(A)** *Hemoperfusion* is a process used to clear blood of substances that bind to plasma proteins or are lipid soluble. When blood is pumped through a cartridge that contains activated charcoal and/or carbon, those two substances compete with plasma proteins to absorb drugs and poisons. Phenytoin is a highly protein bound substance, and hemoperfusion is the *most* effective treatment for removal. Lithium, salicylate, and ethanol are low-molecular-weight substances and, therefore, *hemodialysis* would be the *preferred* method for removal. The semipermeable membrane used during dialysis allows the movement of small molecules and middle-weight molecules from the blood into the dialysate. It is impermeable to larger molecules like phenytoin.

Reference: Alspach, J. G. (ed.). *Core Curriculum for Critical Care Nursing,* 6th ed. St. Louis, Elsevier, 2006, pp 840-841.

3-144. **(C)** In this situation, advocating for the patient occurs through preventing the transfer of infections between patients. The CDC recommends washing with either nonantimicrobial or antimicrobial soap; hence, any soap is effective. According to the CDC, alcohol-based hand rubs are not for visibly soiled hands; therefore, Option A is incorrect. Option B is incorrect because hands should be washed both after the removal of gloves and before the donning of gloves. A 10-minute scrub time is not recommended even for surgical hand antisepsis.

References: Boyce, J., Pittet, D. Guideline for hand hygiene in health-care settings. *Morbid Mortal Wkly Rep*, 51(RR16), 1-44, 2002.

Molter, N. Professional caring and ethical practice. In J. G. Alspach (ed.). *Core Curriculum for Critical Care Nursing*, 6th ed. St. Louis, Elsevier, 2006, pp 1-44.

3-145. **(A)** A narrowed pulse pressure, tachycardia, location of the stab wound, and chest x-ray demonstrating an enlarged cardiac silhouette strongly suggest pericardial tamponade is present. A 10% pneumothorax is not sufficient to cause hypotension, and the condition is treated appropriately with chest tube placement. At least 250 mL of blood is needed in most cases to be visible as a hemothorax on chest x-ray; however, even a 250 mL loss would have been treated appropriately by the 500 mL bolus in the ED. There is no apparent source of excessive bleeding causing hypovolemia on chest x-ray, wound dressing, or in the chest tube collection chamber. Hypovolemia would cause hypotension and tachycardia, but not an enlarged cardiac silhouette.

Reference: American College of Surgeons Committee on Trauma. *Advanced Trauma Life Support for Doctors*, 7th ed. Chicago, American College of Surgeons, 2004.

3-146. **(A)** Part of the pathophysiology of emphysema involves the destruction of alveolar walls with resulting development of large, air-filled structures called "blebs." These areas are at risk for rupturing, which will lead to the development of a pneumothorax. As a result, patient management includes careful monitoring of airway pressures and use of low- to normal-sized tidal volumes. Patients with emphysemia do not demonstrate alveolar/arterial diffusion defects as seen in ARDS, so they typically will respond to increases in FiO_2. There are no standardized strategies for mode of ventilatory management in this patient population.

References: Calverley, P. Chronic obstructive pulmonary diseases. In M. P. Fink, E. Abraham, J. L. Vincent, P. M. Kochanek (eds.). *Textbook of Critical Care*, 5th ed. Philadelphia, Elsevier, 2005.

Ellstrom, K. The pulmonary system. In J. G. Alspach (ed.). *Core Curriculum for Critical Care Nursing*, 6th ed. St. Louis, Elsevier, 2006.

3-147. **(B)** Administration of insulin will help to correct the hyperglycemia associated with steroid administration and stress. This intervention should be followed by administration of IV fluids and electrolytes, as the patient has likely been experiencing polyuria. Low-dose insulin drip will require a greater period of time to correct the metabolic alterations but may be desirable at a later time. While the bicarbonate level is slightly decreased, administration of bicarbonate is not appropriate at this time, as this value will return to normal as fluids and electrolytes are replaced. This level of carbon dioxide may be a normal value for this patient, whose underlying respiratory disease may result in carbon dioxide retention.

References: Newberry, L., Criddle, L. *Sheehy's Manual of Emergency Care*, 6th ed. Philadelphia, Elsevier, 2006, pp 428-431.

Urden, L. D., Stacy, K. M., Lough, M. *Thelan's Critical Care Nursing: Diagnosis and Management*, 5th ed. St. Louis, Elsevier, 2006, pp 605-608.

3-148. **(C)** Although it is common to maintain CSF pressure at 10 mm Hg after thoracic aortic aneurysm repair, there is only about 150 mL of CSF in the system at one time. If CSF is drained too rapidly or in too large a volume, the patient is at risk of subarachnoid hemorrhage. Fluid administration may be used to maintain blood pressure after TAA repair and is used in conjunction with nitroglycerin administration to decrease systolic BP because many of these patients have preexisting hypertension. FFP and platelets are commonly administered to these patients to replace coagulation factors and prevent coagulopathy.

Reference: Bojar, R. M. *Manual of Perioperative Care in Adult Cardiac Surgery*, 4th ed. Berlin, VT, Blackwell, 2005.

3-149. **(C)** NPPV works by increasing inspiratory pressure to expand tidal volume. Increased tidal volume, in turn, enhances alveolar recruitment and diminishes the atelectasis caused by hypoventilation. Care must be exercised in use of NPPV, however, to avoid inadvertently increasing expiratory pressures as well. This is a particular concern for patients with COPD, who already have excessively high expiratory pressures owing to airway collapse on expiration with air-trapping in distal alveoli. Further increases in expiratory pressure from NPPV would then magnify one of the fundamental pathophysiologic effects of COPD. NPPV has minimal effects on V/Q matching and has no effect on mucous production in distal airways.

References: Ellstrom, K. The pulmonary system. In J. G. Alspach (ed.). *Core Curriculum for Critical Care Nursing,* 6th ed. St. Louis, Elsevier, 2006, pp 45-184.

Gronkiewicz, C., Borkgren-Okonek, M. Acute exacerbation of COPD: nursing application of evidenced based guidelines. *Crit Care Nurs Q,* 27, 336-352, 2004.

3-150. **(D)** Forced expiratory volume (FEV$_1$) in 1 second, as an indication of flow, drops a

minimum of 20 mL per year after age 25 years. Option A is incorrect because pulmonary changes observed in older adults include a decrease in maximal inspiratory and expiratory capacity, work capacity, and chest wall compliance secondary to rib cage calcification. Lungs become stiff, and compliance decreases owing to decreased elastic recoil. Options B and C are incorrect because older persons experience a decrease in alveolar surface area and a decline in surfactant production that lead to higher residual lung volumes and air trapping. Auscultation of breath sounds in an older individual reveals decreased air exchange in the lung bases that result from air trapping and decreased lung expansion.

Reference: Forciea, M., Lavizzo-Mourey, R., Schwab, E. P., et al. *Geriatric Secrets,* 3rd ed. Philadelphia, Elsevier, 2004.

Annotated Bibliography

PROFESSIONAL CARING AND ETHICAL PRACTICE

Annis, T. The interdisciplinary team across the continuum of care. *Crit Care Nurse,* 22(5), 76-79, 2002.

This article presents a case study that illustrates how teamwork by the interdisciplinary critical care team and application of the AACN Synergy Model for Patient Care resulted in positive patient outcomes. The article describes the case of a patient who underwent a hemicolectomy for a perforated and necrotic bowel and had a complex postoperative course. The article describes the patient based on the eight characteristics inherent in the model.

Curley, M. A. Q. Patient-nurse synergy: optimizing patient outcomes. *Am J Crit Care,* 7(1), 64-72, 1998.

This article is one of the first published descriptions of the major tenets of the AACN Synergy Model for Patient Care. Although this article is several years old, it remains a useful overview of the AACN Synergy Model for Patient Care.

Ecklund, M., Stamps, D. Promoting synergy in progressive care. *Crit Care Nurse,* 22(4), 60-6, 2002.

This article describes a 26-bed progressive care unit and compares nurses with various levels of experience in relation to the nurse competencies of the AACN Synergy Model for Patient Care and how they would be manifested. It further describes how the AACN Synergy Model for Patient Care was implemented in a pediatric care unit. Two case exemplars are provided.

Hardin, S., Hussey, L. AACN Synergy Model of patient care: case study of a CHF patient. *Crit Care Nurse,* 23(1), 73-76, 2003.

This article applies the AACN Synergy Model for Patient Care to a patient in an ambulatory clinic who is New York Heart Association Class III CHF. The article describes the patient characteristics and nurse competencies needed in this setting.

Hardin, S. R., Kaplow, R. (eds.). *Synergy for Clinical Excellence: The AACN Synergy Model for Patient Care.* Boston, Jones & Bartlett, 2005.

This book describes all aspects of the AACN Synergy Model for Patient Care and each of the patient characteristics and nurse competencies. Case studies illustrate how each patient characteristic and nurse competency is incorporated into clinical practice. Sample test questions are provided for nurses preparing for the adult, pediatric, neonatal CCRN, and PCCN examinations, as are questions consistent with practice of nurse practitioners.

Kaplow, R. Applying the Synergy Model to nursing education. *Crit Care Nurse,* 22(3), 77-81, 2002.

This article provides a clinical exemplar to illustrate the role of the nurse educator in assisting nursing care of a patient in the intensive care unit. The patient is described based on the AACN Synergy Model for Patient Care.

Markey, D. Applying the Synergy Model: clinical strategies. *Crit Care Nurse,* 21(3), 72-6, 2001.

This article presents a case study of a patient who underwent resection of a large retroperitoneal sarcoma, distal pancreatectomy, and splenectomy. The case describes how the patient's clinical condition and course deteriorated throughout her stay in the intensive care unit. It illustrates how the AACN Synergy Model for Patient Care facilitated patient care throughout the patient's postoperative course and enhanced attainment of optimal patient outcomes.

Mullen, J. The Synergy Model as a framework for nursing rounds. *Crit Care Nurse,* 22(6), 66-68, 2002.

This article describes how the AACN Synergy Model for Patient Care can be used as a framework for nursing rounds. The tenets of the model are described, and the patient characteristics and nurse competencies of the model are defined. A case study of a patient with Guillain-Barré syndrome in a pediatric intensive care unit is used to illustrate the model's value in managing care of this patient.

CARDIOVASCULAR

Alspach, J. G. (ed.). *Core Curriculum for Critical Care Nursing* (6th ed.). St. Louis, Elsevier, 2006.

The newly revised Core Curriculum for Critical Care Nursing *is a world-recognized text containing the knowledge essential to critical care nursing practice. The latest edition includes numerous new graphics and tables that enhance the nurse's understanding and ability to think critically through patient situations in the intensive care unit. In addition, the application of the AACN Synergy Model for Patient Care is presented with specific applications demonstrating prioritization of and acuity of patient conditions.*

Baird, M. S., Keen, J. H., Swearingen, P. L. *Manual of Critical Care Nursing* (5th ed.). St. Louis, Elsevier, 2005.

This text is packed with all things critical care. Descriptions of pathophysiologic conditions are concise and logically presented. A great reference book.

Bojar, R. M. *Manual of Perioperative Care in Adult Cardiac Surgery* (4th ed.). Berlin, VT, Blackwell, 2005.

> *A very well-written text on cardiovascular surgery. Includes off-pump, MIDCAB, valve surgery, and surgery for heart failure as well as coronary artery bypass. Postoperative care and potential complications of the particular types of surgery are also presented.*

Camm, A. J., Luscher, T. F., Serruys, P. W. *The ESC Textbook of Cardiovascular Medicine*. Malden, MA, Blackwell, 2006.

> *This text includes best practices in the care of patients with cardiovascular pathologies and contains many ECG tracings and illustrations that complement the text. The text also includes a web site address and access number that allow the reader to access multiple links and images that are very educational and helpful in understanding cardiovascular pathology, diagnostic testing , and current evidence-based treatments.*

Chulay, M., Burns, S. M. *AACN Essentials of Critical Care Nursing*. New York, McGraw-Hill, 2006.

> *This text is for the experienced critical care nurse. It includes AACN protocols, drug tables, and troubleshooting guides for hemodynamic monitoring. and critical thinking case studies.*

Fink, M. P., Abraham, E., Vincent, J., Kochanek P. M. *Textbook of Critical Care* (5th ed.). Philadelphia, Elsevier, 2005.

> *This text covers both adult and pediatric critical care patient conditions and has a web site for continued information searches.*

Kern, M. J. *Interventional Cardiology Handbook*. Philadelphia, Elsevier, 2003.

> *This text includes all aspects of interventional cardiology, including technique, postprocedure care, and postprocedure complications. Although it is primarily geared toward cardiology fellows and interns, it is a valuable resource for cardiovascular nurses who wish to understand the procedural aspects of interventional cardiology procedures.*

Kern, M. J. *Cardiac Catheterization Handbook*. Philadelphia, Elsevier, 2003.

> *This text outlines preprocedure cardiac catheterization and interventional modalities as well as postprocedure care of patients undergoing cardiac catheterization. It also includes the use of drug-eleuting stents and vascular closure devices.*

Woods, S. L., Froelicher, E. S., Motzer, S. U., Bridges, E. J. *Cardiac Nursing* (5th ed.). Philadelphia, Lippincott Williams & Wilkins, 2005.

> *A well-organized text devoted entirely to cardiac anatomy, physiology, pathophysiology, assessment, and management of patients with cardiovascular disorders. Goal-directed nursing care plans with rationales for interventions are provided for many chapters. Acute coronary syndromes, cardiac catheterization, intervention, heart failure, and cardiac surgery are well covered.*

Zipes, D. P., Libby, P., Bonow, R. O., Braunwald, E. (eds.). *Braunwald's Heart Disease: A Textbook of Cardiovascular Medicine* (7th ed.). Philadelphia, Elsevier, 2005.

> *The ultimate reference for current information on cardiovascular pathophysiology and management of cardiovascular pathological conditions.*

PULMONARY

Burns, S. M. Mechanical ventilation of patients with acute respiratory distress syndrome and patients requiring weaning: the evidence guiding practice. *Crit Care Nurse*, 25(4), 14-16, 18, 20-23, 2005.

> *Provides a comprehensive summary of the evidence underlying provision of mechanical ventilation to patients with ARDS as well as weaning. Includes discussion of the acute stage of ventilation, modes of ventilation, use of PEEP, alveolar recruitment, proning, and the weaning process.*

Chulay, M. Respiratory system. In Chulay, M., Burns, S. (eds.). *AACN Essentials of Critical Care Nursing*. New York, McGraw-Hill, 2006.

> *Provides brief overviews of a variety of critical care conditions.*

Ellstrom, K. Pulmonary system. In Alspach, J. G. (ed.). *Core Curriculum for Critical Care Nursing* (6th ed.). St. Louis, Elsevier, 2006.

> *Offers an outline summary of all information essential to care of critical care patients with acute and life-threatening pulmonary disorders, including coverage of physiology, pathophysiology, diagnostic studies, etiology, and medical and nursing management.*

Koran, Z., Howard, P. K. Respiratory emergencies. In *Sheehy's Emergency Nursing Principles and Practice* (6th ed.). St. Louis, Mosby, 2006.

> *A critical care text that focuses on emergency nursing considerations. It provides excellent overviews of emergent conditions as well as clinical foundations for emergency nursing and care of special patient populations.*

O'Steen, D. Orthopedic and neurovascular trauma. In *Sheehy's Emergency Nursing Principles and Practice* (6th ed.). Philadelphia, Mosby, 2006.

> *Provides good coverage of chest and thoracic trauma with emphasis on emergency care considerations.*

Roman, M., Mercado, D. Review of chest tube use. *Med Surg Nurs*, 15(1), 41-43, 2006.

> *This is an excellent review article on chest tubes. It provides a good overview of technique and physiology.*

Yamamoto, L., Schroeder, C., Morely, D., Beiveau, C. Thoracic trauma: The deadly dozen. *Crit Care Nurse Q*, 28(1), 22-40, 2005.

> *This is an excellent article on thoracic trauma that discusses physiology and provides case examples and interventions.*

Yang, J. C. Prevention and treatment of deep vein thrombosis and pulmonary embolism in critically ill patients. *Crit Care Nurse Q*, 28(1), 72-79, 2005.

This review article outlines prevention of deep vein thrombosis and its progression to pulmonary embolism. It discusses current options and recommendations regarding the occurrence of deep vein thrombosis and pulmonary embolism in the intensive care unit population.

NEUROLOGIC

Adams, H., Adams, R., Del Zoppo, G., Goldstein, L. B. Guidelines for the early management of patients with ischemic stroke: 2005 guidelines update. A scientific statement from the Stroke Council of the American Heart Association/American Stroke Association. *Stroke*, 36, 916-923, 2005.
> *This evidence-based document provides recommendations regarding the management of patients with acute ischemic stroke and provides a thorough review of the literature. While a bit dry, it is an essential resource.*

Alspach, J. G. (ed.). *Core Curriculum for Critical Care Nursing* (6th ed.). St. Louis, Elsevier, 2006.
> *This thorough guide for the critical care nurse provides helpful information and references regarding neurological issues in the critically ill patient. Information is succinct and easily identified. Not only is this text helpful for critical care nurses preparing for the CCRN and PCCN examinations, but it also is a valuable clinical resource.*

Bader, M. K., Littlejohns, L. R (eds.). *AANN Core Curriculum for Neuroscience Nursing* (4th ed.). St. Louis, Elsevier, 2004.
> *This is the AANN's comprehensive reference for neuroscience nurses. Information is presented in an outline format. Although it is not as readable as a standard text, it is a great reference and a valuable resource regarding the many details of caring for the neuroscience patient.*

Braimah, J., Kongable, G., Rapp, K., et al. Nursing care of acute stroke patients after receiving rt-PA therapy. *J Neurosci Nurs*, 29(6), 373-383, 1997.
> *Although this article is somewhat dated, it is a nice review of care for the acute ischemic stroke patient.*

Brott, T., Bogousslavsky, J. Treatment of acute ischemic stroke. *New Engl J Med*, 343(10), 710-722, 2000.
> *This review of ischemic stroke treatment is comprehensive and reviews both pathophysiology and treatment options.*

Bullock, R., Chesnut, R. M., Clifton, G., et al. Guidelines for the management and prognosis of severe traumatic brain injury. *J Neurotrauma*, 17, 451-553, 2000. Also accessible on the Internet: http://www2.braintrauma.org/guidelines/downloads/btf_guidelines_management.pdf?BrainTrauma_Session=3b630efb31ea1007e046becce358a93f
> *This is a must-have for anyone caring for patients with severe traumatic brain injury. It is a comprehensive review of the literature in the context of the medical management and prognosis of the head-*

injured patient. Recommendations are graded based on the strength of the data.

Greenberg, M. S. (ed.). *Handbook of Neurosurgery* (6th ed.). New York, Thieme, 2005.
> *This large pocket reference for neurosurgery residents provides a quick-access tool concerning medical and surgical issues surrounding the management of neurosurgical patients. It is a helpful resource regarding almost all aspects of care for this patient population, and it is a great asset for any critical care nurse working with critically ill neurosurgery patients.*

Hickey, J. V. (ed.). *The Clinical Practice of Neurological and Neurosurgical Nursing* (5th ed.). Philadelphia, Lippincott Williams & Wilkins, 2002.
> *This text is a main reference used by neuroscience nurses. It provides many details regarding nursing care of the neuroscience patient. It is arranged topically by disease process.*

Jennett, B., Teasdale, G. Assessment of coma and impaired consciousness. A practical scale. *Lancet*, 2(7872), 81-84, 1974.

Teasdale, G., Jennett, B. Assessment and prognosis of coma after head injury. *Acta Neurochir*, 34, 45-55, 1976.
> *These are the two original publications from Jennett and Teasdale regarding the Glasgow Coma Scale. The tool is used so frequently that it is helpful to read the original descriptions.*

Kirkness, C. J., Mitchell, P. H., Burr, R. L., et al. Intracranial pressure waveform analysis: clinical and research implications. *J Neurosci Nurs*, 32(5), 271-277, 2000.
> *Intracranial pressure monitoring is the most common neurologic monitor used in the intensive care unit. Interpretation of the waveform is a useful aspect of care for this patient population.*

McQuillan, K. A. The neurologic system. In Alspach, J. G. (ed.). *Core Curriculum for Critical Care Nursing* (6th ed.). St. Louis, Elsevier, 2006.
> *This thorough chapter in the essential reference for critical care nurses provides a helpful overview with many neurologic details related to the critically ill patient.*

Robertson, C. Critical care management of traumatic brain injury. In Winn, H. R. (ed.). *Youman's Neurological Surgery* (5th ed.). Philadelphia, Elsevier, 2004.
> *Youman's is one of the primary references used by neurosurgeons. This review of TBI critical care management provides a research-based resource regarding the medical and surgical care of this patient population.*

Wijdicks, E. F. M. *The Clinical Practice of Critical Care Neurology*. New York, Oxford University Press, 2003.
> *This is an advanced, yet very useful, reference regarding neuroscience critical care.*

RENAL

Alspach, J. G. (ed.). *Core Curriculum for Critical Care Nursing* (6th ed.). St. Louis, Elsevier, 2006.

This is a comprehensive text on the essentials of critical care nursing. Each chapter contains a review of anatomy and physiology, pathophysiology, and nursing management. The chapters include all body systems as well as psychosocial, legal-ethical, and special populations.

American Nephrology Nurses Association: *Continuous Renal Replacement Therapy, Nephrology Nursing Guidelines for Care.* Pitman, NJ, American Nephrology Nurses Association, 2005.

This guide presents an overview of CRRT, based on the nursing process, beginning with the pretreatment assessment and ending with termination of therapy. The guide also contains the clinical practice standards for CRRT.

Campbell, D. *How Acute Renal Failure Puts the Brakes on Kidney Function.* 2004. http://nursingcenter.com/prodev/cearticleprint.asp?CE-ID=289404 [www.nursingcenter.com]

This is one of the few recently published nursing articles on acute renal failure. It contains a review of pathophysiology and management of acute renal failure, broken down by each body system. The web site is designed to allow nursing professionals to access continuing education articles. The renal section is very limited.

Chulay, M., Burns, S. M. (eds.). *AACN Essentials of Critical Care Nursing.* New York, Mc Graw-Hill, 2006.

This text provides both beginner and advanced practitioners with the essential foundation for the management of critically ill patients. Section 3 has a series of key reference tables and algorithms that facilitate researching information. Areas included are normal values, pharmacology, ACLS, transfer guidelines, hemodynamic monitoring, ventilator troubleshooting, and cardiac rhythms.

Cohen, S. S. *Trauma Nursing Secrets.* St. Louis, Elsevier, 2003.

Comprehensive book that covers trauma nursing from the prehospital phase through resuscitation. The book is written in a question-and-answer format. The renal section is rather limited.

Kinney M. R., Dunbar S. B., Brunn J., et al (eds.). *AACN Clinical Reference for Critical Care Nursing* (4th ed.). St. Louis, Mosby, 1998.

The clinical reference for critical care nurses in all settings. This text covers research, nursing diagnosis, outcome standards, and nursing interventions in the management of all major disorders.

Krause, R. S. *Renal Failure, Chronic and Dialysis Complications.* 2006. http://emedicine.com/EMERG/topic501.htm [www.emedicine.com]

This article reviews the spectrum of chronic renal failure from pathophysiology and diagnostic testing to treatment guidelines and complications. On the emedicine web site you can access multiple articles related to acute and chronic renal failure and its management. The web site is geared to health professionals.

Lynn-McHale, D., Carlson, K. K. (eds.). *AACN Procedure Manual for Critical Care* (5th ed.). St. Louis, Elsevier, 2005.

The comprehensive manual for procedures in the critical care environment. This manual emphasizes evidence-based practice and incorporates the latest research on the topics presented. The renal section covers CRRT, hemodialysis, peritoneal dialysis, and special procedures—apheresis, plasma pheresis, and plasma exchange.

Merck Manual Home Edition. Disorders of Nutrition and Metabolism: Minerals and Electrolytes. 2003. http://www.merck.com/mmhe/print/sec12/ch155.html [www.merck.com]

This section of the web site discusses multiple electrolytes, hypo- and hyper- states of each electrolyte, and associated diseases, with links to sites on each disease. The site is easy to use and uses layperson terminology to discuss symptoms and management.

Mills, E. (ed.). *Rapid Response to Everyday Emergencies: A Nurse's Guide.* Philadelphia, Lippincott Williams & Wilkins, 2005.

A portable, quick-reference guide to the management of patient care emergencies. Easy to read in a bulleted format, it covers the emergency management of the patient and preventive strategies.

Mosenkis, A. *Medical Encyclopedia: Acute Renal Failure.* 2004. http://www.nlm.nih.gov/medlineplus/print/ency/article/000501.htm [www.nlm.nih.gov]

This article contains the definition, causes, incidence, risk factors, symptoms, tests, treatment, prognosis, and complications of acute renal failure. Although the web site is directed to health care professionals, the simple language allows the article to be understood by the layperson. There is a comprehensive renal section on this web site.

Mushnick, R. *Medical Encyclopedia: Chronic Renal Failure.* 2005. http://www.nlm.nih.gov/medlineplus/ency/article/000471.htm [www.nlm.nih.gov]

This article contains the definition causes, incidence, risk factors, symptoms, tests, treatment, prognosis and complications of chronic renal failure. While the web site is directed to health care professionals, the simplistic language allows the article to be understood by the lay person. There is a comprehensive renal section on this web site.

Nally, J. V. *Acute Renal Failure in the Community Hospital Setting.* 2004 http://www.clevelandclinicmeded.com/diseasemanagement/nephrology/arf/arf.htm [www.clevelandclinicmeded.com]

This article defines acute renal failure and its prevalence, pathophysiology, diagnosis, and treatment. It contains a section on special high-risk groups for the development of acute renal failure. The web site is an excellent source of information on acute and chronic renal failure for health professionals.

Needham, E. *Management of Acute Renal Failure.* 2005. http://www.aafp.org/afp [www.aafp.org]

This article discusses the diagnosis and management of acute renal failure. It contains useful ta-

bles and flow diagrams. The web site, www.aafp. org, contains multiple articles about renal failure and its management. The web site is designed for use by health professionals.

Rothrock, S. G. *Adult Emergency Pocketbook* (3ʳᵈ ed.). Redlands, CA, Tarascon, 2005.

Pocket guide of essential lists, figures, and tables of vital clinical information. Reference section includes dysrhythmia protocols, emergency drug infusions, antibiotic therapy, toxicology, trauma care, and burns.

Urden, L. D., Lough, M. E., Stacy, K. M. (eds.). *Thelan's Critical Care Nursing: Diagnosis and Management* (5ᵗʰ ed.). St. Louis, Elsevier, 2006.

A classic critical care text that centers on each of the systems of the body. Each unit includes anatomy and physiology, assessment, diagnostic procedures, pathology, and patient management. The final section includes nursing management plans.

Urden, L. D., Stacy, K. M., Lough, M. E. (eds.). *Priorities in Critical Care Nursing* (4ᵗʰ ed.). St. Louis, Elsevier, 2005.

This text concerns the collaborative management of critically ill patients using evidence-based practice. The areas covered include cardiovascular, pulmonary, neurologic, renal, gastrointestinal, endocrine, and multisystem alterations. The final unit includes nursing management plans.

ENDOCRINE

Morton, P. G., Fontaine, D. K, Hudak, C. M., Gallo, B. M. *Critical Care Nursing: A Holistic Approach* (8ᵗʰ ed.). Philadelphia, Lippincott Williams & Wilkins, 2005.

With many illustrations, charts, and tables, this text provides easily accessible information. Pathophysiology, guidelines for evidence-based practice, and lists of reliable web sites are provided in each chapter. Case studies and practice questions reinforce concepts presented in the text.

Newberry, L., Criddle, L. *Sheehy's Manual of Emergency Care* (6ᵗʰ ed.). Philadelphia, Elsevier, 2006.

This text provides guidelines for optimal nursing care in a concise format. Emphasis is on rapid detection of complications with appropriate nursing, medical, and surgical interventions.

Pagana, K., Pagana, T. *Mosby's Manual of Diagnostic and Laboratory Tests* (3ʳᵈ ed.). Philadelphia, Elsevier, 2006.

Provides normal, expected laboratory values, as well as detailed explanations of the clinical significance of laboratory values outside the expected norms. Appropriate interventions for correction of alteration of laboratory values are presented, as are potential complications, interfering factors, and related tests.

Urden, L., Stacy, K., Lough, M. *Thelan's Critical Care Nursing: Diagnosis and Management* (5ᵗʰ ed.). St. Louis, Elsevier, 2006.

Comprehensive text for persons working in the acute care setting, but especially for those in critical care areas. Provides pathophysiology, expected medical and surgical interventions, and appropriate nursing care standards according to current, evidence-based practice. Consistently supports theory of the interaction of body systems in failure.

HEMATOLOGY/IMMUNOLOGY

Critical Care Nursing Made Incredibly Easy. Philadelphia, Lippincott Williams & Wilkins, 2003.

Organized by body system, this reference addresses more than 100 critical care disorders with current, detailed information. Through the use of graphics, including tables, charts, and sidebars, essential information is highlighted.

Durston, S. Cirrhosis: Scarred for life. *Nursing Made Incredibly Easy.* Philadelphia, Lippincott Williams & Wilkins, 2004.

This journal article addresses hepatic disease as it pertains to the interaction of all body systems, using plain, understandable explanations of pathophysiology for symptoms experienced by patients. It presents effective nursing interventions to assist in personalized care. Included are charts explaining rating systems for encephalopathy and the Childs-Pugh scale for rating intensity of hepatic disease.

La Pointe, L. A., Von Rueden, K. T. Coagulopathies in trauma patients. *AACN Adv Crit Care*, 13(2), 192-203, 2002.

Provides insight into rationale and currently accepted, evidence-based treatment modalities.

Morton, P. G., Fontaine, D. K., Hudak, C. M., Gallo., B. M. *Critical Care Nursing: A Holistic Approach* (8ᵗʰ ed.). Philadelphia, Lippincott Williams & Wilkins, 2005.

Provides specific, current information pertaining to pathophysiology and treatment of critical illnesses. Provides guidelines for collaborative care, guidelines for evidence-based practice, and multiple illustrations to reinforce text. Accompanying CD-ROM contains animations, a reference for medications used in the critical care unit, thought-provoking practice examinations, a guide to laboratory values, and a procedure guidebook.

Nettina, S. M. *The Lippincott Manual of Nursing Practice* (7ᵗʰ ed.). Philadelphia, Lippincott Williams & Wilkins, 2001.

Latest edition of classic nursing reference providing precise outlines pertaining to disease processes and guidelines for correct and safe performance of procedures.

Newberry, L., Criddle, L. *Sheehy's Manual of Emergency Care* (6ᵗʰ ed.), Philadelphia, Elsevier, 2006.

This text offers guidelines for providing optimal nursing care in a concise format. Emphasis is on rapid detection of complications, appropriate nursing interventions, and expected medical and surgical interventions.

Pagana, K., Pagana, T. *Mosby's Manual of Diagnostic and Laboratory Tests* (3rd ed.). Philadelphia, Elsevier, 2006.

> Provides normal, expected laboratory values, as well as detailed explanations of clinical significance of laboratory values outside the expected norms. Appropriate interventions are presented as well as potential complications, interfering factors, and related tests.

Schell, H., Puntillo, K. A. *Critical Care Nursing Secrets* (2nd ed.). St. Louis, Elsevier, 2006.

> Provides necessary, to the point information including pathophysiology and rationale for alterations in physical assessment and laboratory values, medical, surgical, and nursing interventions. Information is presented in a question-and-answer format.

Urden, L., Stacy, K., Lough, M. *Thelan's Critical Care Nursing: Diagnosis and Management* (5th ed.). St. Louis, Elsevier, 2006.

> Comprehensive text for persons working in the acute care setting, but especially for those in critical care areas. Provides pathophysiology, expected medical and surgical interventions, and evidence-based nursing care standards. Consistently supports theory of the interaction of body systems in failure.

GASTROINTESTINAL

Bacak, B. S., Tweed, E. What is the best way to manage GERD symptoms in the elderly? *J Fam Pract,* 55, 251-258, 2006.

> This is an evidence-based clinical discussion of gastroesophageal reflux disease in the elderly.

Barshes, N. R., Gay, A. N., William, B., et al. Support for the acutely failing liver: a comprehensive review of historic and contemporary strategies. *J Am Coll Surg,* 201, 458-475, 2005.

> A collective medical review of liver failure and treatment strategies.

Beers, M. H., Porter, R. S. *The Merck Manual of Diagnosis and Therapy* (18th ed.). Whitehouse Station, NJ, Merck Research Laboratories, 2006.

> Affords an overview of medical diseases and conditions and their treatment in a clear, concise format.

Carter, S. The surgical team and outcomes management: focus on postoperative ileus. *J Perianesth Nurs,* 21(2A), S2-S6, 2006.

> Article discusses problem of postoperative ileus and the importance of nurses recognizing this condition.

Charles, A., Domingo, S., Goldfadden, A., et al. Small bowel ischemia after roux-en-y gastric bypass complicated by pregnancy: a case report. *Am Surg,* 71(3), 231-235, 2005.

> Provides a case report on an unusual complication of pregnancy. It includes discussion of occurrence and treatment.

Clarke, G., Patel, R., Tsao, S., Blanshard, K. Treatment of refractory post transjugular portosystemic stent-shunt encephalopathy: a novel case of stent luminal reduction. *Eur J Gastroenterol Hepatol,* 16(12), 1387-1390, 2004.

> This is a case report on the use of diameter reduction of TIPS stents in patients with refractory encephalopathy.

D'Arcy, Y. Hot topics in pain management: using NSAIDs safely. *Nursing 2006,* 36, 2006.

> This article describes recent research related to the use of NSAIDs and patient education.

Davila, R. E., Rajan, E., Adler, D. G., et al. American Society for Gastrointestinal Endoscopy (ASGE) guideline: the role of endoscopy in the patient with lower GI bleeding. *Gastrointest Endosc,* 62(5), 656-60, 2005.

> This is a set of evidence-based recommendations from the National Guideline Clearing House.

Dellinger, R. P., Vincent, J. L. The Surviving Sepsis Campaign sepsis change bundles and clinical practice. *Crit Care,* 9(6), 653-4, 2005.

> Details the management and treatment of sepsis that represent the basis of current clinical practice.

Eckert, K. L. Penetrating and blunt abdominal trauma. *Crit Care Nurse Q,* 28, 41-59, 2005.

> Provides an overview of abdominal trauma relating to both penetrating and blunt mechanisms of injury.

Elliot, K. Nutritional considerations after bariatric surgery. *Crit Care Nurse Q,* 26, 133-138, 2003.

> A review article that discusses bariatric surgery, malabsorption, malnutrition, and morbid obesity.

Hudson, K. *Blunt Abdominal Trauma.* Dynamic Nursing Education.com, Feb 2005.

> This is an online continuing education program on blunt abdominal trauma that is interesting and easy to review.

Hurwitz, H., Kabbinaavar, F. Bevacizumab combined with standard fluoropyrimidine based chemotherapy regimens to treat colorectal cancer. *Oncology,* 3, S17-S24, 2005.

Kelley, DM. Hypovolemic shock: an overview. *Crit Care Nurs Q,* 28, 2-19, 2005.

> This is a review article on various types of hypovolemic shock and its sequelae.

Kraft, M. D., et al. Treatment of electrolyte disorders in adult patients in the intensive care unit. *Am J Health Syst Pharm,* 62, 1663-1682, 2005.

> A review article that looks at the treatment of electrolyte disorders in adult patients in the intensive care unit, including guidelines for correcting specific electrolyte disorders.

Krumberger, J., Parrish, C. R., Krenitsky, J. Gastrointestinal system. In Chulay, M., Burns, S. (eds.). *AACN Essentials of Critical Care Nursing.* New York, McGraw-Hill, 2006, p 317.

> A critical care textbook that provides systematic review of gastrointestinal problems and complications.

Krumberger, J. M. How to manage an acute upper GI bleed. *RN,* 68(3), 34-39, 2005.
> *This review article discusses the management of gastrointestinal bleeding.*

Larson, A. M., Curtis, J. R. Integrating palliative care for liver transplant candidates: too well for transplant, too sick for life. *J Am Med Assoc,* 295(18), 2168, 2006.
> *Provides a current view of the need to provide palliative care for those struggling with a life-threatening illness.*

Lim, C. H., Heatley, R. V. Prospective study of acute gastrointestinal bleeding attributable to anti-inflammatory drug ingestion in the Yorkshire region of the United Kingdom. *Postgrad Med J,* 281, 252-254, 2005.
> *This is a cross-sectional study on patients referred for endoscopy for suspected upper gastrointestinal bleeding in one region of the United Kingdom.*

Mackenzie, D. J. Care of patients after esophagectomy. *Crit Care Nurse,* 16-29, Feb 2004.
> *This is an article that reviews the nursing care of patients undergoing esophagectomy and its complications and challenges.*

Maher, A. B. Serotonergic antidepressants and need for blood transfusions. *Orthop Nurs,* 23, 220, 2004.
> *This is a review of a retrospective study investigating the relationship between SSRIs and the need for blood transfusion.*

Mansour, A., et al. Which patients taking SSRIs are at greatest risk of bleeding? *J Fam Pract,* 55, 206-209, 2006.
> *A review of recent research studies looking at different formulations of SSRIs and their complications.*

Marshall, J. S., et al. Roux-en-y gastric bypass leak complications. *Arch Surg,* 138, 520-524, 2003.
> *Describes findings from a research study of 400 morbidly obese patients who underwent gastric bypass and the complications that occurred.*

McMahon, B. J. Epidemiology and natural history of hepatitis B. *Semin Liver Dis,* 25, S3-S8, 2005.
> *Provides a review of the natural history, management, and epidemiology of hepatitis B.*

Pagana, K. D., Pagana, T. *Mosby's Manual of Diagnostic and Laboratory Tests* (2nd ed.). Philadelphia, Elsevier, 2002.
> *This manual of laboratory tests is very easy to use. It explains the test and discusses normal findings, indications, interfering factors, and clinical patient care issues.*

Pakfetrat, M. A pregnant lady with abdominal pain. *Shiraz E-Medical J,* 6, 1-12, 2005.
> *This is a review of a case report of pregnancy and abdominal pain.*

Pastor, C. M., Matthay, M. A., Frossare, J. L. Pancreatitis associated acute lung injury: new insights. *Chest,* 124, 2341-2351, 2003.
> *A review of the pulmonary complications associated with pancreatitis.*

Pirsch, J., Simmons, W. D., Sollinger, H. *Transplantation Drug Manual* (4th ed.). Austin, TX, Landes Bioscience, 2003.
> *This is a comprehensive drug manual for the transplant population.*

Radovich, P. Gastrointestinal system. In Alspach, J. G. (ed.). *Core Curriculum for Critical Care Nursing* (6th ed.). St. Louis, Elsevier, 2006, p 732.
> *This is a comprehensive review of the gastrointestinal system and its complications, diagnoses, and treatments.*

Robertson, M. S., Clancy, R. L., Cade, J. F. *Helicobacter pylori* in intensive care: why should we be interested? *Intensive Care Med,* 29, 1881-1888, 2003.
> *Provides a discussion on the incidence, role, and pathogenesis of* Helicobacter pylori *in gastric mucosal damage.*

Sargent, D. The management and nursing care of cirrhotic ascites. *Br J Nurse,* 15(4), P 212-219, 2006.
> *This is a comprehesive review of the pathophysiology and medical, surgical, and nursing management of ascites in the cirrhotic patient.*

Steward, C. A., Cerhan, J. Hepatic encephalopathy: a dynamic or static condition. *Metab Brain Dis,* 20(3), 193-204, 2005.
> *A review article on the current knowledge of the mechanisms of encephalopathy.*

Trouble down below: understanding small bowel obstruction. *Nursing,* 35, 2005.
> *This is a brief case study review article on small bowel obstruction.*

Whitcomb, D. C. Acute pancreatitis. *N Engl J Med,* 354, 2142-2150, 2006.
> *This article reviews the clinical problem of acute pancreatitis and treatment using evidence-supported strategies; it ends with the author's clinical recommendations.*

Wu, W. K., Cho, C. H. The pharmacological actions of nicotine on the gastrointestinal tract. *J Pharmacol Sci,* 94(4), 2004.
> *This is a research article on the effects of nicotine—specifically, cigarette smoking on the mucosa of the gastrointestinal tract.*

Wyrzykowski, A. D., Feliciano, D. V., George, T. A., et al. Emergent right hemicolectomy. *Am Surg,* 71(8), 653-657, 2005.
> *This is a research article discussing the complications of emergent hemicolectomies.*

Yamada, T. *Handbook of Gastroenterology* (2nd ed.). Philadelphia, Lippincott Williams & Wilkins, 2005.
> *This comprehensive textbook illustrates and discusses all aspects of gastroenterology.*

MULTISYSTEM

Alspach, J. G. (ed.). *Core Curriculum for Critical Care Nursing* (6th ed.). St. Louis, Elsevier, 2006.
> *This new edition of AACN's Core Curriculum for Critical Care Nursing provides information on*

critical care nursing in an outline format. Features new chapters on the AACN Synergy Model for Patient Care, professional care, and ethical practice, as well as on critical care patients with special needs. Includes expanded content on patient transfer and discharge planning, and many new illustrations.

Boswell, S. A., Scalea, T. M. Sublingual capnometry: an alternative to gastric tonometry for the management of shock resuscitation. *AACN Clinical Issues, Adv Pract Acute Crit Care,* 14(2), 176-184, 2003.

This article discusses the advances in technology that enable the clinician to monitor changes, potentially identifying tissue hypoxia much earlier than was previously possible. The ability to monitor PSICO$_2$ via sublingual capnometer may be a valuable aid in the prehospital phase, the emergency department, and the intensive care unit in identifying end points of resuscitation.

Bridges, E. J., Dukes, M. S. Cardiovascular aspects of septic shock: pathophysiology, monitoring and treatment. *Crit Care Nurse,* 25(2), 14-42, 2005.

This article focuses on the cardiovascular aspects of septic shock, including a review of cardiovascular pathophysiology and recommendations for state-of-the-art cardiovascular monitoring and treatment options.

Buchanan Keller, K. The cocaine-abused heart. *Am J Crit Care,* 12(6), 562-566, 2003.

This article is a cardiology casebook that reviews the management of a patient experiencing cardiac symptoms related to cocaine abuse.

Criddle, L. M. Rhabdomyolysis. Pathophysiology, recognition and management: *Crit Care Nurse,* 23(6), 14-32, 2003.

This comprehensive article discusses the pathophysiology of rhabdomyolysis, associated conditions, clinical findings, and treatment strategies for patient management.

Cunneen, J., Cartwright, M. The puzzle of sepsis. Fitting the pieces of the inflammatory response with treatment. *AACN Clinical Issues Adv Pract Acute Crit Care,* 15(1), 18-44, 2004.

This article discusses sepsis as a complex syndrome characterized by simultaneous activation of inflammation and coagulation in response to microbial insult. Conventional treatments as well as new treatment paradigms are reviewed.

Dellinger, R. P., Carlet, J. M., Masur, H., et al. Surviving sepsis campaign guidelines for management of severe sepsis and septic shock. *Crit Care Med,* 32(3), 858-873, 2004.

In 2003, critical care and infectious disease experts representing 11 international organizations developed management guidelines for severe sepsis and septic shock that would be of practical use for the bedside clinician, under the auspices of the Surviving Sepsis Campaign, an international effort to increase awareness and improve outcome in severe sepsis. Evidence-based recommendations can be made regarding many aspects of the acute

management of sepsis and septic shock that are hoped to translate into improved outcomes for the critically ill patient.

Hazinski, M. F., Chameides, L., Elling, B., Hemphill, R., (eds.). 2005 American Heart Association guidelines for cardiopulmonary resuscitation and emergency cardiovascular care. *Circulation,* 112(24), S146-S149, 2005.

This publication presents the 2005 American Heart Association (AHA) guidelines for cardiopulmonary resuscitation and emergency cardiovascular care. The guidelines are based on the evidence evaluation from the 2005 International Consensus Conference on Cardiopulmonary Resuscitation and Emergency Cardiovascular Care Science with Treatment Recommendations.

Lynn-McHale Wiegand, D. J., Carlson, K. K. (eds.). *AACN Procedure Manual for Critical Care* (5th ed.). St. Louis, Elsevier, 2005.

The American Association of Critical-Care Nurses offers comprehensive procedural coverage unique to the critical care environment. Updated edition includes 19 added procedures in a step-by-step format and advanced procedure icons.

Marrs, J. A. Care of patients with neutropenia. *Clin J Oncol Nurs,* 10(2), 164, 2006.

This article describes the causes and complications associated with neutropenia in the oncology patient. Treatment modalities based on the absolute neutrophil count (ANC) and nursing care of this patient population are discussed.

McKinley, M. G. Alcohol withdrawal syndrome. Overlooked and mismanaged? *Crit Care Nurse,* 25(3), 40-49, 2005.

This article describes the pathophysiology involved between alcohol and alterations of neurotransmission in the brain. It defines the relationship between alcohol and thiamine deficiency. The article provides a comprehensive review of the management of patients undergoing alcohol withdrawal syndrome.

Newberry, L., Criddle, L. M. (eds.). *Sheehy's Manual of Emergency Care* (6th ed.). Philadelphia, Elsevier, 2005.

This textbook offers comprehensive coverage of basic and advanced life support, medical emergencies, and emergency care for special populations. New data on elder trauma, emergency operations preparedness, and pain management is included in the text.

Urden, L. D., Stacy, K. M., Lough, M. E. *Thelan's Critical Care Nursing: Diagnosis and Management* (5th ed.). St. Louis, Elsevier, 2006.

Text offers comprehensive examination of trends, issues, and advances in critical care nursing. New edition presents evidence-based collaborative practice features, patient safety alerts, coverage of SARS, and more.

Web site: http://www.acc.org/clinical/guidelines/stemi/Guideline1/index.pdf. May 7, 2006.